AF752319

Psycho-Environmental Variables That Ensure People's Well-Being and Health in Sustainable Indoor Spaces

nova science publishers

www.novapublishers.com

Environmental Science, Engineering and Technology Series

A Design Odyssey in the Built Environment: Functionality, Aesthetics and Heritage
Rashidi Othman, PhD,
Nurlelawati Ab Jalil, PhD,
Norzalifa Zainal Abidin, PhD,
Nurhaya Baniyamin, PhD,
Qurratu Aini Mat Ali, PhD
and Nurul Hamiruddin Salleh, PhD (Editors)
ISBN: 979-8-89530-765-6
eBook ISBN: 979-8-89530-876-9

Radioactivity: Detection, Exposure and Decay
Nataša Sarap (Editor)
ISBN: 979-8-89530-561-4
eBook ISBN: 979-8-89530-712-0

Advancements in Sustainability Systems II
Hussain H. Al-Kayiem, PhD,
Raed A. Jessam, PhD,
Hasanain A. Abdul Wahhab, PhD
and Abdul Salam K. Darwish, PhD (Editors)
ISBN: 979-8-89530-562-1
eBook ISBN: 979-8-89530-654-3

Global Horizons in Agricultural Extension Education: Insights from International Perspectives
R. K. Doharey, PhD, Aman Verma, PhD, Satyapriya, PhD and Amrit Warshini, PhD (Editors)
ISBN: 979-8-89530-446-4
eBook ISBN: 979-8-89530-501-0

Human Capital, Energy and Sustainable Development: Global Empirical Modeling
Raufhon Salahodjaev (Editor)
ISBN: 979-8-89530-444-0
eBook ISBN: 979-8-89530-512-6

Ecological Resilience: Sustainability, Mitigation and Adaptation
Razanah Ramya, PhD,
Muhamad Shafiq Mohd Ali
and Rashidi Othman, PhD (Editors)
ISBN: 979-8-89113-992-3
eBook ISBN: 979-8-89530-034-3

Critical States, Strength and Lifetime of the Matter – Technical Structures, Living Organisms, Environment
Valeriu V. Jinescu, PhD
ISBN: 979-8-89113-962-6
eBook ISBN: 979-8-89530-011-4

Environmental Geotechnics: Waste and Geotechnical Stabilization
Eduardo Pavan Korf,
Pedro Domingos Marques Prietto,
Caroline Müller and Suéllen Tonatto Ferrazzo (Editors)
ISBN: 979-8-89113-651-9
eBook ISBN: 979-8-89113-727-1

More information about this series can be found at
https://novapublishers.com/product-category/series/environmental-science-engineering-and-technology/

Roberto Alonso González Lezcano
Guadalupe Cantarero García
Editors

Psycho-Environmental Variables That Ensure People's Well-Being and Health in Sustainable Indoor Spaces

nova
science publishers
www.novapublishers.com

Copyright © 2025 by Nova Science Publishers, Inc.
DOI: https://doi.org/10.52305/AEHD4416

All rights reserved. No part of this book may be reproduced, stored in a retrieval system or transmitted in any form or by any means: electronic, electrostatic, magnetic, tape, mechanical photocopying, recording or otherwise without the written permission of the Publisher.

We have partnered with Copyright Clearance Center to make it easy for you to obtain permissions to reuse content from this publication. Simply navigate to this publication's page on Nova's website and locate the "Get Permission" button below the title description. This button is linked directly to the title's permission page on copyright.com. Alternatively, you can visit copyright.com and search by title, ISBN, or ISSN.

For further questions about using the service on copyright.com, please contact:
Copyright Clearance Center
Phone: +1-(978) 750-8400 Fax: +1-(978) 750-4470 E-mail: info@copyright.com.

NOTICE TO THE READER

The Publisher has taken reasonable care in the preparation of this book, but makes no expressed or implied warranty of any kind and assumes no responsibility for any errors or omissions. No liability is assumed for incidental or consequential damages in connection with or arising out of information contained in this book. The Publisher shall not be liable for any special, consequential, or exemplary damages resulting, in whole or in part, from the readers' use of, or reliance upon, this material. Any parts of this book based on government reports are so indicated and copyright is claimed for those parts to the extent applicable to compilations of such works.

Independent verification should be sought for any data, advice or recommendations contained in this book. In addition, no responsibility is assumed by the Publisher for any injury and/or damage to persons or property arising from any methods, products, instructions, ideas or otherwise contained in this publication.

The Publisher assumes no responsibility for any statements of fact or opinion expressed in the published contents.

This publication is designed to provide accurate and authoritative information with regard to the subject matter covered herein. It is sold with the clear understanding that the Publisher is not engaged in rendering legal or any other professional services. If legal or any other expert assistance is required, the services of a competent person should be sought. FROM A DECLARATION OF PARTICIPANTS JOINTLY ADOPTED BY A COMMITTEE OF THE AMERICAN BAR ASSOCIATION AND A COMMITTEE OF PUBLISHERS.

Additional color graphics may be available in the e-book version of this book.

Library of Congress Cataloging-in-Publication Data

ISBN: 979-8-89530-831-8 (Hardcover)
ISBN: 979-8-89530-925-4 (eBook)

Published by Nova Science Publishers, Inc. † New York

Contents

Preface

For modern cities to develop in a sustainable manner, a holistic approach to management is required, taking into account social, technological, environmental and economic dimensions. The smart citizen concept places special emphasis on the involvement of the human factor. It is the citizens who must provide information, actively participate in development and co-create their city. The adoption of this smart city model should foster creativity, openness to innovation and change, as well as flexibility, understood as the ability to respond quickly to internal and external needs.

Building a healthy future is inevitable for the health and well-being of current and future generations. Sustainable living environments that improve public health are fundamental to maintaining and improving health and well-being, and contribute to economic development.

This book focuses on current research and studies linking public health and sustainable development. Promoting human health and well-being for a sustainable future requires that development be fair, equitable, and inclusive. Resilient health systems, capable of responding rapidly to emerging diseases while maintaining essential health services, are fundamental to sustainable development. This book will complement existing literature by exploring ways to structure and design strategies for planning and governance to achieve positive health outcomes.

Situations we face include how to control the spread of infectious diseases in an increasingly urbanized world, ensure clean water supplies for healthy populations, build sustainable transportation systems, and implement appropriate fuel policies to ensure clean air, water, and soil.

Sustainable infrastructure development, with a strong awareness of its impact, is crucial; today's buildings account for 30% of global energy consumption and 28% of energy-related carbon emissions. Urban leaders must act with urgency in the face of a global pandemic, climate crisis, economic uncertainty and budget constraints to make urban infrastructure more resilient. Markets are increasingly pressuring cities to reduce carbon emissions, respond to extreme weather events, reduce waste and preserve natural resources, while providing essential infrastructure and resources. Citizens expect this too, and increasingly demand transparency.

"*Psycho-Environmental Variables That Ensure People's Well-Being and Health in Sustainable Indoor Spaces*" offers a broad opportunity to present scientific chapters, both theoretical and practical, on an integrated approach to smart cities, considering the human factor.

Dr. Roberto Alonso González Lezcano

Chapter 1

The Effect of Sound and Music on Emotions: A Case Study of High-Ability and Intellectual Disability Students (Part 1)

Gabriel Caffarena
Roberto Alonso González Lezcano
Ana Jiménez-Perianes
Judit Martínez Martín
Pablo Muñoz Navarro
and Guadalupe Cantarero-García*
Universidad San Pablo-CEU, CEU Universities, Madrid, Spain

Abstract

Music, as a form of non-verbal communication, is an essential tool for exploring cognitive and sensory development in humans. On the other hand, sound, as a trigger for emotions and perceptual sensations, can contribute to the field of plastic arts with very personal results that favor the expression of the individual. This study is part of an experience prior to another complementary activity in which the association of sound, as a non-visual model, to lines, colors or textures, is the object of work. For the proper development of the activity, a specific test is designed on the association of emotions with the perception and auditory reception of sounds and musical compositions. The main objective of the study is to analyze whether responses to this test among students of different ages and profiles are similar. To demonstrate that the emotion triggered by a vibration in the form of harmony, or a dissonance does not distinguish from intellectual quotients. Thus, new paths of social inclusion are opened in which the musical experience demonstrates its universal language.

Keywords: sound analysis, neuro-architecture, accessibility, intellectual disabilities, high abilities

---

* Corresponding Author's Email: gcgarcia@ceu.es

In: Psycho-Environmental Variables That Ensure People's Well-Being and Health …
Editors: Roberto Alonso González Lezcano and Guadalupe Cantarero García
ISBN: 979-8-89530-831-8
© 2025 Nova Science Publishers, Inc.

Introduction

The research described here, titled 'Music and Emotion,' is based on the assumption that the two are closely related. For a musician, holding a workshop on these two topics is not complicated if it focuses on recreational activities. The challenge arises when we want to link music, emotion and accessibility, always without leaving aside the practical aspect of the matter.

An analysis of emotional responses to musical pieces, with very different harmonies, is presented here.

The question that arises is whether the results of the test for the association of the sound or composition with a feeling, with a type of line or with a color, are similar in both profiles.

As a main conclusion, after the study of results, the fact of obtaining results that are not substantially different in response or emotional appreciation is extracted, without being able to distinguish within the entire range of exercises delivered which correspond to the profiles selected for the object activity study.

The association of sound, as a non-visual model, with emotions provides continuity to an established activity linking sounds with colors and strokes. The analysis of these sounds in their basic or complex form (as a musical composition) can therefore generate an artistic, plastic, and abstract image.

This activity stems from collaboration among teachers from various disciplines and psychologists. The specialized musician is also an engineer and teacher in the Biomedical and Telecommunications Engineering Degrees. He exposes the theory of sound applied to the emotional realm through musical vibrations and the harmonies of music composition. As far as architecture is concerned, it is essential to have architects who provide their spatial vision of the space in which the activity takes place since the acoustic reverberation will vary depending on whether it is an exterior or interior space, large or small, and the height of itself and the construction materials will affect the perception of said sound. Psychologists design an appropriate test for the given activity to be able to evaluate or measure intellectual development factors from the perception of sounds to the identification of emotion.

This workshop is developed within a singular university environment such as the Form Analysis classroom of the Degree in Architecture and provides students with a differential experience since it is offered to students of two very different profiles: on one hand, twelve-year-old gifted children (IQ above 130) and, on the other hand, adults over eighteen years of age with intellectual disabilities (IQ limit 85) and on the autism spectrum. Students also present disparate knowledge bases on auditory-musical, graphic and spatial perception, which enriches the experience.

The hypothesis that arises is whether the graphic results will be visually distant, for which a test system (prior to the representation) is established to associate the sound or composition with a type of emotion.

Analytical Framework

Literature Review

If we consider music and painting as part of creativity due to their artistic, expressive, and emotional connections and neural functioning, we can compare how two groups—gifted students and students with disabilities—respond to musical stimuli. Despite their differences, both groups produce pictorial responses primarily based on sensory perception. If we take into account the sensory profile of high-ability students, where structural differences at a neurophysiological level determine certain over-excitabilities and high sensitivity, it leads us to analyze the brain images that show the difference in functioning and processing in comparison with normative groups. The high-capacity brain invests more time in the development of the cerebral cortex during childhood compared to its chronological peers, which specializes, creates new connections and facilitates learning, allowing greater myelination of the structures and better metabolism of energy.

A longitudinal research study with neuroimaging analysis (Shaw et al., 2006) determined that in this process of maturation of the cortex of the individuals with high abilities in the sample, it had a higher index of plasticity and some quantitative and qualitative differences in the density of gray and white matter in the frontal areas, with a higher resulting neuronal density. A greater density of white matter in high-ability students can explain an increase in processing speed and the number of connections between different brain areas. As a result, these students tend to solve problems differently, exhibit a greater ability to associate ideas and recall memories, possess better executive functioning, and demonstrate high levels of abstract and creative thinking. (Duncan, 2001).

Another characteristic domain associated with high abilities is creativity in general, and music in particular (Winner, 2000), (Mrazik and Dombrowski, 2010), related to neuroanatomical support and the inferior parietal cortex of the right hemisphere. The frontal lobes, especially the right hemisphere, are linked to the resolution of creative tasks, cooperating both intra- and inter-hemispherically (Camfield, 2005). According to Soria-Urios, Duque and García-Moreno (2011), music involves cortical and subcortical areas of the brain, being capable of provoking different emotional responses. With music therapy you can work on anxiety, stress or depression, very important emotions to manage in our society.

In this activity, in which students of different intellectual levels participated, and two highly creative actions were carried out simultaneously, such as the pictorial interpretation of sound, the relationship between intelligence and creativity could be raised. Ferrando, Prieto, (Ferrandi and Sánchez 2005) carried out research whose results showed little relationship between the constructs intelligence and creativity. On the other hand, (Chibas Ortiz 2005), adds that, although creativity and intelligence are not coincident concepts, a minimum of intelligence is necessary to be able to create. In students with intellectual disabilities, creativity allows them to develop their expression, stimulates them cognitively, helps them communicate physically, visually and plastically and promotes their meaningful learning. According to (Jaén López 2013), creativity allows the discovery and relationship between existing elements, taking into account previous learning.

In this way, we can relate both the creative part of the workshop and the emotional part, with the different intellectual levels and ages of the students, under the same study, where the brain behavior of each subject will be linked to their skills and previous experiences, generating more similarities than differences.

Sound begins with the vibration of the air that is captured by our ears and interpreted by our brain. If we paint the vibration at a point in space, we obtain a representation of the sound. The vibration of the air is transmitted to the eardrum and the cochlea (in the inner ear) transforms the vibration into electrical and nerve signals. People generate sounds with their vocal cords, and these consist of tone, intensity and timbre. We also associate two of these characteristics with color (tone that implies frequency and intensity that implies volume or power) (Figure 1).

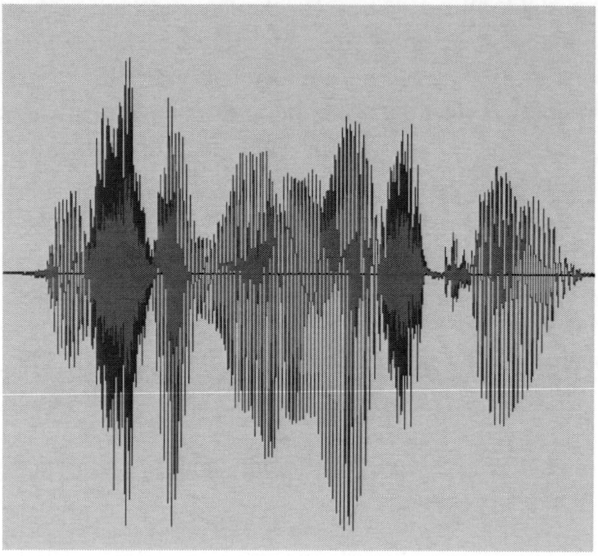

Figure 1. Source by Caffarena: Sound waves produced by the author talking obtained through Audacity software.

The brain is what links music with emotion and the areas of the brain that interpret music are connected to the areas that emit dopamine, endorphins and oxytocin. For this reason, ancestral dances and songs have a significant role in cultures by uniting socially. Music is associated with memory and related emotions. In turn, music is related to spatial accessibility and according to the study by Harbin Institute of Technology University College of London, speakers were placed in a square to guide traffic through it and it was found that people did not leave the path when walking, they walked and they concentrated near the speaker and they walked more slowly and calmly (Meng et al. 2018) (Figure 2).

Among researchers there is disagreement on defining what primary emotions are and they do not even agree that they really exist. There are trends that revolve around Ekman studies (Ekman, 1992) who affirms that there are central emotions, which affect four facial expressions: fear, anger, sadness and joy. Both Ekman and Goleman express their agreement in considering the essential ones related to relevant cases of our emotional life and establish as main emotions: fear, anger, sadness, joy, love, surprise, aversion and shame. Based on this, they define emotions derived from the previous ones such as fear related to anxiety, apprehension, fear, worry, concern, restlessness, uncertainty, nervousness, anguish, fright, terror, phobia, and panic.

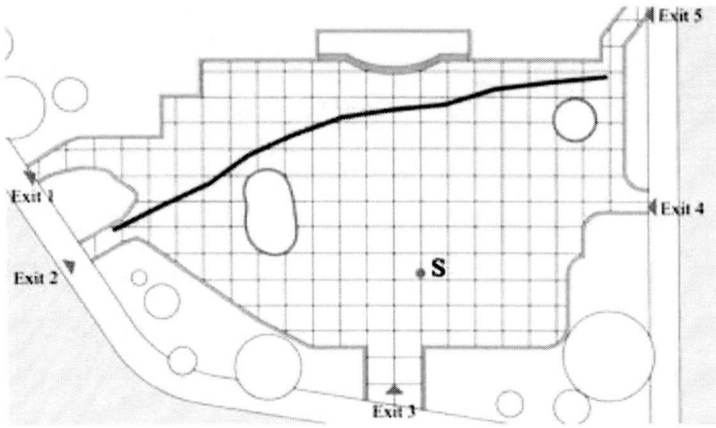

Figure 2. Source by Meng et al. 2018 (Creative Commons Attribution License (CC BY).

Thus, the researcher (Damasio, 1994) identifies the differences between emotions in the early stages of life and emotions in adulthood, which are generated from early emotions, establishing the term primary emotions to the first and emotions secondary to those of adulthood.

There are two types of emotions: The perceived emotion → the one we think the author feels. The induced emotion → the one we feel when listening to music. The effect that music has on emotions has been studied. In general, each person's experience is different:

- Personal situation
- Environment in which music is heard
- Personality
- Musical preference

This makes it difficult to have a general "recipe" to influence people's mood. The reality is that music has a meaning that is communicated to those who listen to it. According to Meyer studies, there are two main opposing tendencies: those who propose that musical meaning is found in the perception of the relationships perceived in the musical work, and those who consider that music communicates other meanings among which they find the emotional states of the list (Meyer, 1956).

If we research in the origins of music, researchers like Honing addressed theories referent to the purpose of music but there is disagreement on whether the fundamentals are biologic, evolutionary or sociological. The Darwinian point of view explores the idea of music as part of the mating ritual; a way to attract partners. Also, music seems to be connected to language and it seems to precede vocalization and also to be a tool for parents to teach infants to talk, while promoting parental bond. Moreover, music is seen as a cohesive force for communities that celebrate or mourn singing and dancing. Recent research pursues a multicomponent perspective (Honing et al.,2015). As well Drott addresses music's role in social movements, using work in mediation, assemblage, and actor-network theories to address the complex, contradictory, and contentious status that music often assumes within political protest (Drot 2018). And some studies show how the movement of people while going from home to work gets less erratic in the presence of music. Meng tested the ability of music to reduce random movements in the streets (Meng et al., 2018).

According to music and therapy, the research by Trimble & Hesdorffer the music can be seen as a way to stimulate the brain aiming at improving the health status of a person. There are studies showing that music can be used to recover from motor impairments (strokes, Parkinson's disease, etc.) improve the state in mood disorders. There is evidence that music can reduce epilepsy seizure frequency. (Trimble & Hesdorffer 2017). Recent studies reaffirm that music is the language of emotions. Han's paper gives a detailed survey of music emotion recognition. Starting with some preliminary knowledge of music emotion recognition, this paper first introduces some commonly used evaluation metrics. Then a three-part research framework is put forward. The authors including some commonly used datasets, emotion models, feature extraction, and emotion recognition algorithms (Han et al., 2022). According to other research studies about psychotherapeutic pain management through music and touch is effective, harmless, comprehensive and inexpensive compared to pharmacological treatment. The authors made a psychotherapeutic proposal based on music and touch to reduce pain in neonates (Sandoval et al., 2018). According to the acoustic environment, Meng focused in this as one of the factors influencing emotion, however, existing research has mainly focused on the effects of noise on emotion, and on music therapy, while the acoustic and psychological effects of music on interactive behavior have been neglected. Therefore, this study aimed to investigate the effects of music on communicating emotion including evaluation of music, and values of pleasure, arousal, and dominance, in terms of sound pressure level and musical emotion (Meng et al., 2020). As well other studies determined the benefits of the use of sound resources in cognitive functions or skills, with the aim of promoting the inclusion of music as a resource in the study and therefore in learning. The authors conducted a literature review in which it was found that the human brain has shown greater stimulation when listening to and making music, the brain of musicians was more developed than that of other people, when making music the two brain hemispheres are activated, one responsible for movement when playing the instrument and the other responsible for creativity, emotions and evoked feeling, music influences cognitive skills and functions, promoting the retention of information through patterns of sounds and rhymes, attention and concentration are also improved in conjunction with language (Llanga et al., 2019).

Goal

The main objective of the workshop is: Understand and develop the perception of sound and music through emotions.

Secondary objectives that arise are:

1. Establish synergies in musical artistic understanding and psychology.
2. Share an inclusive experience with students of different ages and intellectual abilities.

The aim is to awaken internal sensitivity and verbally express the emotions that the sounds, or where appropriate, the musical pieces or compositions suggest to us. The graphic results on the artistic representation, which subsequently emerge from a complementary activity, will be recorded and analyzed to establish parallels between different student profiles. The hypothesis states that the results measured in highly gifted students will not be different from those of students with intellectual disabilities.

Method

Students are introduced to the concept of 'sound' and how sound is used to create music. The concept 'sound wave' is exposed and how various classical musical instruments (piano and guitar) allow them to produce sound waves. Likewise, an introduction to the fundamentals of music is established, talking about rhythm, tone, timbre and harmony and how they relate to the ability to influence mood and produce emotions. Also, the activity discusses the use of digital technologies for the creation of music. This tool will help us understand the role of space in music and will allow us to compare the effect of acoustics. The use of computer systems to compose music can serve as an introduction to music for those people who have a lot of respect for regulated music, classical instruments, etc. Therefore, it is understood that it can be of great interest to students.

In a second section, musical fragments of classical works and electronic music are projected and analyzed. Finally, we proceed to give a few touches on academic studies that relate music to concentration, anxiety, happiness and even the way we walk through urban spaces. The possibilities that music offers to help people face certain situations or navigate within a building or outdoor urban space are discussed. Given the time limitations, only the essence of each of the topics that are discussed.

In order to achieve the results of the objectives set out here, the study method has been based on THREE PHASES clearly defined and described below.

PHASE 1: Selection of Sounds, Space, Participants, and Faculty of the Activity

1.1. Analysis of sounds and music composition. First, it is necessary to introduce an analysis of different sounds previously created, played and registered by a pianist and taken to a TEST (Figure 3.) specifically designed for this research that links sound to emotions. This first part, on which we focus the research presented here, is led by the team made up of musicians, engineers, architects and psychologists.

1.2. The importance of the placement selection. The activity takes place in a specific classroom as it is the singular place of Form Analysis classroom in the Escuela Politécnica Superior EPS of San Pablo CEU University in Madrid. The classroom space architectural design consists of double height which enhances the echo and a very high acoustic reverberation.

1.3. The selected participants. 16 San Pablo CEU University between 18-30 years old students (average 25 years old) with intellectual disabilities (IQ between 70 and 85) and 8 students (QI above 130) from the San Pablo CEU Sanchinarro School.

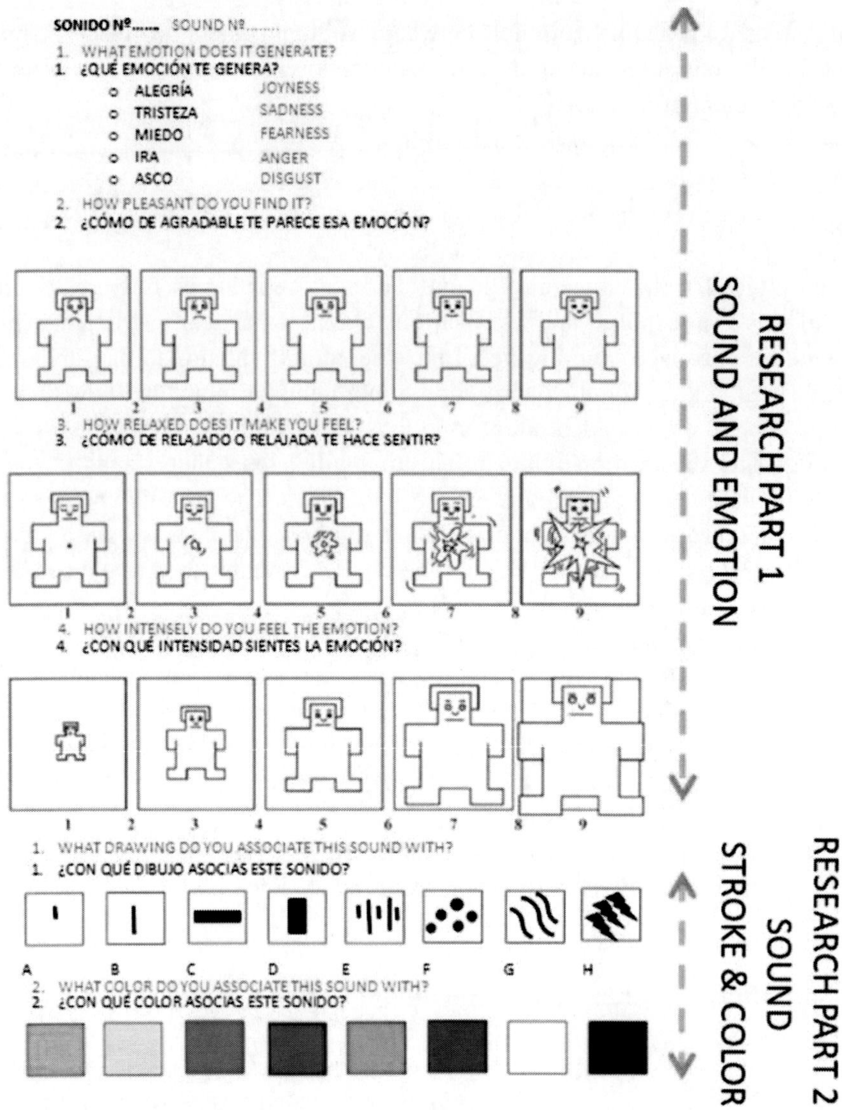

Source: Picture provided by authors.

Figure 3. TEST. Definition of PART 1 (sound and emotion) based in 'Self -Assessment Manikin, SAM; Lang (1980) and definition of PART 2 (graphic response about sound and its association with stroke and color. This takes part of a complementary research).

1.4. The selected faculty team of the activity. Organizing team of the multidisciplinary collaborative workshop:

- The workshop is run by: 1 musician and professor of the Information Technology Department, 1 architect professor of the subjects of Form Analysis, Natural Drawing and Artistic Drawing in the Degree of Architecture, Interior Architecture and Digital Art.
- Participating: 1 professor, PhD in education and architecture, from the San Pablo CEU Sanchinarro School, 1 technical architect and PhD student in Architecture and Trainer of people with intellectual disabilities, 1 psychologist from the SOU

(University Guidance Service) and a PhD Psychologist doctorate in Medicine and 1 Professor and Director of the Master of Energy Efficiency. 2 architects and professors of Form Analysis, Natural Drawing and Artistic Drawing courses of the Architecture Degree.

PHASE 2: Case Study. Secondly, a Specific Activity Is Carried out in Order to Pursuit Results and Introduce New Conclusions to the Statement of the Art

2.1. Firstly, the pianist leads the session, and the students take the TEST for associative analysis of sounds with emotions.
The projected sounds are:
- SOUND 1: 1 high-frequency note on piano
- SOUND 2: 1 low-frequency note on piano
- SOUND 3: 1 high-frequency note (same as before) on violin
- SOUND 4: 1 low-frequency note (same as before) on violin
- RHYTHM 5. 1 rhythm (dynamic-happy-fun-bright-lively…)
- RHYTHM 6: 1 rhythm (sad-funereal-slow-paused-dark-dark)
- COMPOSITION 7: 1 evocative musical composition (open)
- COMPOSITION 8: 1 evocative musical composition (open)

2.2. Material used. The University provides pencils and 8 TESTs on colored printed paper (Figure 1) for each student (one for each sound).

2.3. TEST results. The student will express her answer personally on TEST, choosing the appropriate one and without writing text. Students will focus on answering the questions that the TEST suggests, which are the following:
- What emotion does it generate?
- How pleasant do you find it?
- How relaxed does it make you feel?
- How intensely do you feel the emotion?

Finally, to conclude this research, the answers to the first 4 questions of the TEST posed above and presented here inTables 1, 2, 3 and 4 will be matched with the results of both student profiles (over 18 years with intellectual disabilities and those under 18 years of age with high intellectual abilities). A survey will also be provided to students so that students can express their degree of satisfaction and draw conclusions, as well as possible improvements to the activity.

Results and Discussion

The association of sounds and music with emotions for neuronal effects favors connections in areas of the brain and helps to recognize or name our state of mind. Sharing results between students with two very different profiles is an enriching experience that would not arise for students in another common situation in their life experience. Proposing this activity to students of different ages provides differential feedback and to that we add that the cognitive abilities of the students who receive the information are 60% different (from 80 to 130 IQ). If we also add to this that knowledge about music will depend on your previous learning background, we can give diverse results which add complexity to the conclusions. Hence, the method combines the answers in a single TEST in order to facilitate reliable conclusions (Figure 4).

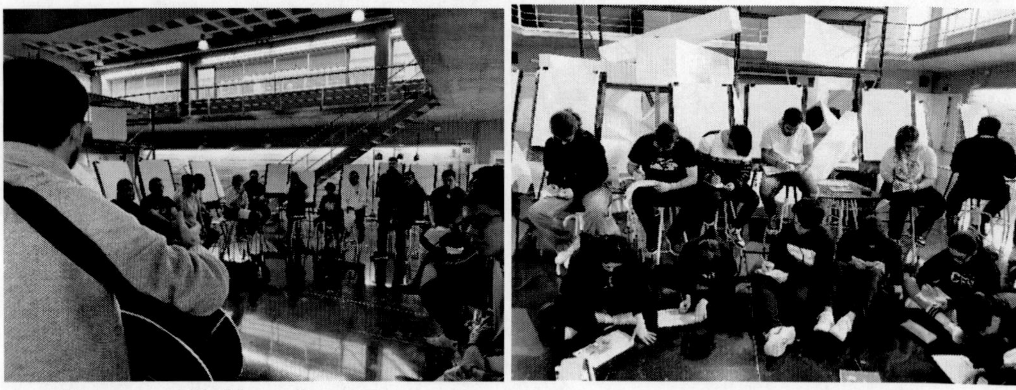

Source: Picture provided by author.

Figure 4. Sounds TEST response process.

Case Study Results and Psychological Discussion

The association of emotion with different low- or high-pitch sounds leads the student to choose the appropriate tool for its perception. A total of 24 TEST results were collected (8 from highly gifted students and 16 from students with intellectual disabilities) (Tables 1, 2, 3 and 4).

Table 1. Test results about EMOTIONS associated to SOUNDS according to the emotion that generates to the student.
Note: column DN = Don't Know is NS/NC (in Spanish NS = no sabe/NC = no contesta)

		EMOCIÓN QUE GENERA EL SONIDO/ EMOTION THAT GENERATES YOU						
		A	B	C	D	E	NS/NC	
SOUND 1	ID STUDENTS	6	3	3	1	2		conclusive result
	HC STUDENTS	1	3	4				no conclusive result
SOUND 2	ID STUDENTS	1	2	9	4			conclusive result
	HC STUDENTS		1	4	3			conclusive result
SOUND 3	ID STUDENTS	10	2		1	2	1	conclusive result
	HC STUDENTS	5	2		1			conclusive result
SOUND 4	ID STUDENTS	4	1	5	4	1	1	no conclusive result
	HC STUDENTS	2	2	1	2	1		no conclusive result
SOUND 5	ID STUDENTS	9	2	2	2	1		conclusive result
	HC STUDENTS	3	1	2	2			conclusive result
SOUND 6	ID STUDENTS	2	3	6	3	1	1	conclusive result
	HC STUDENTS		1	4	3			conclusive result
SOUND 7	ID STUDENTS	12	1		2	1		conclusive result
	HC STUDENTS	6	1		1			conclusive result
SOUND 8	ID STUDENTS	2	3	3	4	3	1	no conclusive result
	HC STUDENTS	1	1	2	1	2		no conclusive result

A= ALEGRIA-JOYNESS/ B=TRISTEZA-SADNESS/ C= MIEDO-FEARNESS /D=IRA-ANGER/E=ASCO-DISGUST

DN= DON'T KNOW

Source: Table provided by authors.

Table 2. Test results according to how pleasant the sound is for the student. Note: column DN = Don't Know is NS/NC (in Spanish NS = no sabe/NC = no contesta)

¿CÓMO DE AGRADABLE TE PARECE? / HOW PLEASANT SEEMS TO YOU?

		1	2	3	4	5	6	7	8	9	NS/NC	
SOUND 1	ID STUDENTS			3	1	9	1			1	1	conclusive result
	HC STUDENTS			1	2	4		1				conclusive result
SOUND 2	ID STUDENTS		1	5	1	4	2			1	2	no conclusive result
	HC STUDENTS		3	2	2				1			no conclusive result
SOUND 3	ID STUDENTS	1	1	1	1	2	1	5	1	3		no conclusive result
	HC STUDENTS	1			1	3		2		1		no conclusive result
SOUND 4	ID STUDENTS	1	1	4	1	4	1	2	1	1		no conclusive result
	HC STUDENTS		1	2	2		1	2				no conclusive result
SOUND 5	ID STUDENTS	1		2		3		3	1	6		conclusive result
	HC STUDENTS		1		1	1	3	2				no conclusive result
SOUND 6	ID STUDENTS	4		2	2	5	1	1		1		conclusive result
	HC STUDENTS	1	1	1	4			1				conclusive result
SOUND 7	ID STUDENTS	1		3				5	1	6		conclusive result
	HC STUDENTS			1				2	4	1		conclusive result
SOUND 8	ID STUDENTS	2	1	5	3	3	1			1		conclusive result
	HC STUDENTS		1	3	1	2						conclusive result

1: NO, NOT REALLY - 9 : YES, A LOT
DN= DON'T KNOW

Source: Table provided by authors.

Table 3. Test results about according to how relaxed the sound is for the student. Note: column DN = Don't Know is NS/NC (in Spanish NS = no sabe/NC = no contesta)

¿CÓMO DE RELAJADO/A TE HACE SENTIR? / HOW RELAXED IT MAKES YOU FEEL?

		1	2	3	4	5	6	7	8	9	NS/NC	
SOUND 1	ID STUDENTS	1		2		7	1	3			2	conclusive result
	HC STUDENTS	1		5				2				conclusive result
SOUND 2	ID STUDENTS	1		3		6	2	1		1	2	no conclusive result
	HC STUDENTS	1		1		1	1	4				no conclusive result
SOUND 3	ID STUDENTS	1		4		5		3		1	2	conclusive result
	HC STUDENTS	1	1	1		2	1	2				conclusive result
SOUND 4	ID STUDENTS	2	2	3	1	3	2		1		2	no conclusive result
	HC STUDENTS	1			1	2	2	1	1			no conclusive result
SOUND 5	ID STUDENTS			2		5	1	2			2	conclusive result
	HC STUDENTS				2			4	1	1		conclusive result
SOUND 6	ID STUDENTS	3		1	3	3	1	1		2	2	no conclusive result
	HC STUDENTS		1	1		2	2	1		1		no conclusive result
SOUND 7	ID STUDENTS	3		2		2	2		2	3	2	no conclusive result
	HC STUDENTS	1	2	2		1			1	1		no conclusive result
SOUND 8	ID STUDENTS	1	1	3	2	4	1	1		1	2	no conclusive result
	HC STUDENTS				1	2	2		2	1		no conclusive result

1: YES, A LOT- 9 : NO, NOT REALLY
DN= DON'T KNOW

Source: Table provided by authors.

As psychological discussion we could point up:

Primary emotions such as fear, joy, sadness, anger, and disgust are fundamental to the human experience and play an important role in emotional cognition.

The emotion that has occurred the least in the study, in both groups, is disgust. This emotion has a protective function against possible threats or harmful situations. This is why it can be difficult to associate this emotion with a specific sound.

In relation to Sound 1 (see table of results), the ID students have marked joy as the emotion to highlight compared to the HC students who have fundamentally selected fear and sadness. This could be due, on the one hand, to the aspects on which one group has been able to focus its attention, such as the intensity, harmony, amplitude or frequency of the sound, and another group to the personal or experiential association that could generate other, different emotional responses. On the other hand, the influence of the different areas that can be activated at the brain level is considered.

Table 4. Test results about according to how intense the sound is for the student. Note: column DN = Don't Know is NS/NC (in Spanish NS = no sabe/NC = no contesta)

¿CON QUÉ INTENSIDAD SIENTES LA EMOCIÓN? / HOW INTENSELY DO YOU FEEL THE EMOTION?

		1	2	3	4	5	6	7	8	9	NS/NC	
SOUND 1	ID STUDENTS		1	2	3	7		1			2	conclusive result
	HC STUDENTS			3	1	2		2				no conclusive result
SOUND 2	ID STUDENTS			4	1	5		3		1	2	conclusive result
	HC STUDENTS			1		1	3		3			no conclusive result
SOUND 3	ID STUDENTS	2	1	2	1	4	1	1	1	1	2	no conclusive result
	HC STUDENTS	2		1	2			1	2			no conclusive result
SOUND 4	ID STUDENTS		1	4	3	4	1	2				no conclusive result
	HC STUDENTS	1		1	2	1		2	1			no conclusive result
SOUND 5	ID STUDENTS		1	1		3	2	3	1	4	1	no conclusive result
	HC STUDENTS					2	2	2	1	1		no conclusive result
SOUND 6	ID STUDENTS	2	1	5	1	3	1			2	1	conclusive result
	HC STUDENTS					2	2	1	2	1		no conclusive result
SOUND 7	ID STUDENTS			1		3	2	2	1	5	2	conclusive result
	HC STUDENTS					1	1	5	1			conclusive result
SOUND 8	ID STUDENTS			3	2	2	1	4		2	2	no conclusive result
	HC STUDENTS				1	1	2	1	1	2		no conclusive result

1: NO, NOT REALLY - 9 : YES, A LOT
DN= DON'T KNOW

Source: Table provided by authors.

When listening to music and feeling, several areas of the brain are activated, each with a specific and related function. Some of these main areas are:

- *The prefrontal cortex*: associated with higher cognitive processing, including planning, decision making, and emotional regulation. Music can activate the prefrontal cortex, influencing interpretation and emotional response to music.
- *The limbic system (amygdala):* This system is responsible for emotions, motivation, and reward. Music can activate the nucleus accumbency, which releases dopamine, a neurotransmitter associated with pleasure. The amygdala is a key structure in emotional processing and memory formation. It is known to respond to emotional stimuli, including music, and plays an important role in generating emotional responses to music.
- *The nucleus Accumbency*: related to motivation and reward processing. If sound activates this system, it can contribute to the feeling of pleasure, well-being, and happiness when listening to specific music.
- *The cingulate cortex*: involved in emotional regulation and attention. Music can affect your activity, which can influence the emotional response and attention you pay to the sound.
- *The insula:* involved in emotional awareness and the perception of the body's internal sensations, thus contributing to the emotional experience associated with music.
- *The hippocampus:* associated with memory and the encoding of emotional events, influencing the formation of emotional memories associated with music.

- *The cerebellum:* in addition to being involved in motor control and coordination, it is also related to emotional regulation. It is an important area for coordination when playing instruments or dancing.

The activation of the different areas will depend on several factors such as the type of music or familiarity with them. This is why in the present study different sounds and melodies have been taken into account that have been presented in a similar way to both groups.

In relation to this, it can be noted that the own elaboration of sounds or compositions could be predetermined by the emotion aroused in the composer, generating a specific result (selection expectation) associated with a specific emotion. Therefore, a control measure could be carried out for future research.

On the other hand, as shown in the results (Figure 1), the sounds represented by a musical note generated a much clearer emotional response than the sounds formed by a melody, with the exception of sound 4, which presents a more ambiguous response, in both groups, as does sound 8 characterized by a melody. This may be related to the brain structures that have been activated in each participant. The melody can activate more brain areas related to memories, interoception, motivation or other more complex variables that influence emotions in an individualized way, according to the person's experience.

The Self-Assessment Manikin test (SAM; Lang, 1980) is a quick and easy instrument to evaluate emotional responses in different subjects (Bradley & Lang, 1994). However, it is considered important to be able to use another instrument since some participants had difficulties when seeing and interpreting the image in relation to the emotion it represented. It would be interesting to replicate the same study with another instrument for measuring visual pictograms.

Without a doubt, if we simplify the relationship between music and Intelligence Quotient (IQ), we find that the relationship is not simple, it is a complex concept that can not only be measured with tests, but that many other variables can influence. As Rubia-Vila (2018) points out before the year, they have the ability to perceive music in such a way that there are studies that consider it to be an innate ability. In their review, Custodio and Cano (2017) present, in some studies, a positive correlation between musical ability and IQ, while others have not found any significant relationship. For example, people with Williams Syndrome show outstanding aptitudes in specific areas, such as music, despite having an IQ between 50 and 70. This leads to the hypothesis that musical ability is independent of IQ and as reflected in the results obtained in the present study. That is why it could be considered an aptitude independently of intellectual capacity.

These studies need to continue to determine the possible relationship between music and possible cognitive areas.

This study leads us to propose the relationship between synesthesia and IQ. Synesthesia can be defined as a neurological phenomenon in which the stimulation of one sense causes the automatic and involuntary experience of another sensation in another sense (Pinto Prieto, 2021; Callejas, 2012). In this case, a sound generates a specific emotion. This is called emotional-musical synesthesia.

This type of synesthesia occurs when the person experiences an automatic and involuntary association between emotions and musical characteristics, such as tone, rhythm, timbre, among others.

For example, an emotional-musical synesthetic person could experience primary emotions, such as joy, sadness, or secondary emotions such as happiness and nostalgia, when listening to certain sounds or musical melodies (Pinto Prieto, 2021; Callejas, 2012). As we have pointed out before, there are different areas of the brain associated with emotion, such as the amygdala and the limbic system, that may also be active when people experience emotional-musical synesthesia.

Some studies have suggested that people with synesthesia may have an above-average IQ. However, it is important to note that the relationship between synesthesia and IQ is complex and can be influenced by a variety of factors, such as the specific type of synesthesia, cultural context, family environment, and other genetic and neurobiological factors. Therefore, more studies are needed to delve deeper into this relationship and study the different variables that can influence them.

Conclusion

The way the brain works when we listen to music or paint is a complex and fascinating topic. The interaction of multiple areas of the brain is involved, including those related to perception, emotion, memory, creativity and attention. Music and visual art can have a significant impact on mood, creativity, and mental health due to this complex brain interaction.

One of the simplest and most common reasons for music's presence in our lives is that it helps us express emotions, evoke memories, release tension, and influence our mood. Some theoretical as well as practical and psycho-pedagogical approaches have achieved surprising results through music, not only in stimulating creativity and fostering people's emotional expression and well-being, but also in developing cognitive skills and human values.

Both music and painting offer opportunities for expression, personal development and creativity for people with intellectual disabilities and people with high abilities, each adapted to their individual needs and abilities. Brain functioning is highly adaptive and is influenced by a variety of genetic and environmental factors.

The entire analysis of brain structure discussed in this article has to do with the relationship between neuronal functioning in both study groups, in which, working on the emotional interpretation of sounds, results that are both similar and disparate are obtained. Analyzing as a connection point the creative skills, which link music and painting, with the emotional ones, which relate the different intellectual levels of our students, we can specify a series of similarities in these two parameters: creativity and emotions.

Despite differences in the level of intellectual functioning, there are creative similarities in people with intellectual disabilities and people with high abilities: creative diversity can manifest itself in many different ways, such as visual art, music, writing, dance and further; originality, since both can be creative and original in their approach to problems and projects; lateral thinking, or the ability to see unusual connections between ideas or concepts; inspiration from personal experience and emotions, everyday life, relationships and emotions are common themes in creativity; challenge and motivation for creative projects, which can contribute to your personal and emotional development and to find creativity as a way to explore your interests and challenge your intellect; creative therapy, which can help in the expression of emotions, problem solving and improving emotional well-being.

It is important to recognize that creativity is a universal human quality that can flourish in different circumstances and levels of intellectual ability. Fostering creativity in all individuals, regardless of intellectual capacity, is essential for personal growth and self-expression.

Despite their intellectual differences, we can also contemplate emotional similarities between the two groups object of this study, such as: the experience of basic emotions, such as joy, sadness, anger, fear and love in a similar way, being a fundamental part of the human experience; the need for affection and relationships, love and belonging, such as family and social relationships, which are important for your emotional well-being; the response to emotional experiences, such as stress, success, loss and happiness, can influence emotional state and mental health; emotional development, a process that occurs throughout life experiencing emotional changes as they mature and can learn to manage and express their emotions in a healthier way over time; emotional communication, with a variety of forms of communication, such as verbal expression, non-verbal expression and social interaction, to convey and understand your emotions; emotional resilience when facing challenges and overcoming difficulties in their lives. Recognizing and understanding these similarities is important to promote empathy, inclusion, and emotional support in all individuals, regardless of their intellectual ability.

It can be concluded that both students with an IQ of 80 and those with an IQ above 130 actively react to sounds, expressing their emotions through their responses, memories, experiences, and painting skills, all while maintaining the freedom to express their feelings.

Some experiences of analytical work of an auditory and visual-spatial nature, with this student profile or in synergy with other profiles, have opened new avenues of research. These are:

- Researching from the area of Psychology with people with cognitive disabilities through artistic and spatial tools provided by architects.
- Encouraging people of different intellectual profiles to interact in common experiences and expecting similar results.
- Favoring the analysis of the understanding of sound, vibration and timbre of sounds as well as rhythms and compositions in people of different intellectual profiles.

The paths opened in this chapter are some such as:

We could use music to help people move down the street or move around a building.
We could use music to deal with daily situations that cause us stress or discomfort.

Research results suggests that people frequently use music to regulate their emotions. However, little is known about what kinds of music may regulate affective states. More broadly, energetic and rhythmic music was positively associated with using all examined forms of musical emotion regulation, suggesting this dimension of music is especially useful in modulating emotions. These results highlight the potential use of music as a tool for emotion regulation. Future research can extend our findings by examining the efficacy of different types of music at modulating emotional states.

Acknowledgments

This research is made possible thanks to the participation of students with intellectual disabilities from the CF-CAAU Universal Accessibility Support Consultant Training Course funded by the FONCE Foundation and the European Social Fund (2018-2023).

References

Alonso Peña, José Ramón and Bueno, Marta (2020). "La música mejora nuestra concentración" La ciencia busca la respuesta. The conversation. Available online: https://theconversation.com/la-musica-mejora-nuestra-concentracion-la-ciencia-busca-la-respuesta-142231 (accessed on 28 March 2022).

Bradley, M. & Lang, P. (1994). Measuring emotion: The self-assessment manikin and the semantic differential. *Journal of Behavior Therapy and Experimental Psychiatry*, 25, 49-59. https://doi.org/10.1016/0005-7916(94)90063-9.

Callejas, A. (2012). *Synesthesia: the color of words, the flavor of music, the place of time.* Alliance.

Cantarero-García, G. et al. (2021). "Taller de representación gráfica de sonidos para alumnos de edades y capacidades diferentes." Madrid, Spain: CEU Ediciones. p. 257-258 ISBN: 978-84-18463-23-5.

Camfield, D. (2005). Neurobiology of creativity. En Stough, C. (Ed.), *Neurobiology of exceptionality* (pp. 53-72). New York: Kluwer Academic/Plenum Publishers.

Custodio, N., & Cano-Campos, M. (2017). Effects of music on cognitive functions. *Journal of Neuro-psychiatry*, 80(1), 60-69.

Damasio, A. (1994): *Descarte's error. Emotion, reason and the human brain*, pp. 155–195, Traducción 2006, Barcelona, Crítica.

Drott, E. (2018). Musical Contention and Contentious Music; or, the Drums of Occupy Wall Street. *Contemporary Music Review*, 37(5–6), 626–645. https://doi.org/10.1080/07494467.2017.1402461.

Duncan, J. (2001). An adaptive coding model of neural function in prefrontal cortex. *Nature reviews neuroscience,* 2(11), 820-829. https://doi.org/10.1028/3509757.

Ferrando, M., Prieto, M. P, Ferrandiz, C., Sanchez, C. (2005). Inteligencia y Creatividad. *Revista Electrónica de Investigación Psicoeducativa* Nº Vol 3. 21 -50.

González-García, H., Pelegrín, A., & Trinidad Morales, A. (2019). Influencia de la ira en el nivel de competición, éxitos y deportistas profesionales. *Ansiedad y Estrés*, *25*(2), 105–110. https://doi.org/10.1016/j.anyes.2019.08.003.

Han, D., Kong, Y., Han, J., & Wang, G. (2022, December 1). A survey of music emotion recognition. *Frontiers of Computer Science*. Higher Education Press Limited Company. https://doi.org/10.1007/s11704-021-0569-4.

Honing, H., ten Cate, C., Peretz, I., & Trehub, S. E. (2015). Without it no music: Cognition, biology and evolution of musicality. *Philosophical Transactions of the Royal Society B: Biological Sciences*. Royal Society of London. https://doi.org/10.1098/rstb.2014.0088.

Launay, J., & Pearce, E. (2015). Choir singing improves health, happiness–and is the perfect icebreaker. *The Conversation*, *28*.

Available online: https://www.ox.ac.uk/research/choir-singing-improves-health-happiness-%E2%80%93-and-perfect-icebreaker.

Llanga, E., & Insuasti, J. P. (2019). La influencia de la música en el aprendizaje. *Atlante: Cuadernos de Educación y Desarrollo*, 1–11. Retrieved from https://www.eumed.net/rev/atlante/2019/06/musica-aprendizaje.html.

Jaén López, C. (2013). Cómo trabajar la creatividad en niños con discapacidad. *Revista Internacional de audición y lenguaje, logopedia, apoyo a la integración y multiculturalidad.* RIALAM vol 2 Nº 4 Recuperado http://rialaium.web.node.es recuperado (pp. 33-51).

Meng, Q., Zhao, T., & Kang, J. (2018). Influence of music on the behaviors of crowd in urban open public spaces. *Frontiers in Psychology*, *9*(APR). https://doi.org/10.3389/fpsyg.2018.00596.

Meng, Q., Jiang, J., Liu, F., & Xu, X. (2020). Effects of the musical sound environment on communicating emotion. *International Journal of Environmental Research and Public Health, 17*(7). https://doi.org /10.3390/ijerph17072499.

Mestre Navas, J. M. & Fernandez Berrocal, P. (2007). Manual of emotional intelligence. Pyramid.

Meyer, L. (1956): Emotion and meaning in music, University of Chicago, "Emoción y significado en la música," Tradución de TURINA, J. L. (2001), Madrid, Alianza Editorial.

Mrazik, M. & Dombrowski, S. C. (2010). The neurobiological foundations of giftedness. *Roeper Review,* 32(4), 224-234. doi: 10.1080/02783193.2010.508154.

Pinto Prieto, J. D. (2021). *Living synesthesia.* https://repositorio.uniandes.edu.co/entities/publication/ 37b0c8bb-3a34-4548-ac14-9eeca4e40565.

Rodríguez, S. (2017). *La música puede incrementar la empatía.* Available online: http://www.newvewe.com/ blog/la-musica-puede-incrementar-la-empatia

Rubia-Vila F. J. (2018). Neurobiological bases of music. RANM ANNALS. Royal National Academy of Medicine of Spain, 135(02). http://dx.doi.org/10.32440/ar.2018.135.02.supl01.art03.

Sandoval, V. G., Pimazzoni, D. N., Trejo, B. D., & Muñíz, J. G. (2018). Manejo psicoterapéutico del dolor: a través de la música y el tacto en neonatos: el Método Sentire. Estudios Sobre Las Culturas Contemporáneas, 24(47), 9–40. Retrieved from http://0-search.ebscohost.com.llull.uib.es/login.aspx% 3fdirect%3dtrue%26AuthType%3dcookie%2cip%2cuid%26db%3da9h%26AN%3d131273120%26lang %3des%26site%3dehost-live.

Shaw P., Greenstein D., Lerch J., Clasen L., Lenroot R., Gogtay N., et al. (2006). Intellectual ability and cortical development in children and adolescents. *Nature*, 440: 676-9.

Soria-Urios, G., Duque, P., y García-Moreno, J. (2011). Música y cerebro (II): evidencias cerebrales del entrenamiento musical. *Revista de neurología,* 53(12): 739. doi: 10.33588/rn.5312.2011475.

Trimble, M., & Hesdorffer, D. (2017). Music and the brain: the neuroscience of music and musical appreciation. *BJPsych. International*, *14*(2), 28–31. https://doi.org/10.1192/s2056474000001720.

Winner, E. (2000). The origins and ends of giftedness. *American psychologist,* 55(1), 159-169. doi: 10.1037/0003-066X.55.1.159.

Biographical Sketches

Dr. Gabriel Caffarena, PhD

Affiliation:

Universidad San Pablo-CEU, CEU Universities, Institute of Technology, Madrid, Spain.
Licenses/Registration: Senior Member, IEEE

Educational Credentials:

- 2008: PhD Cum Laude at Telecommunication Engineering School (ETSIT), Universidad Politécnica de Madrid (UPM).
- 1998: Telecommunication Engineering Degree, Telecommunication Engineering School (ETSIT), Universidad de Málaga (UMA), Spain.

Business Address:

Information Technology Department, Institute of Technology, Universidad San Pablo-CEU, CEU Universities, Campus de Montepríncipe, 28668, Madrid, Spain.

Research:
Selected Publication and Recent Research: ORCID CODE: 0000-0002-2902-3869.

Teaching Experience: 18 years

- 2021-2023: Associate Professor. Universidad San Pablo CEU.
- 2012-2020: Profesor Adjunto. Universidad San Pablo CEU.
- 2010-2011: Profesor Colaborador Doctor. Universidad San Pablo CEU.
- 2003-2009: Assistant Professor. Universidad Politécnica de Madrid.

Professional Experience: 25 years

- 2023-present: Chip Development Manager. Vodafone.
- 2000-2001: Network Support Engineer. Imperial College London.
- 1998-2000: Neuroscience Research Technician. University College London.

Professional Appointments:

- 2017-2022: Master in Biomedical Engineering Coordinator. Universidad San Pablo CEU.

Honors:

- 2019: Teaching Quality Award. University San Pablo CEU
- 2019: First Innovation CEU Universities Award
- 2010: Ángel Herrera Research Award.
- 2010: Best PhD Thesis Award. Universidad Politécnica de Madrid.
- 2013: Best Paper Award. IADIS.
- 2004: Best Paper Award. ReConFig.

Selected Publications from the Last 3 Years:

1. Caffarena, G. (2022). Wordlength Optimization of Fixed-Point Algorithms. In: Bosio, A., Ménard, D., Sentieys, O. (eds) *Approximate Computing Techniques*. Springer, Cham. https://doi.org/10.1007/978-3-030-94705-7_9. ISBN: 978-3-030-94704-0.
2. Abraham Otero, Paulo Félix, David G. Márquez, Constantino A. García, Gabriel Caffarena (2022). "A fault-tolerant clustering algorithm for processing data from multiple streams," *Information Sciences,* Volume 584, 2022, Pages 649-664, ISSN 0020-0255.
3. Desai, M. P., Caffarena, G., Jevtic, R., Márquez, D. G., Otero, A. A Low-Latency (2021). "Low-Power FPGA Implementation of ECG Signal Characterization Using Hermite Polynomials," *Electronics* 2021, 10, 2324. https://doi.org/10.3390/electronics10192324,

Dr. Roberto Alonso González Lezcano, PhD

Accredited as Full Professor by AQU-Catalunya (March 2023). Tenured Professor at the Department of Architecture and Design, area of Building Systems, within the Institute of Technology of Universidad CEU San Pablo. Coordinator of the subjects Building Systems as well as Electrical and Lighting systems. Professor Accredited by ANECA in the figures of Tenured Professor. Two six-year research period by CNEAI (last period 2016-2021). Coordinator of the post-graduate degree of Energy Efficiency and Sustainability in Buildings and Coordinator of the Laboratory of Building Systems within Universidad CEU San Pablo. Coordinator of line 2: Innovation, Construction and Technology, in the Doctoral Program of Composition, History and Techniques in Architecture and Urbanism. Extraordinary Doctorate Award. San Pablo CEU University. 57 impact articles in the last 5 years. H Index:17. Editor of 8 JCR-indexed journals (140 edited articles, indexed in the JCR). Principal Investigator of the ARIE Group: Architecture, Efficient Installations. CEU San Pablo University. Angel CV date 08/11/2023 CURRICULUM VITAE (CVA) IMPORTANT – The Curriculum Vitae cannot exceed 4 pages. Instructions to fill this document are available in the website. 2 Herrera Award for the best research work in the area of Architecture and Engineering in the year 2022 at CEU San Pablo University, for the utility model "Indoor LED luminaire emitting the full visible light spectrum", developed and exploited by the company Pentaluz. 29 books published, 22 of them in the last 5 years. Coordinator and co-author of the collections of Abecé of Building Systems (Munilla-Lería Eds.) consisting of 5 volumes. Building Systems in Building Design (Asimétricas Eds.) consisting of 7 volumes. 2023 Editor at Building Research and Information (indexed in the JCR) at Recent Patent on Engineering (indexed in Scopus and WoS). 2020-2022 Editor of the books " Intersecting Health, Livability, and Human Behavior in Urban Environments" ISBN: 9781668469248 "Advancing STEM Education and Innovation in a Time of Distance Learning " ISBN: 9781668450536, "Urban Sustainability and Energy Management of Cities For Improved Health and Well-Being" ISBN: 9781668440308, "Advancements in Sustainable Architecture and Energy Efficiency" ISBN 9781799870234 and "Health and Well-Being Considerations in the Design of Indoor Environments" ISBN 9781799872795, indexed in WoS, Clarivate Analytics, Book Citation Index, Scopus, SPI. 2021 Editor of the Topic "Energy Efficiency, Environment and Health". (100 articles edited) MDPI Publishing. Journals indexed in the JCR involved in the Topic: Energies, IJERPH, Peocesses, Buildings and Atmosphere. Deadline: January 29, 2023. Editor at Nova Science Publishers of the book "Sustainable and Healthy Building Environments" indexed in WoS, Clarivate Analytics, Book Citation Index, Scopus, SPI. ISBN: 9798886974010. 2020-2022 Editor of the JCR Sustainability journal of the Special issue "Indoor Environment Quality and Health in Energy-Efficient Buildings", (9 articles edited) Deadline February 28, 2022, "Sustainable Building and Indoor Air Quality" (17 articles edited). Editor in the JCR Energies journal of the Special Issue "Energy Efficiency and Indoor Environment Quality" (10 articles edited). Since 2016 Reviewer of the journals Energy and Building, Building and Environment, Sustainable Cities and Society, Engineering Structures, Building Research and Information, International Journal of Ventilation de Taylor, Journal of Housing and the Built Environment, Journal of the Brazilian Society of Mechanical Sciences and Engineering, Journal of Environmental Chemical Engineering, Sustainability, International Journal of Environmental Research and Public Health, Energies, Materials, Journal of Engineering Technology, (480 reviews in 51 journals in total) etc ... all indexed in JCR. Top 10% Reviewers of the last two years. Energy and

Building journal indexed in the JCR. 2019. Architecture and Solidarity Award of the 1st Housing Excellence Awards of the newspaper La Razón for the VEM Project financed by Airbus Defense and Space and developed at the CEU San Pablo University. Award won due to the VEM project developed with AIRBUS company. 2015. Member of the Team Crew and Advisor of the Universidad Autónoma de Occidente and Universidad de San Buenaventura in the MIHOUSE Project team in the Solar Decathlon Latin American and Caribbean 2015 contest held in Cali, Colombia.

Dr. Ana Jiménez-Perianes, PhD

Affiliation:
Universidad San Pablo-CEU, CEU Universities, Psychology Department, Madrid, Spain.
Licenses/Registration:
Registered Psychologist, Official Psychologist Association of Madrid (COPM) Member N.21528.

Educational Credentials:

- Licenciada en Psicología (Universidad CEU San Pablo)
- Doctora por la Facultad de Medicina (Universidad CEU San Pablo)
- Máster en Medicina molecular Aplicada. Daño Celular, Envejecimiento, Bioprotección y Oncogénesis (Universidad CEU San Pablo).
- Máster en Criminal Profiling (UDIMA).
- Máster en Comportamiento no Verbal y Detección de la Mentira (UDIMA).
- Máster en Psicología Legal y forense (UNED).
- Máster en Formación para Profesor de Educación Secundaria Obligatoria y Bachillerato (Universidad CEU San Pablo).
- Experto en Psicología Infanto-Juvenil: Aspectos Clínicos, Evolutivos y Educativos (Universidad de Granada)
- Experto en Diagnóstico y Educación de los Alumnos con Alta Capacidad (UNED).
- Experto profesional en Análisis del perfil criminológico y la futura detección de criminales violentos (UNED).
- Perito Judicial Experto en ciberdelincuencia y conducta criminal en la web (UNED).
- Perito Judicial Experto en acoso escolar y ciberacoso (UDIMA).
- Perito Judicial Experto en Pericia Grafológica (UNED).

Business Address:
Psychology Department, Universidad San Pablo-CEU, Campus de Monteprincipe, 28668, Madrid, Spain.

Research:
Selected Publication and Recent Research: ORCID CODE: 0000-0003-3169-8547.

Teaching Experience: 17 years

- 2018-present: Profesor Adjunto. Universidad San Pablo CEU.
- 2017-2018: Profesor Colaborador Doctor. Universidad San Pablo CEU.
- 2007-2017: Profesor Colaborador. Departamento de Psicología (Universidad San Pablo CEU).

Professional Experience: 16 years

- Psicóloga en práctica privada en psicología forense y psicología sanitaria.
- Escuela de padres.
- Psicóloga infanto-juvenil. Especialista en niños y adolescentes con alta capacidad intelectual.

Professional Appointments:

- Profesora Adjunta del área de Personalidad, Evaluación y Tratamiento psicológico (PETRA) del Departamento de Psicología, Facultad de Medicina, de la Universidad CEU San Pablo (Madrid).
- Directora del Máster Universitario en Psicología Jurídica y Forense de la Universidad CEU San Pablo.
- Coordinadora de alumnos del Máster Universitario Oficial en Psicología General Sanitaria de la Universidad CEU San Pablo.
- Coordinadora de la asignatura "Evaluación y diagnóstico en psicología de la salud" del Máster Universitario en Psicología General Sanitaria de la Universidad CEU San Pablo.
- Directora de la revista de Behavior & Law Journal.

Honors:

- International Affiliate Membership #00196253 de la American Psychological Association (APA-USA).
- Miembro del Panel Internacional de Expertos en salud mental de la Organización Mundial de la Salud (OMS), para el desarrollo de la 11ª edición de la Clasificación Estadística Internacional de Enfermedades y Problemas Relacionados con la Salud (CIE-11), subapartado de Trastornos mentales y del comportamiento. Global Clinical Practice Network (GCPN) World Health Organization [https://gcp.network/es/].
- Psicóloga General Sanitaria Habilitada por la Consejería de Sanidad de la Comunidad de Madrid.

Selected Publications from the Last 3 Years:

1. Vargas Hernández, J., & Jiménez Perianes, A. (2022). Videojuegos. En L. Aguacil y A. Piñas (eds). *Las adicciones en la adolescencia y en la juventud*. Guía práctica para padres y educadores. Dykinson.

2. Jiménez Perianes, A., & Cima Muñoz, A. (2022). Las necesidades educativas especiales, una responsabilidad especial: el caso de los alumnos con altas capacidades intelectuales. En P. Santos Rodriguez (Ed.). Libertad y responsabilidad educativas, (235-247). Tirant lo Blanch. Garcia-Adasme SI, Cárdenas-Rebollo JM, Jimenez-Perianes A, Lalinde M, Jimeno S, Ventura PS, Díaz A, López-Escobar A. (2021). Pediatric home confinement due to COVID-19: Somatic and anxiety spectrum consequences. *J Clin Nurs* (21-22):3238-3248. doi: 10.1111/jocn.15829. Epub 2021 May 6. PMID: 33960054; PMCID: PMC8242703.
3. Cedenilla Vecina, M. & Jiménez-Perianes, A. (2020). Aproximación teórica al síndrome de Munchausen por poderes. *Behavior & Law Journal*, 6, 1-11. https://doi.org/10.47442/blj.v6.i1.77
4. Jiménez-Perianes, A. (2020). *Glosario en términos en psicopatología*. Madrid: CEU Ediciones

Dr. Judit Martínez Martín, PhD

Affiliation:

Profesora de la especialidad de Dibujo y Educación Plástica y Visual.
Máster Universitario en Formación para Profesor de ESO y Bachillerato
Universidad San Pablo CEU. Facultad de Humanidades y Ciencias de la Comunicación
Profesora del Departamento de Artes Plásticas del IES Príncipe Felipe de la Comunidad de Madrid.

Licenses/Registration:

Registered Architect, Official Architects´ Association of Madrid (COAM) Member N.

Educational Credentials:

- 2023: curso Altas Capacidades: conocimiento y desarrollo óptimo. Fundación Avanza.
- 2022-24: Microsoft Educator Expert
- 2021: Bachillerato Internacional. Certificado del IB de prácticas directivas. Certificado avanzado del IB de investigación en prácticas directivas.
- 2021: Master en Dirección, Innovación y Liderazgo de Centros Educativos. Universidad Camilo José Cela. Madrid
- 2017: Premio Extraordinario de Doctorado, convocatoria 2015-2016
- 2016: PhD. Cum Laude at Facultad de Educación. Universidad Nacional de Educación a Distancia (UNED)
- 20011: Master de Calidad en la Construcción MC2

Diploma de estudios avanzados. DCTA
Architecture School of Madrid (ETSAM), Universidad Politécnica de Madrid (UPM), Spain.

- 2009: Especialista en Dirección Técnica de Obras (ETSAM, UPM, Madrid)
- 2008: Especialista en Dirección y Gestión de la Edificación (ETSAM, UPM, Madrid)

- 2002: Diploma of Architect, Architecture School of Madrid (ETSAM), Universidad Politécnica de Madrid (UPM), Spain. (Professional Degree in Architecture).

Business Address:
Facultad de Humanidades. Universidad SAN Pablo CEU. Pº Juan XXIII, 10. 28040. Madrid

Research:
Selected Publication and Recent Research: ORCID CODE: 0000-0003-4803-3189

Teaching Experience: 20 años

- 2023: profesora del Departamento de Artes Plásticas del IES Príncipe Felipe. Madrid
- 2012-2023: profesora de ESO y Bachillerato Internacional, directora del Departamento de Artes, coordinadora de innovación tecnológica. Coordinadora del Aula IDEA de Altas Capacidades. Colegio CEU San Pablo Sanchinarro. Madrid.
- 2009-2012: investigadora del Grupo TISE. DCTA. ETSAM. UPM. Madrid
- 2003-2005: directora y profesora de la Escuela Taller Benigno Murcia. Catalogación del Patrimonio Histórico de Ceuta. Ciudad Autónoma de Ceuta, INEM y Fondo Social Europeo.

Professional Experience: 10 años

- 2009-2012: responsable de Actividades del Solar Decathlon Europe 2010 y 2012.
- 2008: directora de proyectos en Prefabricados Castelo, SA.
- 2007: colaboradora en Riaño Arquitectos
- 2006: colaboradora en Beriot- Bernardini Arquitectos. Madrid
- 2002: colaboradora en Pérez Marín Arquitectos. Ceuta

Professional Appointments:

Honors:

Selected Publications from the Last 3 Years:

1. 2023: Dart4City Manual de Profesores (Montes, N., Zapatera, A., Martínez, J., Rainero, S., Zannetti, A., Marathefti, M., Kofteros, A., Gallon, K., Pacheco, G., Mancuso, A.) https://dart4city.eu/wpcontent/uploads/2023/04/manual-profesores-ESP-WEB.pdf.

Dr. Guadalupe Cantarero-García, PhD

Affiliation:
Universidad San Pablo-CEU, CEU Universities, Institute of Technology, Madrid, Spain.
Licenses/Registration: Registered Architect, Official Architects´ Association of Madrid (COAM) Member N. 15576

Educational Credentials:

- 2014: PhD. Cum Laude at Architecture School of Madrid (ETSAM), Universidad Politécnica de Madrid (UPM).
- 2006: Executive Master of Management EMM at Architecture School of Madrid (ETSAM), Universidad Politécnica de Madrid (UPM).
- 2001: Master of Management in Art Exhibitions. Architecture Center. Antonio Camuñas Foundation.
- 2001: Diploma of Architect, Architecture School of Madrid (ETSAM), Universidad Politécnica de Madrid (UPM), Spain. (Professional Degree in Architecture).
- 1997: Erasmus scholarship at the Urban French Institut. (Institut Francais d'Urbanisme, Paris.

Business Address:
Architecture and Design Department, Institute of Technology, Universidad San Pablo-CEU, CEU Universities, Campus de Monteprincipe, 28668, Madrid, Spain.

Research:
Selected Publication and Recent Research: ORCID CODE: 0000-0003-3169-8547.

Teaching Experience: 19 years
- 2025-present: Profesor Titular. Universidad San Pablo CEU.
- 2019-2025: Profesor Adjunto. Universidad San Pablo CEU.
- 2014-2019: Profesor Colaborador Doctor. Universidad San Pablo CEU.
- 2007-2014: Profesor Colaborador. Escuela Politécnica Superior (Universidad San Pablo CEU).

Professional Experience: 28 years

- 2005-present. Founder CEO. Cantarero Arquitectos- Architecture Studio.
- 2000-2005: Architect in the Heritage Department. Fundación Universitaria San Pablo CEU.
- 1999-2000: Practices at Enrique Porto Rey architecture and urbanism.
- 1998: Practices at Pinillos Arquitectos.
- 1997: Practices at Jean Pierre Buffi Architects, Paris.

Professional Appointments:

- 2015-2021: Degree in Architecture Coordinator and 2022 NAAB Team renewal Coordinator
- 2018-2021: Director of the Laboratory of Smart Cities, Universidad San Pablo CEU
- 2019-2022: CEU UNE Projects Ambasssador, Universidad San Pablo CEU
- Executive Master of Management EMM at Polytechnic School of Madrid ETSAM
- Member and referee of the Common Ground Publishers and referee of RITA RedFundamentos
- Member of the research group "Madrid and Landscape" Financed projects: REF: HAR2014-57843-R and REF: PID2019-110693RB-I00
- 2018-2022: Director of the Financed UNIDIVERSIDAD Project in Universidad San Pablo CEU.

Honors:

- 2007: Chamartín Inmobiliaria First Award: Singular Building
- 2010: Ángel Herrera Solidarity Award.
- 2019: First Innovation CEU Universities Award
- 2019: Ángel Herrera First Award to the Best Research Team PA&P Project.
- 2023: Ángel Herrera First Award to the best Collaborative Online International Learning Project.
- 2025: CEU University First Award in Innovation Project: 'Anatomía Artística Exchange'

Selected Publications from the Last 3 Years:

1. Cantarero-García, Guadalupe. (2020). "Formación inclusiva universitaria para alumnos con discapacidad intelectual como consultor de apoyo de Accesibilidad Universal" *Innovación docente e investigación en Ciencias, Ingeniería y Arquitectura,* Ed: Dykinson, pp 129-138. ISBN: 978-84-1324-559-1.
2. Cantarero-García, Guadalupe (2022) "Análisis espacial inclusivo para alumnos de arquitectura y estudiantes con discapacidad intelectual" en María del Mar Simón Márquez, José Jesús Gázquez Linares, Ana Belén Barragán Martín, África Martos Martínez, *Innovación Docente e Investigación en Ciencias, Ingeniería y Arquitectura: Experiencias de cambio en la Metodología Docente*, Cap. 19 Ed. DYKINSON, pp. 213-224, ISBN: 978-84-1122-865-7.
3. Cantarero-García, Guadalupe. (2023) Marina Mollá y Roberto A. González-Lezcano "Smart citizen in architecture and landscape. Method design based on spatial intelligence and universal accessibility learning by students with intellectual disabilities," *Frontiers,* 2023, doi 10.3389/fbuil.2023.1094760.

Chapter 2

Graphic Representation of Sound and Music: A Case Study of High-Ability and Intellectual Disability Students (Part 2)

Guadalupe Cantarero-García*
Fátima Sarasola Rubio
and Rocío Santo-Tomás Muro
Universidad San Pablo-CEU, CEU Universities, Madrid, Spain

Abstract

Observation and analysis of forms are the basis for graphic language learning: drawing. Graphic expression, as a means of non-verbal communication, is considered essential for exploring human cognitive and sensory development. Sound, as a trigger for emotions and perceptual sensations, can contribute to the field of plastic arts by producing highly personal results that enhance individual expression.
The main objective of the study is to understand and develop the perception of sound and music and represent it graphically to provide new conclusions about the graphic response according to different ages and intellectual abilities. In this way, new paths are opened not only from the synergy of both artistic experiences: musical and graphic, but also from the space and time shared by students with different cognitive profiles.

Keywords: sound analysis, drawing, accessibility

Introduction

This activity emerges from a collaboration between architecture and middle school faculty members. The presence of specialized professors in each discipline, along with psychologists, is necessary to evaluate and measure factors of intellectual development, from sound perception to its graphic representation.

* Corresponding Author's Email: gcgarcia@ceu.es

In: Psycho-Environmental Variables That Ensure People's Well-Being and Health …
Editors: Roberto Alonso González Lezcano and Guadalupe Cantarero García
ISBN: 979-8-89530-831-8
© 2025 Nova Science Publishers, Inc.

This workshop takes place in a unique university environment, specifically within the Form Analysis classroom of the Architecture Degree in Architecture Form Analysis classroom space and provides students with a differential experience since it is offered to students of two very different profiles: on one hand, twelve-year-old children of high abilities and, on the other hand, adults over eighteen years of age with intellectual disabilities (IQ limit 85 Intellectual Quotient) and on the autism spectrum. Students also present different knowledge bases on auditory-musical, graphic and spatial perception, which enriches the experience.

The research question that arises is whether the graphic results will be visually distant. A test system (prior to the representation) is established to associate the sound or composition with a type of line and its density, a color, or a texture, as well as a later representation on paper using brushes of different thicknesses and acrylics.

Analytical Framework

Literature Review

Perception and Its Graphic Representation

When we talk about observation in the architectural field, we might include all the senses in order to understand the model of analysis from other perspectives rather than the merely visual dimension. In the Architectural Graphic Expression Area, specifically in the 'Form Analysis' course, we teach students to analyze using this 'global observation' approach. This encourages the analysis of concepts inherent to the form such as volume and color (generated by light, shadow), fullness and emptiness (which form in the interaction with other elements), proportion and scale (in the formal comparison with other annexed elements) etc. but avenues of auditory attention are also opened thanks to experiences like the one presented here.

Numerous architects are concerned with broadening the concept of 'perception' to the realm of the sensory and not limiting it to the visual field. The last decade has seen the creation of new lines of architectural research that move in between the discipline of the psychology of space and the intersections created with neuroscience and psychology.

At the beginning of the 21st century, architects such as Juhani Pallasmaa combined their research on sensory perception in architecture with the field of neuroscience, a discipline that emerged in the 1950s. Ramón y Cajal is considered the father of this discipline (csic.es/es/legado-cajal) already integrated into the project of studios such as Dominican Interior Designers (dominicaninteriordesigners.com/neuroarquitectura-disenar-para-la-mente) and studies how the spaces we inhabit affect our physical health, mental and emotional in order to project cities, buildings and interiors that improve our well-being and quality of life.

The concept to be discussed: *neuroscience*, is currently being taken up again. A trigger is estimated due to the confinement we experienced during the global COVID19 pandemic in 2020. Currently, the *neuroscience* concept is directly applied to the spatial perception area as *neuroarchitecture* and has to do with spatial perception and sensory. For many architects, he has determined a before and after in the way of understanding architecture as a trigger for ideas through observation and, in this case that concerns us, analysis. Pallasmaa speaks of 'acoustic intimacy' and remembers that sight isolates while sound includes:

"Sight is directional while sound is omnidirectional. The sense of sight implies exteriority, but sound creates a sensation of interiority" (Pallasmaa, 2006).

Professor Javier Seguí refers to imagination as: "the internal event in which new possibilities, personal roles or sequences of behavior appear, projected on a mental screen as a visual, auditory, verbal or composite "figuration" of various sensory components (olfactory + tactile, etc.), based on complex associations in which past events ("memory states") are integrated with schemes of current events" (Seguí, 2008).

Previous Studies with People with Disabilities

Although human beings inherently possess visuospatial abilities, the ability to recognize sounds and represent them graphically is neither well understood nor extensively measured. (It is necessary for architects and psychologists to work together to study these concepts and their effect on the cognitive development of people with intellectual disabilities or borderline intelligence and people on the autistic spectrum.

Recent studies indicate that individuals with ASD (Autism Spectrum Disorder) exhibit heightened responses due to early detection of frequency deviation (pitch discrimination) and reduced habituation (prolonged processing of deviation) when exposed to new sounds. This means that they do not respond well to or tolerate unusual or new sounds that they have never heard before.

Projects such as Sonus TEA study strategies against noise for people with autism, making it easier to understand why some sounds can cause physical discomfort and frustration (fundacionconectea.org).

The experiences developed in these workshops are considered innovative and differential and have been tested for more than thirty years with university students, in the course Form Analysis at CEU University, to understand intangible concepts and in specific some cases with six years old students (see Figure 1), but the state of the art does not include similar experiences with students with intellectual disabilities nor with high capabilities students. These workshops open, as well, new research lines that combine both different student profiles and multidisciplinary teaching teams from different areas of knowledge and different evaluations in the field of spatial perception. These vary depending on the selection of the place that offers different concepts to work on (framing, light-shadow, routes, flows, natural and urban elements of the landscape, etc.).

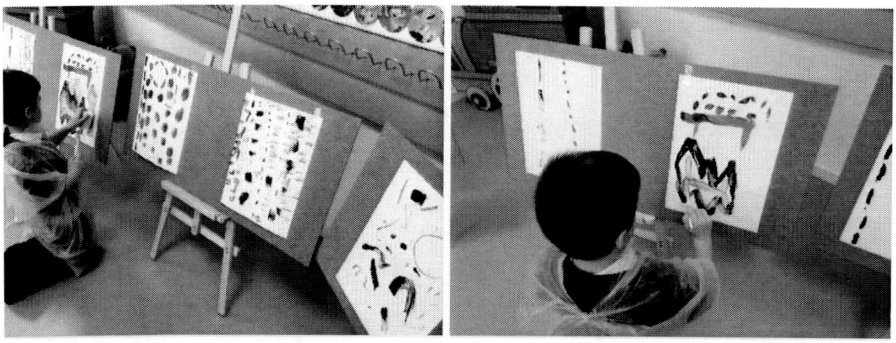

Source: Picture provided by authors.

Figure 1. Previous experiences of sounds and music with 6 years old students (2019).

This chapter introduces this activity for the first time as innovative due to the profile of the students who develop it (Intellectual Disability Students). According to the International DSM-5 diagnostic classification (APA, 2013), people with borderline intellectual ability (V62.89; R41.83) obtain a Total Intellectual Quotient (IQ) score, measured through updated standardized tests, in the range between 70 and 79, which means that they are below the intelligence score considered average or normative (IQ 80-120). Moreover, according to the ICD-10 classification (World Health Organization - WHO), the necessary criteria for the person's possible difficulties to be considered as typical of a mild intellectual disability (two standard deviations below the mean; IQ < 70) is not met. (psisemadrid.org/inteligencia-limite/) (sanidad.gob.es/estad Estudios/estadisticas/normalizacion/CIE10/CIE10ES_2018_diag_pdf_20180202.pdf).

The experience is carried out in the unique setting of the University's Form Analysis Classroom, where students, registered in the Youth Guarantee System (www.sepe.es) and selected by psychologists and special trainers, participate in the non-visual experience introduced here.

As of 2017, students with this intellectual profile are experiencing inclusion. "The Strategy for Disability 'Inclusion' lays the foundation for transformation in the United Nations Charter on Human Rights and Development". (https://www.un.org/es/our-work/protect-human-rights) by enrolling at the University as students of the Universal Accessibility Support Consultant Training Course (called in Spanish: Curso de Formación Consultor de Apoyo de Accesibilidad Universal CF-CAAU) of the financed project UNIDIVERSITY granted by FONCE and the European Social Fund which promotes training programs for employment aimed exclusively at young people with intellectual disabilities. In 2018, the San Pablo CEU University was notified favorably of the possibility of training students with this profile as support facilitators in the evaluation of an architectural or urban space through the personal sensitivity of appreciating or perceiving the space in its positive or negative points.

Goal

The main objective of the workshop is to understand and develop the perception of sound and music through graphic language representation on paper.

The following secondary objectives emerge from the workshop are:

1. To establish synergies in the artistic understanding of music and graphics.
2. To share an inclusive experience with students of different ages and intellectual abilities.

The aim is to awaken inner sensitivity and to express graphically the emotions suggested by sounds or, where appropriate, musical pieces or compositions. The graphic results are recorded and analyzed in order to establish parallels between different student profiles. The hypothesis is that the results measured in highly able pupils will not differ much from those of pupils with intellectual disabilities.

Method

In order to achieve the results of the objectives set out here, the study method has been based on THREE PHASES clearly defined and described below.

PHASE 1: Selection of Sounds, Space, Participants, and Faculty of the Activity

1.1 Analysis of sounds and music composition. First, it is necessary to introduce an analysis of different sounds previously created, played and registered by a pianist and taken to a specifically designed TEST for other research, linking sound to emotions.

1.2 The importance of the placement selection. The selected placement activity takes place in a specific classroom as it is the singular place of Form Analysis classroom at Escuela Politécnica Superior EPS of San Pablo CEU University in Madrid.

1.3 The selected participants are: 16 students with intellectual disabilities (IQ between 70 and 85) and 8 highly gifted students from Colegio San Pablo CEU Sanchinarro.

1.4 Organizing a selected team of the multidisciplinary collaborative workshop:

- Directors: 3 PhD architects, (authors of this research) and professors of the subjects of Form Analysis, Natural Drawing and Artistic Drawing in the Degree of Architecture, Interior Architecture and Digital Art.
- Participating: 1 PhD musician and professor of the Information Technology Degree. Member of the Biomedical Engineering Laboratory, 1 architect and Professor of Drawing at the San Pablo CEU Sanchinarro Middle School, 1 technical architect and a PhD student in Architecture and Trainer of people with intellectual disabilities, 1 psychologist from the University Guidance Service (called in Spanish SOU Servicio de Orientación Universitaria) and PhD student in Psychology and 1 Professor and Director of the Master of Energy Efficiency.

PHASE 2: Case Study. Secondly, a Specific Activity Is Carried Out in Order to Pursuit Results and Introduce New Conclusions to the Statement of the Art

2.1 Firstly, the pianist conducts the graphic session, and it is developed after carrying out the TEST of associative analysis of the same sounds with emotions. The last part of this TEST presents two relevant factors to this research, which have to do with strokes and color. Then, they develop 8 drawings based on the same sounds presented in the relationship with these with emotions:

- 4 drawings representing separate sounds in notes (bass and treble) played on piano and violin.
- 2 drawings representing rhythms.
- 2 drawings representing musical compositions.

The students represent graphically the same musical triggers used in the previous part of the workshop. They focus on the results of strokes and colors, selecting the most appropriate one for what each sound suggests to them.

1. SOUND 1: 1 high-pitched piano note
2. SOUND 2: 1 high-pitched piano note
3. SOUND 3: 1 high note (same as before) on violin
4. SOUND 4: 1 low note (same as before) on violin
5. RHYTHM 5. 1 rhythm (dynamic-cheerful-funny-brilliant-bright-lively...)
6. RHYTHM 6: 1 rhythm (sad-funereal-slow-slow-paused-dark-dark-dark...)
7. COMPOSITION 7: 1 evocative musical composition
8. COMPOSITION 8: 1 evocative musical composition

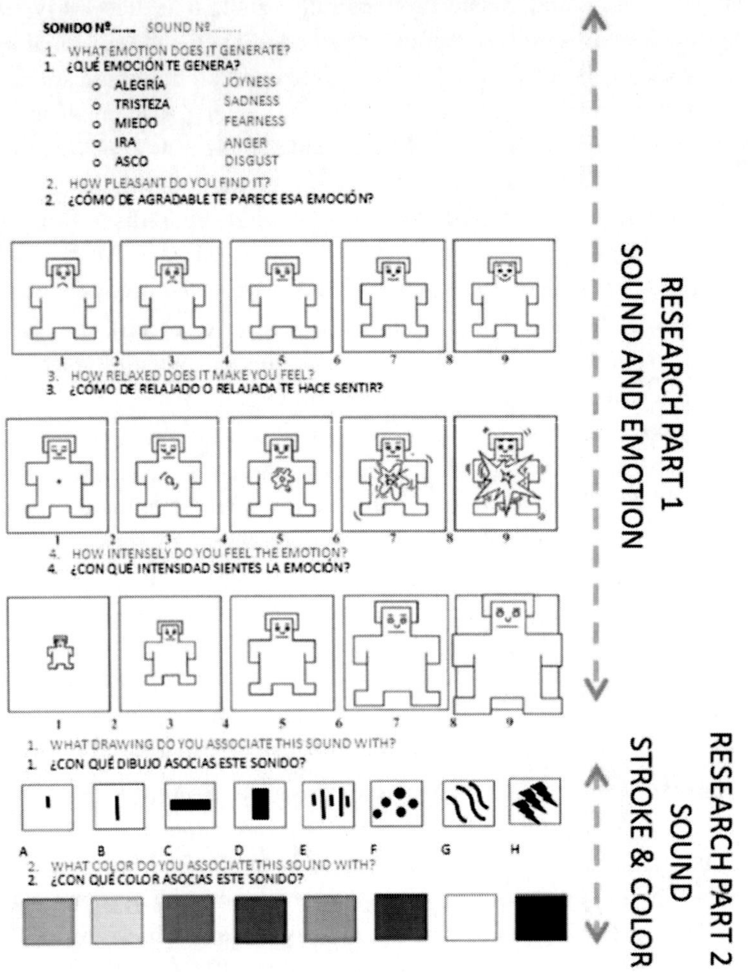

Source: Picture provided by authors.

Figure 2. General TEST. Source: Self-Assessment Manikin, Sam and Lang, 1980. Test completed by trace and color assessment provided by authors and defined in the Research Part 2 TEST employed for this research and provided by authors: Question 1. "What drawing do you associate this sound with?" Question 2. "What color do you associate this sound with?"

2.2. Technique used: The University provides the artistic material for the work on easel, on white DINA-1 paper, with acrylic and gouache technique in basic colors of cyan blue, cadmium yellow, magenta red pigments plus black and white pigments. Also, plastic pots for water, rags and brushes plus color mixing palettes.

2.3. Graphic results: The student expresses graphically on paper their response with different brushes and strokes to the sounds. The length, density, texture, and color of these sounds offer us information about the understanding of low, high, continuous, discontinuous, harmony, rhythm, silence and other abstract concepts.

Finally, to conclude this research, the results of the TEST (see Figure 2), are compared with the graphical results of both profiles of students (over 18 years old with intellectual disabilities and under 18 years old with high intellectual abilities).

Students expressed their degree of satisfaction and encourage conclusions as well as possible improvements of the activity on a survey. The TEST presented here as images responds to the easy reading system required for students of borderline intelligence. Easy reading is a 'Method that includes a set of guidelines and recommendations related to the writing of texts, the design and layout of documents and the validation of their comprehensibility, intended to make information accessible to people with comprehension difficulties. reader' (https://www.plenainclusion.org/discapacidad-intelectual/recurso/lectura-facil/)

Results and Discussion

The experience that this workshop brings to the students is differential because this workshop is offered to pupils of different ages, cognitive abilities and different knowledge bases and graphic and auditory-musical perception, in a unique environment such as the Analysis of Forms classroom (see Figure 3).

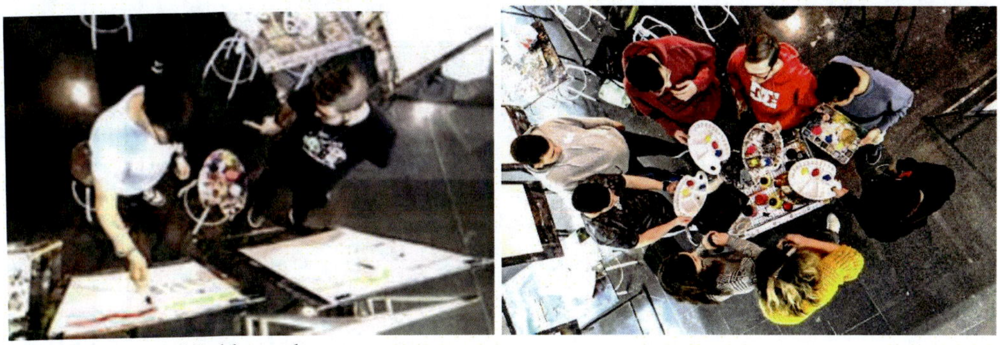

Source: Picture provided by authors.

Figure 3. Sounds graphic representation process.

Case Study Results

The association of color and stroke with different low or high-pitched sounds leads the student to choose the right tool for the perception of that sound.

We collected a total of 24 DINA 1 results (8 from highly able students and 16 from students with intellectual disabilities). As a point of improvement for the next activity, we note that the order of representation of sounds was implemented differently for the two types of students and that for the highly able students the DINA-1papers were structured as a grid of 8 sounds reading vertically from top to bottom (see Figure 4).

S1	S5
S2	S6
S3	S7
S4	S8

Source: Figure provided by authors.

Figure 4. Structure followed by high capabilities students.

The results for highly able pupils are shown below (see Figure 5) for further analysis, discussion, and conclusions:

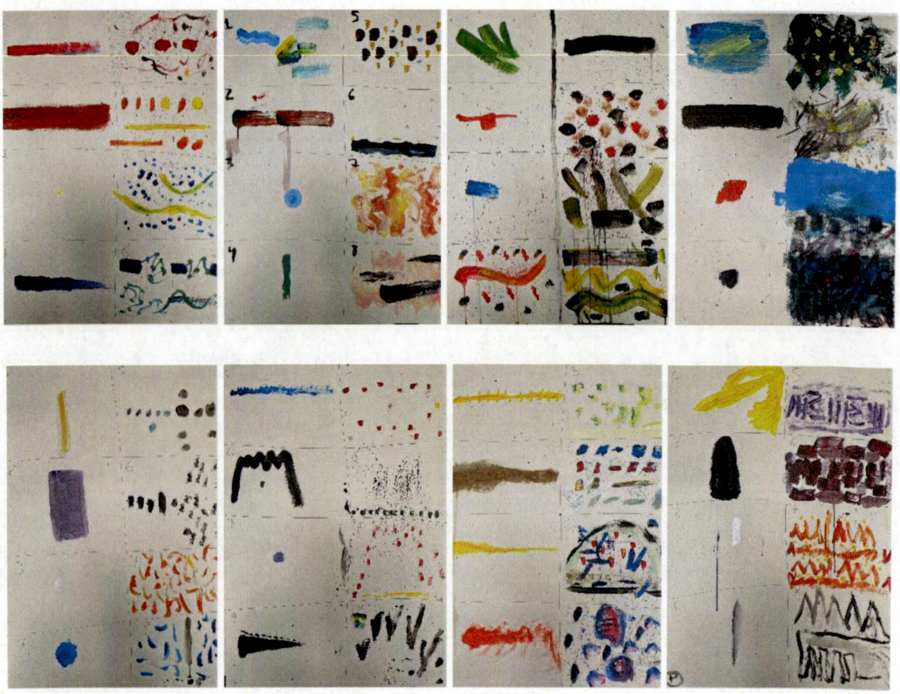

Source: Picture provided by authors.

Figure 5. High capabilities students' graphic result.

The DINA-1 of students with intellectual disabilities were structured as a grid of 8 reading sounds from left to right and from top to bottom (see Figure 6).

S1	S2
S3	S4
S5	S6
S7	S8

Source: Figure provided by author.

Figure 6. Structure followed by limited intellectual coefficient students.

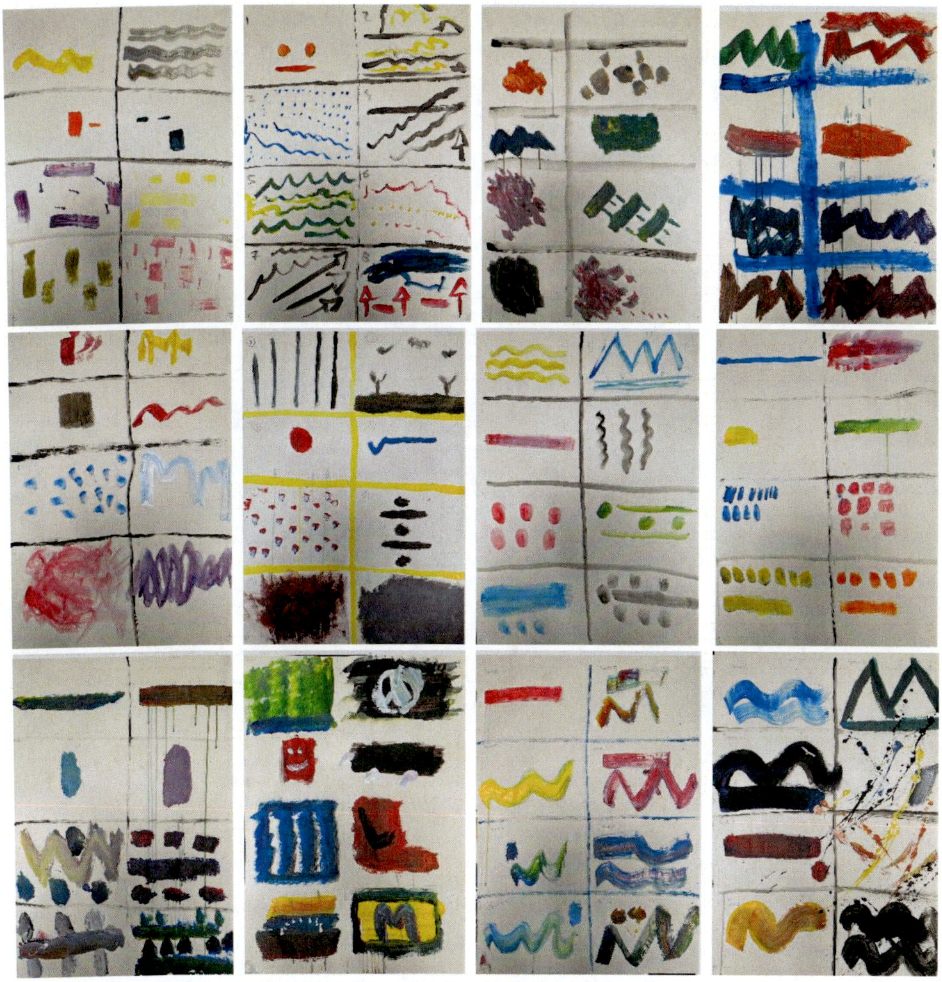

Source: Picture provided by authorsTest Results about strokes and color.

Figure 7. Limited intellectual coefficient students' graphic results.

Table 1 of results on strokes offers clearer conclusions than Table 2 of color since both highly able students and students with intellectual disabilities respond in a homogeneous and similar way.

Six of the eight sounds are conclusive in their response:

- sound 1 = stroke B
- sound 2 = stroke D
- sound 3 = stroke A
- sound 4 = stroke C
- sound 7 = stroke E
- sound 8 = stroke H

Sounds 5 and 6 offer conclusions by student profile since:

- Sound 5 is mostly associated with E by students with intellectual disabilities.
- Sound 5 is mostly associated with H by students with high abilities.
- Sound 6 is mostly associated with E by students with intellectual disabilities.
- Sound 5 is mostly associated with F by students with high abilities.

Table 1. Test results about strokes associated to sounds.
Note: column DN = Don't Know is NS/NC (in Spanish NS = no sabe/NC = no contesta)

	WHICH STROKE DO YOU LINK THE SOUND WITH? ¿CON QUÉ DIBUJO ASOCIAS ESTE SONIDO?	A	B	C	D	E	F	G	H	DN	
SOUND 1	ID STUDENTS	2	5	4		1			1	3	conclusive result
	HC STUDENTS		3	2	1			1	1		conclusive result
SOUND 2	ID STUDENTS			2	8	1			1	4	conclusive result
	HC STUDENTS			1	6				1		conclusive result
SOUND 3	ID STUDENTS	6	1	2	1	1		2		3	conclusive result
	HC STUDENTS	6						2			conclusive result
SOUND 4	ID STUDENTS	1	1	4	3	1	1	1	2	2	conclusive result
	HC STUDENTS		1	4	2						conclusive result
SOUND 5	ID STUDENTS				2	7	1	2	3	1	no conclusive result
	HC STUDENTS					1	2		5		no conclusive result
SOUND 6	ID STUDENTS	2			2	6		3	1	2	no conclusive result
	HC STUDENTS						5		3		no conclusive result
SOUND 7	ID STUDENTS	1		1	1	5		4	1	3	conclusive result
	HC STUDENTS					4	1	2	1		conclusive result
SOUND 8	ID STUDENTS		1		3	3	1		6	2	conclusive result
	HC STUDENTS					1	1		6		conclusive result

ID=INTELLECTUAL DISABILITY / HC= HIGH CAPABILITY

A= DOT/ B= VERTICAL LINE/ C= HORIZONTAL THICK STROKE/D=VERTICAL THICK STROKE/ E=RITHM short and long vertical lines /F=DOTS/G=WAVES/H=STRAIGHT AND IRREGULAR RAYS
DN= DON'T KNOW

Source: Table provided by authors.

Table 2 of results on color offers fewer clear conclusions than Table 1 of strokes since:

- High ability pupils respond more randomly.
- Students with intellectual disabilities respond more homogeneously.

Table 2. Test results about colors associated to sounds.
Note: column DN = Don't Know is NS/NC (in Spanish NS = no sabe/NC = no contesta)

		WHICH COLOR DO YOU LINK THE SOUND WITH? ¿CON QUÉ COLOR ASOCIAS ESTE SONIDO?	BLU	YLL	MAG	RED	GR	PR	WH	BL	DN	
SOUND 1	ID STUDENTS		2	1		1	1	1	3	3	4	no conclusive result
	HC STUDENTS		2	1		2			2	1		no conclusive result
SOUND 2	ID STUDENTS				2	1	2	1	1	6	3	conclusive result
	HC STUDENTS		1			2	1			4		conclusive result
SOUND 3	ID STUDENTS		3		4	2			4	1	2	tie result
	HC STUDENTS		1	2	1		1		3			conclusive result
SOUND 4	ID STUDENTS			4	1	2	1	3	1	2	2	no conclusive result
	HC STUDENTS		1					6		1		conclusive result
SOUND 5	ID STUDENTS		1	2		5	4			2	2	tie result
	HC STUDENTS		1		1	2	1	1		2		tie result
SOUND 6	ID STUDENTS		2		1	2	2	3		4	2	no conclusive result
	HC STUDENTS		1			1	2	2		2		tie result
SOUND 7	ID STUDENTS		6	3	1	1	2			1	2	no conclusive result
	HC STUDENTS			2	1	2			2	1		no conclusive result
SOUND 8	ID STUDENTS		1	2	1	3				7	2	conclusive result
	HC STUDENTS		1			1	1	1		4		conclusive result

ID=INTELLECTUAL DISABILITY / HC= HIGH CAPABILITY
BLU= BLUE/ YLL= YELLOW/ MAG= MAGENTA/ RED/GR=GREEN/ PR= PURPLE/ WH=WHITE/ BL=BLACK
DN= DON'T KNOW

Source: Table provided by authors.

Enquiry for Students Results

In order to complete and deepen the students' opinion on the activity carried out and provide more information on points of improvement in successive workshops, a survey to collect data on satisfaction and quality was deemed necessary.

Enquiry model entitled: music emotions and graphic representation of sounds.

Offered to: students contain (without differentiating both study profiles):

- Language: Spanish
- Enquiry time average12:57 min.
- People responding to the enquiry: 14/24 students did the enquiry
- Welcome and introduction to the topic: *"This activity arises from a synergy between architecture and engineering teachers. The presence of specialized teachers in each discipline as well as psychologists is necessary to be able to evaluate or measure intellectual development factors from the perception of sounds to graphic representation."*

1. *Question: Did you like the activity?*
   Answer: 1-5 star rating with 5 being the highest rating
   Result: 4.57/5
2. *Question: Do you think it is important for creative development?*
   Answer: 1–5-star rating with 5 being the highest rating
   Result: 4.64/5

3. *Question: Do you think creative development is important for your life?*
   Answer: 1–5-star rating with 5 being the highest rating
   Result: 4.36/5
4. *Question: Have you done any painting activities related to sounds before?*
   Answer: 1–5-star rating with 5 being the highest rating
   Result: 2.93/5
5. *Question: The activity was easy for me*
   Answer: Yes/No
   Result: yes: 12 students/14 responses
6. *Question: The teachers have presented the activity clearly*
   Answer: Yes/No
   Result: yes: 13 students/14 responses
7. *Question: Would you recommend the activity to a family friend?*
   Answer: 1–5-star rating with 5 being the highest rating
   Result: 4.21/5
8. *Question: Tell us how we can improve*
   Answer: 11 written responses

Conclusion

The human need to express emotions through art leads to abstract representation. The conclusions presented here summarize how this moment marked a new way of learning.

Drawing, as a form of graphic expression, facilitates the communication of ideas and the representation of both visual and non-visual models. By visual models we mean all those that can be observed, that are tangible and exist, by non-visual models we mean those that are not tangible, such as sounds and aromas.

The main conclusion drawn from this study is that the results from these two student profiles are not substantially different (in quality and use of the technique) not being able to distinguish (within the entire range of exercises delivered) which correspond to the profiles selected for the activity study object.

The theme of the workshop unleashes a series of questions that go beyond a mere physical analysis but also a psychological one that raises the awareness of the citizen for a total inclusion and feedback of the common learning between students and teachers.

The experience of graphic representation based on sounds as a non-visual model has been part of the teaching method of the subject 'Form Analysis' within the Degree in Architecture and taught exclusively by architects.

- Both students with intellectual disabilities and highly able students generated for the first time the association of sounds to a color, a line, a shape, or a specific density.
- At the same time, innovations present in this experience as it is developed in a university space and combination of profiles of students with intellectual disabilities and students with high abilities from school education.

Some experiences of auditory and visuospatial analytical work, with this learner profile or in synergy with other profiles, have opened new lines of research. (See Figure 8) These are:

- The research from the area of psychology with people with cognitive disabilities through artistic and spatial tools provided by architects.
- To encourage people of different intellectual profiles to interact in common experiences and expect similar results.
- To promote the analysis of the understanding of sound, vibration and pitch of sounds as well as rhythms and compositions in people of different intellectual profiles.

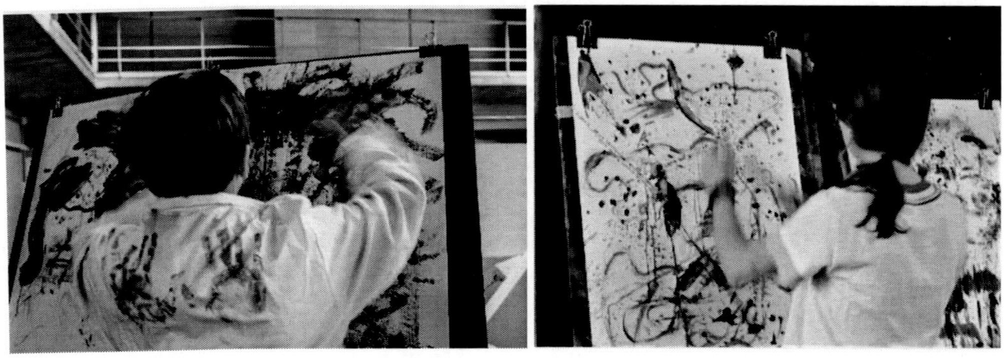

Figure 8. Other activities students' graphic results according to music compositions.

Acknowledgments

This research was possible thanks to the participation of students with intellectual disabilities in the CF-CAAU Training Course in Universal Accessibility Support Consultant funded by the FONCE Foundation and the European Social Fund (2018-2023).

References

Arnheim, R. (1995). *Arte y percepción visual: psicología del ojo creador*. Madrid: Alianza, 1995; 1a ed., 13a reimp.]. http://search.ebscohost.com/login.aspx?direct=true&db=cat01072a&AN=CEU.204828&lang=es&site=eds-live.

Cantarero-García, G. et al. (2021). "Taller de representación gráfica de sonidos para alumnos de edades y capacidades diferentes." Madrid, Spain: CEU Ediciones. p. 257-258 ISBN: 978-84-18463-23-5.

Gardner, H. (1983). *Multiple intelligences: New horizons*. New York, NY: Ed. Basic Books.

Goleman, (1995). *Emotional Intelligence*. New York, NY: Ed. Bantam Books.

Rebernik, N., Osaba, E., Bahillo, A., & Montero, D. (2017). A Vision of a Smart City Addressing the Needs of Disabled Citizens. In Proceedings Accessibility 4.0, Conference Paper, Málaga 27th (pp. 70-79).

Roselli, M. (2015). Desarrollo neuropsicológico de las habilidades visoespaciales y visoconstruccionales. *Revista Neuropsicología, Neuropsiquiatría y Neurociencias*, 15(1), 175-200.

Pallasmaa, J. (2006). *Los ojos de la piel.* Barcelona, Ed. Gustavo Gili. (p. 50-51).

Seguí, J. (2008). Anotaciones para un imaginario del dibujar. *EGA Revista de Expresión Gráfica Arquitectónica*, 13(13), 70. https://doi.org/10.4995/ega.2008.10270.

Biographical Sketches

Dr. Guadalupe Cantarero-García, PhD

See CV in Chapter 1

Dr. Fátima Sarasola Rubio, PhD

Affiliation:
Universidad San Pablo-CEU, CEU Universities, Institute of Technology, Madrid, Spain.

Education:

- 2016: PhD. Thesis in Architecture, Institute of Technology, CEU San Pablo Madrid.
- 2005: Diploma of Advanced Studies in the "Drawing, History and Construction" programme, Department of "Ideación Gráfica Arquitectónica" D.I.G.A, Architecture School of Madrid (ETSAM).
- 2000: Diploma of Architect, Architecture School of Madrid (ETSAM), Spain. (Professional Degree in Architecture).

Business Address:
Architecture and Design Department, Institute of Technology, Universidad San Pablo-CEU, CEU Universities, Campus de Monteprincipe, 28668, Madrid, Spain.

Research:

- 2020-present: Member of the research group "LECOBI" (PC06/0720)
- 2015-2016: Member of the research group "Arquitectura Española Contemporánea" ("Contemporary Spanish Architecture") of the Institute of Technology (USPCEU). Took part in the the R&D Research project "Espacios para la Enseñanza", which received a USP and Banco del Santander grant (ref: USP BS APP6 2015).

Selected Publication and Recent Research: ORCID CODE: 0000-0003-0149-2046.

Teaching Experience: 28 years

- 2020-present: Profesor Adjunto. Architecture and Design Department, Institute of Technology, Universidad San Pablo-CEU.
- 2016-2020: Profesor Colaborador Doctor. Architecture and Design Department, Institute of Technology, Universidad San Pablo-CEU
- 2008-2016: Profesor Colaborador. Architecture and Design Department, Institute of Technology, Universidad San Pablo-CEU.
- 2007-2008: Lecturer in Form Analysis, Projects and Architectural Drawing. JC Architecture Academy, Madrid.
- 1995-2007: Lecturer in Form Analysis, Projects and Architectural Drawing. Nova Architecture Academy, Madrid.

Professional Appointments:

- 2018- present: Architectural Form Analysis and Life Drawing Coordinator
- 2000-2007: Co-owner of Nova Architecture academy

Honors:

- 2023: First award for Scientific Dissemination Activity, University San Pablo-CEU.
- 2022: Second award for Educational and Teaching Innovation of the University San Pablo-CEU.
- 2020: CEU Ángel Herrera Award for Best Teaching Work of the Institute of Technology, University San Pablo CEU.
- 2019: First award for Teaching Innovation, University San Pablo-CEU.

Publications from the Last 3 Years:

1. Sarasola Rubio, F. (2022) El dibujo de la invención: las patentes y modelos de utilidad de J. A Coderch, R. De la Hoz, A. De la Sota, M. Fisac y F. J Sáenz de Oíza de los años cincuenta y sesenta: Universidad Politécnica de Cartagena, 261-264. ISBN: 978-84-17853-51-8.
2. Sarasola Rubio, F. (2022) Graphic Analysis of the Patents and Utility Models Registered by Spanish Architects Between 1950 and 1970, *Springer Series in Design and Innovation,* 23, 312-321, doi: 10.1007/978-3-031-04640-7_32.
3. Sarasola Rubio, F. (2021) El proyecto pedagógico de Jorge Oteiza desde la Arquitectura, En: *Escuelas y prácticas educativas experimentales de arte en el País Vasco*. 1957-1979 / coord. por Artium, Centro-Museo Vasco de Arte Contemporáneo, Fundación Museo Jorge Oteiza, 138-148, ISBN 9788412396553.
4. Sarasola Rubio, F. (2021) Arquitectos e inventores. Las patentes inéditas de Alejandro de la Sota, Francisco Javier Sáenz de Oíza y Rafael de la Hoz, CEU Ediciones, Colección: Lecciones Magistrales, Depósito legal: M-6465-2021.

Dr. Rocío Santo-Tomás Muro, PhD

Affiliation:
Universidad San Pablo-CEU, CEU Universities, Institute of Technology, Madrid, Spain.

Education:

- 2021: PhD. Thesis in Architecture, Institute of Technology, Universidad San Pablo-CEU, Madrid.
- 2016: Diploma of Architect, Universidad San Pablo-CEU, Madrid.

Business Address:
Architecture and Design Department, Institute of Technology, Universidad San Pablo-CEU, CEU Universities, Campus de Monteprincipe, 28668, Madrid, Spain.

Research:

- 2016-present: Member of the research group "Patrimonio, Arquitectura & Paisaje (PA&P)" (Universidad San Pablo-CEU)
- 2019: Research Stay at Newcastle University ((School of Architecture, Planning & Landscape)

Selected Publication and Recent Research. Orcid: 0000-0002-8577-7008.

Teaching Experience:

- 2021-present: Profesor Colaborador Doctor. Architecture and Design Department, Institute of Technology, Universidad San Pablo-CEU
- 2016-2020: FPI Contract. Architecture and Design Department, Institute of Technology, Universidad San Pablo-CEU
- 2014-2015: Teacher Assistant in Form Analysis. Architecture and Design Department, Institute of Technology, Universidad San Pablo-CEU

Professional Appointments:

- 2021- present: Architectural Form Analysis and Life Drawing Lecturer. Universidad San Pablo CEU.
- 2016-2020: FPI Predoctoral Contract. Universidad San Pablo CEU.
- 2016: URBANMATTER STUDIO
- 2016: GÁLVEZ-WIECZOREK Studio
- 2015: BDG Architectura + Design Studio

Honors:

- 2023: Extraordinary Doctorate Award, CEINDO, University San Pablo-CEU.
- 2022: MENTION. Doctoral Thesis AWARD, COAM
- 2022: Second award for Educational and Teaching Innovation of the University San Pablo-CEU.
- 2020: CEU Ángel Herrera Research Award Research in the field of Architecture and Engineering for the book: *Paisajes de aproximación a la ciudad de Madrid*, together with the other members of the PA&P Research Group.
- 2015: Accésit, CEU San Pablo Personal Creativity Competition
- 2015: Finalist, RESilience Innovation Award
- 2014: Mutua Madrileña Community Service AWARD for the implementation of a "Guest house" on the campus of the University of Makeni, (Sierra Leone, Africa).
- 2010: Edinburgh Summer University Course AWARD.

Publications:

1. Rodríguez Romero, Eva J., Santo-Tomás Muro, Rocío y González Truco, Iván (2023). "Aprendiendo a valorar el paisaje urbano cotidiano: técnicas participativas con estudiantes" en Pinilla Gómez, Raquel y Criz Carvajal, Isleni: *Estudios de innovación docente como punto de encuentro de ciencias humanísticas y sociales*. Madrid: Dykinson, pp. 718-737.
2. Santo Tomás Muro, Rocío; Rodríguez Romero, Eva J., and Sáenz De Tejada Granados, Carlota (2021): "Análisis perceptivo de la infraestructura verde urbana en Madrid a partir del software NVIVO" in *New Trends in Qualitative Research*, vol. 9. Investigación cualitativa en Ciencias Sociales: Avances y Desafíos, Ludomedia, pp 344-354.
3. Sáenz De Tejada Granados, Carlota; Santo-Tomás Muro, Rocío and Rodríguez Romero, Eva. 2021. Exploring landscape preference through photo-based Q methodology. Madrid seen by suburban adolescents. *International Research in Geographical and Environmental Education*. Taylor and Francis Ltd. 30(3), pp. 255-278.
4. Guadalupe Cantarero García, Rocío Santo-Tomas Muro (2018) "Madrid en la pintura. Reflexiones compositivas sobre las miradas artísticas del siglo XX y XXI." Ed: Conarquitectura. En VVAA: *Paisajes de aproximación a la ciudad de Madrid*. pp. 223-236. ISBN 9788494776854.

Chapter 3

The Impact of Indoor Environmental Quality on Physical Well-Being

Sunil K. Sansaniwal[1,*]
and Julia K. Day[2]
[1]Energy, Green Transition and Climate Change Division, NITI Aayog, Government of India, New Delhi, India
[2]Integrated Design and Construction Lab, School of Design and Construction, Washington State University, Pullman, Washington, USA

Abstract

Indoor Environmental Quality (IEQ) has emerged as a key factor influencing the overall well-being of individuals who spend most of their time indoors. This chapter discusses the multifaceted aspects that contribute to IEQ and elucidates its profound impact on the physical health of individuals. Based on the complex interplay of key IEQ elements (air quality, thermal comfort, lighting, noise levels and ergonomics) as discussed in the available literature, the chapter unravels their profound influence on human physical well-being. Valuable insights are gained into the cumulative impact they have on occupants' overall experience within indoor spaces. The chapter emphasizes the importance of implementing effective strategies to enhance IEQ. It highlights the critical role of purposeful design and diligent maintenance in creating indoor environments that actively promote optimal well-being for occupants. The chapter recognizes the pivotal role that designers, architects and facility managers play in creating and sustaining indoor environments that prioritize the health and satisfaction of the individuals who inhabit them. Moreover, this chapter offers a detailed understanding of the multifaceted nature of IEQ and highlights its impact on occupants' physical well-being.

Keywords: indoor environmental quality, occupant's well-being, healthy survival, sustainable built environment

* Corresponding Author's Email: sansani4u@yahoo.com

In: Psycho-Environmental Variables That Ensure People's Well-Being and Health …
Editors: Roberto Alonso González Lezcano and Guadalupe Cantarero García
ISBN: 979-8-89530-831-8
© 2025 Nova Science Publishers, Inc.

Introduction

The quality of the indoor environment plays a crucial role in occupant well-being, as people spend a significant portion of their lives indoors, particularly in homes, offices and academic institutions [1]. Therefore, understanding its impact on physical health is essential. Researchers, architects and policymakers recognize the need to explore the relationship between Indoor Environmental Quality (IEQ) and well-being [2]. IEQ encompasses key factors such as air quality, thermal comfort, lighting, acoustics and ergonomics, all of which contribute to overall comfort and health in built environments [1, 3]. Each of these elements affects physiological, psychological and cognitive well-being [4]. Air quality is a fundamental aspect of IEQ, focusing on pollutant levels, allergens and ventilation efficiency. Poor indoor air quality—caused by inadequate ventilation, high pollutant concentrations, or allergens—can introduce contaminants like volatile organic compounds (VOCs), formaldehyde, particulate matter and biological agents such as mold and dust mites. These pollutants contribute to respiratory issues, allergies, cognitive impairment and cardiovascular diseases [5]. Insufficient ventilation recirculates contaminants, further degrading air quality [6]. Research shows that improving ventilation, minimizing pollutant sources and maintaining appropriate humidity levels significantly enhance indoor air quality and occupant well-being [7].

Thermal comfort is another critical factor influencing occupant health. It refers to an individual's satisfaction with indoor temperature, humidity and airflow. Proper insulation, HVAC systems and personalized thermal controls contribute to achieving optimal comfort [8]. Extreme temperatures can cause discomfort, fatigue, reduced productivity & increased stress. Symptoms like headaches, drowsiness and difficulty concentrating often arise from poor thermal conditions, emphasizing the need for maintaining ideal temperature settings [9-10]. Lighting, both natural and artificial, significantly affects visual and non-visual functions. Poor lighting can cause eye strain, fatigue and circadian rhythm disruptions, leading to sleep disorders and mood disturbances. A well-designed lighting system improves visual comfort, mood and productivity [11]. Studies highlight the importance of light quality, intensity, color temperature and daylight availability in occupant health, underscoring the need for lighting strategies that prioritize well-being [12-13].

Acoustics influence indoor comfort by shaping sound transmission, absorption and ambient noise levels [14]. Noise control is vital for maintaining a comfortable and healthy indoor environment. Excessive noise leads to stress, reduced concentration and long-term health effects. Effective sound insulation, background noise control and sound privacy help create a space conducive to well-being [15]. Research highlights the link between noise exposure and health outcomes, emphasizing the importance of noise mitigation strategies [16-18]. Ergonomic design, including furniture layout, accessibility and user-friendly features, directly impacts physical health and comfort. Proper ergonomics reduce the risk of musculoskeletal disorders, improve posture and encourage movement, contributing to overall well-being [19]. Studies show that ergonomic design principles enhance occupant comfort and accessibility, reinforcing the importance of designing spaces that promote health and productivity [20].

Understanding the connection between IEQ and occupant well-being is essential for architects, designers, building owners and policymakers in developing healthier and more sustainable indoor environments. Optimizing IEQ not only improves physical health but also enhances productivity, satisfaction and overall quality of life. This chapter explores the impact of IEQ on physical well-being in detail.

Literature Review

Definition and Components of IEQ

IEQ refers to the overall quality of the indoor environment within a building or enclosed space, encompassing various physical and environmental factors that can affect the comfort, health and well-being of occupants. IEQ extends beyond mere functionality and addresses the holistic experience of individuals in indoor settings. IEQ takes into account several interrelated factors that contribute to the overall indoor experience, including thermal comfort, indoor air quality, lighting, acoustics and ergonomics, as explained below [9, 14]:

A. *Thermal Comfort:* It reflects an individual's satisfaction with the thermal environment, typically assessed subjectively. This satisfaction depends on environmental factors such as room air temperature, mean radiant temperature, floor surface temperature, relative humidity and air velocity, along with personal factors like metabolic rate and clothing insulation [9]. Thermal comfort is crucial in both air-conditioned and naturally ventilated spaces, significantly affecting building energy performance and occupant health [21]. Among IEQ elements, it has the highest weighting factor [22-23]. High heat gain and a delayed response to overheating increase the risk of thermal discomfort, especially during summer in tropical regions [1]. Factors such as excessive glazing, open-plan layouts, low ceilings and electrical appliances further elevate this risk [24]. Climate change exacerbates thermal discomfort in buildings. However, simple measures like occupant-controlled ventilation (e.g., opening windows, using fans and adjusting blinds) can improve productivity [25]. Thermal comfort standards, including ASHRAE 55-2017 and ISO 7730-2005, define temperature ranges based on international research. However, a recent review [8] of thermal comfort studies in India found that comfort temperature ranges in the region are significantly higher than those recommended by global standards. This variation is mainly due to socio-cultural factors and local adaptive behaviors, highlighting the need for region-specific thermal comfort standards based on local research.
B. *Indoor Air Quality:* IAQ is determined by the concentration of indoor air pollutants and the rate of ventilation. Contaminants originate from various sources, including indoor activities like cooking, heating and cleaning; emissions from building materials and household appliances; and human behaviors such as painting and smoking [5, 26]. IAQ is influenced by chemical and physical factors, including gaseous pollutants (e.g., CO_2, CO, TVOC, CH_2O), inhalable and respirable particulate matter ($PM_{2.5}$ and PM_{10}) and microbial counts. Many pollutants come from outdoor air and can enter buildings through natural or mechanical ventilation systems [27]. Therefore, an adequate supply of fresh outdoor air is crucial for maintaining good IAQ. In densely populated regions, declining ambient air quality has made it increasingly important to ensure acceptable IAQ for occupant health and well-being. Poor IAQ is particularly harmful to

vulnerable groups, such as children, the elderly and individuals with pre-existing lung or heart conditions [28]. Globally recognized IAQ standards include ASHRAE 62.1-2019 [29] and ASHRAE 62.2-2022 [30].

C. *Lighting:* Visible light is part of the electromagnetic spectrum that enables human vision and exhibits both particle and wave properties, with its wave aspect influencing color frequency [31]. Proper lighting is essential for occupant health and productivity, as inadequate lighting can cause visual discomfort and affect key bodily functions, including the circadian clock, nervous system and alertness. Excessive light intensity can lead to glare, while insufficient lighting can cause eye strain [32]. Therefore, maintaining appropriate light levels is crucial to preventing eye strain and vertigo. The required light intensity varies depending on the activity within a space. For instance, classrooms and offices need higher brightness levels than bedrooms or living rooms [33]. Light intensity can be managed through natural daylighting via windows and artificial lighting. Darkened windows help control daylight, while dimmers allow adjustments to artificial lighting [34]. Visual comfort is evaluated based on brightness, illumination, luminous spectrum and glare. A uniform distribution of light within a workspace is essential, as uneven lighting can create more glare and discomfort compared to consistent illumination [35].

D. *Acoustics:* It Acoustics refers to sound quality and its role in improving a space's functionality while minimizing unwanted noise [36]. It is categorized into room acoustics and building acoustics. Room acoustics focus on sound quality factors such as privacy, speech intelligibility and effective communication in office spaces. Building acoustics, on the other hand, aim to prevent noise from traveling between rooms, ensuring minimal disturbances in adjacent areas. Common indoor noise sources include HVAC systems, poor soundproofing materials and external noise [36]. Acoustic comfort is particularly important in institutional buildings where concentration is crucial for learning. In office environments, sound privacy enhances occupant satisfaction and work productivity [37]. Poor acoustics can negatively impact health, well-being and efficiency, making proper sound isolation essential. Buildings should adhere to acoustic standards that align with their design and function. Humans perceive sound within a frequency range of 20 Hz to 20,000 Hz [38]. Acoustic engineering plays a key role in ensuring compliance with building performance standards. Thoughtful acoustic design can enhance occupant comfort and productivity while maintaining the building's aesthetic appeal [39].

E. *Ergonomics*: It Ergonomics focuses on designing environments that support comfort and align with natural human movements. Its primary aim is to create spaces that are not only functional for living or working but also enhance occupant well-being [19]. By reducing fatigue and improving energy levels, ergonomics plays a key role in boosting productivity. It also positively impacts mental health by minimizing stress and anxiety caused by physical discomfort [40]. Ergonomics involves optimizing the design and arrangement of furniture, equipment and the overall physical environment to enhance human performance and well-being. Important factors include seating comfort, desk and workstation design and proper equipment positioning to reduce the risk of musculoskeletal disorders and improve ergonomic efficiency [20].

Impact of IEQ on Human Physical Well-Being

As people spend most of their time indoors, the quality of the indoor environment directly affects their health, fitness and overall well-being. IAQ is especially important for physical health, as poor IAQ characterized by pollutants, allergens and volatile organic compounds (VOCs) can cause respiratory issues such as allergies, asthma and other breathing problems [1]. Long-term exposure to indoor pollutants can also lead to chronic health conditions. Elevated CO_2 levels indoors can cause Sick Building Syndrome and impair cognitive function, which is particularly concerning for students, as it can negatively impact learning ability [41-42]. To ensure good IAQ, indoor CO_2 levels should not exceed outdoor levels by more than 650 ppm [43]. Particulate matter also plays a significant role in air quality and can cause various health issues when inhaled. There is ongoing debate about whether smaller particles ($\leq$5 μm) have a greater impact on human health [41, 44-45]. The widespread use of modern products has led to higher indoor concentrations of VOCs and formaldehyde, which degrade air quality and harm occupant health. These compounds have been linked to serious health issues, including cancer, skin rashes, headaches and eye irritation [46-47].

Occupational exposure to high SO_2 levels can cause respiratory distress, heart and lung diseases, nasal irritation and severe health risks [48]. The permissible exposure limit for SO_2 indoors should not exceed 13,000 μg/m^3 over an 8-hour period [49]. Common indoor sources include smoking, kerosene heating, cooking, poorly vented appliances and malfunctioning chimneys. NO_2, a toxic gas from the nitrogen oxides (NO_x) family, is another major indoor air pollutant. Other nitrogen oxides such as NO, HNO_3 and HONO can also be found indoors in measurable amounts. The primary sources of NO_2 are similar to those of SO_2. In some cases, indoor NO_2 and SO_2 levels exceed outdoor levels due to emissions from home appliances. Acute and chronic exposure to NO_2 concentrations (370–9,400 μg/m^3) can severely impact the immune system, blood chemistry and liver function [50]. The Occupational Safety and Health Administration recommends that indoor CO (carbon monoxide) levels should not exceed 50 ppm over an 8-hour period. Prolonged exposure to high CO levels can damage the central nervous system, lungs and cardiovascular system [51]. In naturally ventilated indoor spaces, CO concentrations should remain below 30 ppm under normal conditions [51]. O_3 (ozone), while beneficial in the upper atmosphere for UV protection, acts as an indoor air pollutant at ground level. Long-term exposure to high O_3 concentrations can cause lung damage. Office buildings often have higher indoor O_3 levels, mainly due to air cleaners, photocopiers and laser printers. Outdoor O_3 also contributes to indoor levels, accounting for 30–70% of outdoor concentrations, depending on ventilation and ozone removal rates [52]. To ensure good indoor air quality, it is essential to implement proper ventilation, air filtration and pollution control measures [53].

Indoor thermal conditions play a crucial role in physical well-being. Extreme temperatures can significantly affect comfort, sleep quality and energy levels. Uncomfortable thermal conditions may lead to fatigue, reduced productivity and difficulty performing physical tasks [9]. Temperature imbalances and poor heat transfer contribute to thermal stress, which can cause unsafe work behaviors, decreased productivity and safety risks. Prolonged exposure to thermal stress can also have lasting biological effects on the body [54]. This is particularly important in industrial settings, military operations and athletic activities, where exposure to extreme temperatures can severely impair work performance. In cold environments, the body experiences reduced physical function, including weakened muscle strength and endurance due to lower core and muscle temperatures [55]. Cold exposure, especially in the hands, can significantly impact fine motor skills and manual tasks. Studies show that gradual cooling is more damaging than rapid cooling at the same hand temperature [56-57]. Research also highlights the minimum hand and finger temperatures needed to maintain tactile sensitivity and dexterity [9]. Maintaining optimal thermal comfort not only improves physical well-being but also enhances comfort, energy efficiency and overall health [58].

Improper lighting, whether too bright or too dim, can cause visual discomfort and affect key bodily functions, including the circadian rhythm, nervous system and alertness [32]. Glare from excessive brightness can strain the eyes, while insufficient lighting can lead to eye strain and hinder visual perception, making tasks more difficult and increasing the risk of accidents. To prevent eye strain and vertigo, it is essential to maintain proper light intensity. A uniform light distribution within a task area enhances visual comfort, as uneven lighting can create distracting brightness variations [35]. Well-designed lighting systems that ensure adequate illumination while minimizing glare contribute to visual comfort, safety and overall well-being [59]. For office environments, most studies recommend light levels between 300 and 500 lx on the work plane [60-62]. The EN 12464-1:2011 standard provides guidelines for appropriate indoor lighting levels across different building types and services [60].

Excessive indoor noise can negatively affect physical well-being, leading to stress, fatigue and high blood pressure. Prolonged exposure can also disrupt sleep patterns, impair concentration and slow physical recovery. Common indoor noise sources include HVAC systems, poor sound insulation in building materials and noise from nearby lecture spaces. These disturbances impact not just hearing but also overall health, potentially causing headaches, hypertension, sleep disturbances and psychosomatic illnesses. Reducing noise through soundproofing, strategic design and noise control measures can significantly enhance occupant well-being [63-64]. In office settings, sound privacy is essential for satisfaction and productivity [65]. The use of both external and internal sound insulation has become a standard practice in modern buildings. Beyond IEQ requirements, acoustic comfort also influences energy performance. For example, occupants may close windows to block outdoor noise, reducing natural ventilation and increasing cooling demand [66].

The design and arrangement of furniture, equipment and workspaces significantly impact physical well-being. Poor ergonomics can cause musculoskeletal disorders, including back pain, neck strain and repetitive strain injuries. Ergonomically designed workstations, adjustable furniture and proper body positioning help maintain good posture, reduce injury risks and enhance comfort and well-being [19, 67]. Global standards play a crucial role in regulating healthy indoor environments. Standards such as ASHRAE 55-2017 [67], ISO 7730-2005 [68] and CEN EN 16798-2019 [69] provide frameworks for analyzing indoor conditions and promoting physical activity. Access to fitness areas, exercise facilities and open spaces encourages movement, improving cardiovascular health, muscle strength, flexibility and overall fitness [63]. Safety is a top priority in indoor spaces to prevent accidents and injuries. Features like adequate lighting, non-slip surfaces, well-maintained equipment and clear pathways contribute to a secure environment. A safe indoor space reduces accident risks, promotes physical well being and enables safe physical activity [2]. Additionally, the indoor environment affects access to healthy resources. Clean drinking water, nutritious food options and wellness spaces support physical health. Thoughtfully designed cafeterias, food preparation areas and relaxation zones foster a healthier indoor environment that enhances overall well-being [70-71].

Methodology

Research Design

This research follows a comprehensive and systematic approach, using the Biopsychosocial Model as its theoretical framework to examine the relationship between IEQ parameters and occupants' physical well-being [72]. A cross-sectional study design is typically used, enabling data collection at a specific point in time to analyze associations between IEQ factors and well-being, providing key insights into their potential effects. Random sampling helps ensure a representative sample, allowing findings to be generalized to a larger population [73]. Data collection relies on precise measurement tools for each IEQ parameter, including air quality monitors, thermal comfort analyzers, lux meters, sound meters and validated well-being questionnaires. These tools capture both objective and subjective indicators for a comprehensive assessment [1]. The process involves site visits, surveys and obtaining informed consent to maintain data integrity and ethical standards. Statistical analyses, such as correlation and regression, are used to assess the impact of IEQ on physical well-being while controlling for potential confounding variables [74]. This structured research design ensures a detailed evaluation and generates valuable insights for developing healthier indoor spaces.

Data Collection Methods

Various methods for collecting data to study the impact of IEQ on human health are as follows:

1. *Surveys and Questionnaires*: They are effective tools for gathering self-reported data from occupants. They can capture occupants' perceptions regarding the indoor environment and their well-being outcomes. The design of surveys and questionnaires includes relevant questions about IEQ parameters and physical well-being [75].
2. *Environmental Monitoring*: This involves deploying monitoring devices to collect data on variables such as indoor air quality (CO2, PM2.5, PM10, VOCs, CH2O, CO, O3, etc.), lighting levels (illuminance, uniformity of lighting, color temperature, etc.), thermal comfort (temperature, humidity, air flow, floor surface temperature, etc.), acoustics (noise levels, sound quality, etc.) and ergonomic factors (workstation design, furniture ergonomics, etc.). Measuring devices should be properly calibrated and strategically deployed to ensure accurate measurements [76].
3. *Physiological Measurements*: This assesses occupants' physical responses to the indoor environment. It includes the monitoring of heart rate, blood pressure, cortisol levels and skin conductance. Physiological measurement provides objective data on both physiological stress responses and the physiological well-being of occupants [77].
4. *Wearable Devices*: They collect real-time data on occupants' physical activity, sleep patterns and stress levels. Wearable devices such as fitness trackers or smart watches can provide valuable insights into how the indoor environment affects occupants' daily behaviors and physical well-being [78].
5. *Observations:* Conduct structured or unstructured observations to collect qualitative data about occupants' behaviors, interactions with the indoor environment and

responses to different IEQ parameters. These observations provide rich contextual information and also complement other data collection methods [79].

6. *Interviews and Focus Groups*: They help in gathering in-depth insights into occupants' experiences, perceptions and specific issues related to the indoor environment and its impact on their well-being. They uncover nuanced factors that quantitative measures may not capture [80].
7. *Existing Databases and Records*: Utilizing existing databases and records regarding occupant well-being outcomes such as healthcare records, absenteeism rates, or productivity metrics can provide valuable indicators of the impact of IEQ on physical well-being [81].

Data Analysis Methods

The choice of data analysis methods should align with the nature of the collected data and the research objectives. Combining quantitative and qualitative techniques provides a comprehensive understanding of how IEQ affects occupants' physical well-being, offering valuable insights for policy, design and interventions. Descriptive statistics, such as mean, median, standard deviation and frequency distributions, help summarize data, offering a clear overview and identifying trends [82]. Correlation analysis examines relationships between IEQ parameters and occupant well-being, assessing both the strength and direction of associations. Pearson correlation measures linear relationships, while Spearman's rank correlation identifies monotonic relationships [83]. Regression analysis evaluates the impact of IEQ parameters while accounting for confounding variables. Depending on the dependent variable, either multiple regression or logistic regression can determine the influence of specific IEQ factors on physical well-being [84]. Comparative analysis helps assess differences between groups based on IEQ exposure levels. Techniques such as t-tests, ANOVA and non-parametric tests identify variations in well-being outcomes across different IEQ conditions [85].

Mediation and moderation analyses help uncover the mechanisms and boundary conditions influencing the relationship between IEQ and well-being. Mediation analysis identifies whether certain variables explain this relationship, while moderation analysis examines whether it is affected by other factors [86]. Factor analysis detects latent variables within the data, revealing interconnections among different IEQ parameters and their combined effects on well-being [87]. For qualitative data collected through interviews and open-ended surveys, techniques such as thematic analysis help code, categorize and identify patterns to extract meaningful insights [88]. Data visualization enhances the presentation of findings through charts, graphs and visual representations, illustrating the relationships between IEQ parameters and well-being outcomes. This improves understanding and makes key findings easier to communicate [89].

Strategies to Improve IEQ

Several effective strategies can enhance IEQ and improve the physical well-being of building occupants.

A. *Ventilation:* Ensure a fresh air supply through mechanical systems or open windows, depending on environmental conditions [90-92].
B. *Air Quality Management*: Regular maintenance and cleaning of HVAC systems prevent dust, mold and pollutants. High-efficiency air filters help remove contaminants from indoor air [93].
C. *Natural Light:* Designing spaces with large windows and open layouts enhances well-being and reduces energy consumption. Task lighting and adjustable lighting further improves comfort and productivity [94-95].
D. *Nature & Views:* Access to natural elements and greenery reduces stress and boosts well-being [96].
E. *Temperature & Humidity*: Maintain indoor conditions around 25°C and 30-60% relative humidity. Smart HVAC systems adapt to changing conditions and occupant preferences [97].
F. *Noise Reduction:* Use sound-absorbing materials (e.g., acoustic panels) and soundproof spaces to minimize distractions [98].
G. *Biophilic Design:* Incorporate natural elements like plants, wood and water features to enhance connection to nature and overall well-being [98].
H. *Ergonomics:* Provide adjustable furniture and ergonomic workstations to support physical health and reduce musculoskeletal issues [99].
I. *Color & Materials*: Use soothing colors to create a calming or energizing atmosphere. Select low-VOC paints, finishes and materials to reduce indoor air pollution [100].
J. *Odor Control*: Prevent unpleasant odors through proper waste disposal and regular cleaning. Use natural, non-irritating air fresheners when needed.
K. *Wellness Programs*: Encourage physical activity and stress management with exercise spaces and wellness initiatives.
L. *Occupant Engagement*: Educate occupants on IEQ's importance and involve them in decision-making. Allow workspace customization for lighting, temperature and comfort.
M. *Building Maintenance*: Implement a robust maintenance schedule to ensure optimal system performance [101].
N. *Green Building Standards*: Certifications like LEED uphold high IEQ standards [102].

Conclusion

The IEQ significantly impacts occupants' physical well-being, with factors like air quality, lighting, thermal comfort, acoustics and ergonomics working together to shape health outcomes. Their combined effects are greater than any single factor alone, highlighting the need for thoughtful indoor space design. To deepen our understanding of IEQ's impact on health, research should explore multiple avenues. Longitudinal studies can establish causal relationships and reveal long-term effects, while intervention studies can clarify how specific IEQ adjustments directly influence well-being. Including diverse occupant groups ensures more inclusive indoor environments. Advances in IoT and wearable sensors provide real-time data for precise analysis and cost-effectiveness studies can guide decision-making on IEQ improvements. These insights should shape guidelines and standards that prioritize healthier indoor environments. Encouraging multidisciplinary collaboration will enhance our understanding of IEQ and well-being, driving data-driven innovations that improve occupants' health and quality of life.

References

[1] Sansaniwal SK, Kumar S, Jain N, Mathur J, Mathur S. Towards implementing an indoor environmental quality standard in buildings: A pilot study. *Building Services Engineering Research and Technology*. 2021 Jul;42(4):449-83.

[2] Altomonte S, Allen J, Bluyssen PM, Brager G, Heschong L, Loder A, Schiavon S, Veitch JA, Wang L, Wargocki P. Ten questions concerning well-being in the built environment. *Building and Environment*. 2020 Aug 1;180:106949.

[3] Arif M, Katafygiotou M, Mazroei A, Kaushik A, Elsarrag E. Impact of indoor environmental quality on occupant well-being and comfort: A review of the literature. *International Journal of Sustainable Built Environment*. 2016 Jun 1;5(1):1-1.

[4] Rohde L, Larsen TS, Jensen RL, Larsen OK. Framing holistic indoor environment: Definitions of comfort, health and well-being. *Indoor and Built Environment*. 2020 Oct;29(8):1118-36.

[5] Datta A, Suresh R, Gupta A, Singh D, Kulshrestha P. Indoor air quality of non-residential urban buildings in Delhi, India. *International Journal of Sustainable Built Environment*. 2017 Dec 1;6(2):412-20.

[6] Paleologos KE, Selim MY, Mohamed AM. Indoor air quality: pollutants, health effects and regulations. In *Pollution assessment for sustainable practices in applied sciences and engineering* 2021 Jan 1 (pp. 405-489). Butterworth-Heinemann.

[7] Ige J, Pilkington P, Orme J, Williams B, Prestwood E, Black D, Carmichael L, Scally G. The relationship between buildings and health: a systematic review. *Journal of public health*. 2019 Jun 1;41(2):e121-32.

[8] Sansaniwal SK, Mathur J, Garg V, Gupta R. Review of studies on thermal comfort in Indian residential buildings. *Science and Technology for the Built Environment*. 2020 Jul 2;26(6):727-48.

[9] Sansaniwal SK, Mathur J, Mathur S. Review of practices for human thermal comfort in buildings: present and future perspectives. *International Journal of Ambient Energy*. 2022 Dec 31;43(1):2097-123.

[10] Bueno AM, de Paula Xavier AA, Broday EE. Evaluating the connection between thermal comfort and productivity in buildings: A systematic literature review. *Buildings*. 2021 Jun 7;11(6):244.

[11] De Carli M, De Giuli V, Zecchin R. Review on visual comfort in office buildings and influence of daylight in productivity. *Indoor Air*. 2008 Aug 16;2008:17-22.

[12] Katabaro JM, Yan Y. Effects of lighting quality on working efficiency of workers in office building in Tanzania. *Journal of environmental and public health*. 2019 Nov 14;2019.

[13] Hwang T, Kim JT. Effects of indoor lighting on occupants' visual comfort and eye health in a green building. *Indoor and Built Environment*. 2011 Feb;20(1):75-90.

[14] Sansaniwal SK, Mathur J. Development and validation of ISHRAE Indoor Environmental Quality Standard. *The Fifth International Conference on Efficient Building Design*, Beirut, Lebanon 2022.

[15] Mewomo MC, Toyin JO, Iyiola CO, Aluko OR. Synthesis of critical factors influencing indoor environmental quality and their impacts on building occupants health and productivity. *Journal of Engineering, Design and Technology*. 2023 Feb 3;21(2):619-34.

[16] Clark C, Crumpler C, Notley H. Evidence for environmental noise effects on health for the United Kingdom policy context: a systematic review of the effects of environmental noise on mental health, wellbeing, quality of life, cancer, dementia, birth, reproductive outcomes and cognition. *International journal of environmental research and public health*. 2020 Jan;17(2):393.

[17] Jafari MJ, Khosrowabadi R, Khodakarim S, Mohammadian F. The effect of noise exposure on cognitive performance and brain activity patterns. *Open access Macedonian journal of medical sciences*. 2019 Sep 9;7(17):2924.

[18] Zhang X, Zhou S. Building a City with Low Noise Pollution: Exploring the Mental Health Effect Thresholds of Spatiotemporal Environmental Noise Exposure and Urban Planning Solution. *International Journal of Environmental Research and Public Health*. 2023 Feb 27;20(5):4222.

[19] Attaianese E. Ergonomics of built environment ie how environmental design can improve human performance and well-being in a framework of sustainability. *Ergonomics International Journal*. 2017;1(1):1-8.

[20] Engelen L. Does active design influence activity, sitting, wellbeing and productivity in the workplace? A systematic review. *International Journal of Environmental Research and Public Health*. 2020 Dec;17(24):9228.

[21] Djongyang N, Tchinda R and Njomo D. Thermal comfort: A review paper. *Renewable and Sustainable Energy Reviews* 2010; 14(9):2626-2640.

[22] Wong LT, Mui KW and Hui PS. A multivariate-logistic model for acceptance of indoor environmental quality (IEQ) in offices. *Building and Environment* 2008; 43(1):1-6.

[23] Cao B, Ouyang Q, Zhu Y, Huang L, Hu H, Deng G. Development of a multivariate regression model for overall satisfaction in public buildings based on field studies in Beijing and Shanghai. *Building and environment*. 2012 Jan 1;47:394-9.

[24] Barbosa S and Alberto KC. Effect of the double skin façade material on the thermal performance of the educational building in tropical climate. *Architectural Science Review* 2019; 62(3):206-215.

[25] Indraganti M. Thermal comfort in apartments in India: Adaptive use of environmental controls and hindrances. *Renewable Energy* 2011; 36(4):1182-1189.

[26] Al-Hemoud A, Gasana J, Al-Dabbous A, Alajeel A, Al-Shatti A, Behbehani W, Malak M. Exposure levels of air pollution (PM2. 5) and associated health risk in Kuwait. *Environmental research*. 2019 Dec 1;179:108730.

[27] Cincinelli A and Martellini T. Indoor air quality and health. *International Journal of Environmental Research and Public Health* 2017; 14(11):1286.

[28] Kelly FJ and Fussell JC. Improving indoor air quality, health and performance within environments where people live, travel, learn and work. *Atmospheric Environment* 2019; 200:90-109.

[29] ANSI/ASHRAE 62.1. Ventilation for acceptable indoor air quality. *Atlanta: American Society of Heating, Refrigerating and Air-conditioning Engineers,* 2022.

[30] ANSI/ASHRAE 62.2. Ventilation and acceptable indoor air quality in residential buildings. *Atlanta: American Society of Heating, Refrigerating and Air-conditioning Engineers*, 2019.

[31] Fincher W and Boduch M. Standards of human comfort: relative and absolute. Center for Sustainable Development, University of Texas at Austin, 2009.

[32] ISHRAE Standard 100001:2016. *Indoor environmental quality*. India: Indian Society of Heating, Refrigeration and Air-conditioning.

[33] Barrett P, Davies F, Zhang Y, Barrett L. The impact of classroom design on pupils' learning: Final results of a holistic, multi-level analysis. *Building and Environment*. 2015 Jul 1;89:118-33.

[34] Frontczak M. Human comfort and self-estimated performance in relation to indoor environmental parameters and building features. Ph. D Thesis, Technical University of Denmark, Lyngby, Denmark, 2012.

[35] Suk JY. Luminance and vertical eye illuminance thresholds for occupants' visual comfort in daylit office environments. *Building and Environment* 2019; 148:107-115.

[36] Benjamin AO and Alibaba HZ. Achieving Acoustic Comfort in the Architectural Design of a Lecture Hall. *International Journal of Civil and Structural Engineering Research* 2019; 6(2):161-184.

[37] Lee YS. Office layout affecting privacy, interaction and acoustic quality in LEED-certified buildings. *Building and Environment*. 2010 Jul 1;45(7):1594-600.

[38] Quehl J. Comfort studies on aircraft interior sound and vibration (Doctoral dissertation, Universität Oldenburg).

[39] Wang K. The aesthetic principles of soundscape in architectural design and built environment (Doctoral dissertation, Texas A&M University).

[40] Deouskar N. The impact of ergonomics on the productivity of people. *International Journal of Marketing & Financial Management*. 2017;5(6):59-63.

[41] Jaber AR, Dejan M and Marcella U. The Effect of Indoor Temperature and CO_2 Levels on Cognitive Performance of Adult Females in a University Building in Saudi Arabia. *Energy Procedia* 2017; 122:451-456.

[42] Bakó-Biró Z, Clements-Croome DJ, Kochhar N, Awbi HB, Williams MJ. Ventilation rates in schools and pupils' performance. *Building and environment*. 2012 Feb 1;48:215-23.

[43] ANSI/ASHRAE Standard 62.1-2013. Ventilation for acceptable indoor air quality. *Atlanta: American Society of Heating, Refrigerating and Air-conditioning Engineers*, 2013.

[44] Deng Q, Deng L, Miao Y, Guo X, Li Y. Particle deposition in the human lung: Health implications of particulate matter from different sources. *Environmental research*. 2019 Feb 1;169:237-45.

[45] Nezis I, Biskos G, Eleftheriadis K, Kalantzi OI. Particulate matter and health effects in offices-A review. *Building and Environment*. 2019 Jun 1;156:62-73.

[46] Li Y, Cakmak S and Zhu J. Profiles and monthly variations of selected volatile organic compounds in indoor air in Canadian homes: Results of Canadian national indoor air survey 2012–2013. *Environment International* 2019; 126:134-144.

[47] Salthammer T. Formaldehyde sources, formaldehyde concentrations and air exchange rates in European housings. *Building and Environment* 2019; 150:219-232.

[48] Occupational safety and health administration. S*ulfur Dioxide: General Descriptio*n, USA 2012.

[49] Centers for disease control and prevention. Toxic Substances Portal: Sulfur Dioxide. Agency for Toxic Substances and Disease Registry, USA 2009.

[50] Zhang X. Particles Matter, Nitrogen Dioxide and Sulfur Dioxide. In: *Indoor Environmental Quality and Health Risk toward Healthier Environment for All,* Singapore, 2020: pp. 217-235.

[51] Occupational safety and health administration. *Carbon monoxide*. U.S. Department of Labour, Washington DC, USA 2012.

[52] Weschler CJ and Shields HC. Indoor ozone/terpene reactions as a source of indoor particles. *Atmospheric Environment* 1999; 33(15):2301-2312.

[53] Capolongo S, Settimo G. Indoor air quality in healing environments: impacts of physical, chemical and biological environmental factors on users. *Indoor air quality in healthcare facilities*. 2017:1-1.

[54] Ramsey JD, Burford CL, Beshir MY, Jensen RC. Effects of workplace thermal conditions on safe work behavior. *Journal of safety Research*. 1983 Sep 1;14(3):105-14.

[55] Pilcher JJ, Nadler E, Busch C. Effects of hot and cold temperature exposure on performance: a meta-analytic review. *Ergonomics*. 2002 Aug 1;45(10):682-98.

[56] Kiess HO, Lockhart JM. Effects of level and rate of body surface cooling on psychomotor performance. *Journal of Applied Psychology*. 1970 Aug;54(4):386.

[57] Lockhart JM, Kiess HO, Clegg TJ. Effect of rate and level of lowered finger surface temperature on manual performance. *Journal of Applied Psychology*. 1975 Feb;60(1):106.

[58] Lan L, Lian Z, Pan L. The effects of air temperature on office workers' well-being, workload and productivity-evaluated with subjective ratings. *Applied ergonomics*. 2010 Dec 1;42(1):29-36.

[59] Kim DH, Mansfield KP. A cross-cultural study on perceived lighting quality and occupants' well-being between UK and South Korea. Energy and Buildings. 2016 May 1;119:211-7.

[60] EN12464-1. Light and lighting – Lighting of work places. *Indoor work places*. Brussels, Belgium: European Committee for Standardization; 2011.

[61] Franzetti C, Fraisse G and Achard G. Influence of the coupling between daylight and artificial lighting on thermal loads in office buildings. *Energy and Buildings* 2004;36(2):117-126.

[62] David M, Donn M, Garde F, Lenoir A. Assessment of the thermal and visual efficiency of solar shades. *Building and Environment.* 2011 Jul 1;46(7):1489-96.

[63] Rocca M. Health and well-being in indoor work environments: a review of literature. In2017 IEEE International Conference on Environment and Electrical Engineering and 2017 *IEEE Industrial and Commercial Power Systems Europe (EEEIC/I&CPS Europe)* 2017 Jun 6 (pp. 1-6). IEEE.

[64] Salonen H, Lahtinen M, Lappalainen S, Nevala N, Knibbs LD, Morawska L, Reijula K. Physical characteristics of the indoor environment that affect health and wellbeing in healthcare facilities: A review. *Intelligent Buildings International*. 2013 Jan 1;5(1):3-25.

[65] Li W and Drisdelle L. Evaluation of an Indoor Open Space's Acoustical Quality–A Case Study. *Canadian Acoustics* 2019; 47(3):48-49.

[66] ISO 16283-1:2014. Acoustics—Field measurement of sound insulation in buildings and of building elements — Part 1: Airborne sound insulation. Geneva, Switzerland: International Organization for Standardization, 2014.

[67] Mansor R, Sheau-Ting L. Criteria for occupant well-being: A qualitative study of Malaysian office buildings. *Building and environment*. 2020 Dec 1;186:107364.

[68] ANSI/ASHRAE 55-2017. Thermal environmental Conditions for Human Occupancy. Atlanta: American Society of Heating, *Refrigerating and Air-conditioning Engineers*, 2017.

[69] EN ISO7730-2005. Moderate thermal environments-Determination of the PMV and PPD indices and specification of the conditions for thermal comfort. Geneva: International Standards Organisation, 2005.

[70] CEN EN 16798-2019. Energy performance of buildings-Part 1: Indoor environmental input parameters for design and assessment of energy performance of buildings addressing indoor air quality, thermal environment, lighting and acoustics.

[71] Srinivasan S, O'fallon LR, Dearry A. Creating healthy communities, healthy homes, healthy people: initiating a research agenda on the built environment and public health. *American journal of public health*. 2003 Sep;93(9):1446-50.

[72] Marberry SO, Guenther R, Berry LL. Advancing human health, safety and well-being with healthy buildings. *Journal of Hospital Management and Health Policy*. 2022 Jun 25;6.

[73] Pinto M, Pastorinho MR, Lanzinha J, Monteiro M. Model for Health Risk Assessment in Portuguese Housing Spaces. *Environments*. 2022 Jun 6;9(6):69.

[74] Barragán-Landy M, Sousa S, Romero F, Leão C. A Proposed Representative Sampling Methodology. In *20th European Conference on Research Methodology for Business and Management Studies*: ECRM 2020 Jun 1 (p. 8).

[75] Sansaniwal SK, Mathur J, Mathur S. Quantifying occupant's adaptive actions for controlling indoor environment in naturally ventilated buildings under composite climate of India. *Journal of Building Engineering*. 2021 Sep 1;41:102399.

[76] Franke M, Nadler C. Towards a holistic approach for assessing the impact of IEQ on satisfaction, health and productivity. *Building Research & Information*. 2021 May 19;49(4):417-44.

[77] Tiele A, Esfahani S, Covington J. Design and development of a low-cost, portable monitoring device for indoor environment quality. *Journal of Sensors*. 2018 Mar 4;2018.

[78] Diamond LM, Otter-Henderson KD. Physiological measures. *Handbook of research methods in personality psychology*. 2007:370-88.

[79] Abboushi B, Safranek S, Rodriguez-Feo Bermudez E, Pratoomratana S, Chen Y, Poplawski M, Davis R. A review of the use of wearables in indoor environmental quality studies and an evaluation of data accessibility from a wearable device. *Frontiers in Built Environment*. 2022 Feb 18;8:787289.

[80] Wang C, Zhang F, Wang J, Doyle JK, Hancock PA, Mak CM, Liu S. How indoor environmental quality affects occupants' cognitive functions: A systematic review. *Building and environment*. 2021 Apr 15;193:107647.

[81] Oh HJ, Jeong NN, Sohn JR, Kim J. Personal exposure to indoor aerosols as actual concern: Perceived indoor and outdoor air quality and health performances. *Building and Environment*. 2019 Nov 1;165:106403.

[82] Parkinson T, Parkinson A, de Dear R. Continuous IEQ monitoring system: Context and development. *Building and Environment*. 2019 Feb 1;149:15-25.

[83] Fisher MJ, Marshall AP. *Understanding descriptive statistics*. Australian critical care. 2009 May 1;22(2):93-7.

[84] Chok NS. Pearson's versus Spearman's and Kendall's correlation coefficients for continuous data (Doctoral dissertation, University of Pittsburgh).

[85] Chatterjee S, Hadi AS. *Regression analysis by example*. John Wiley & Sons; 2013 May 30.

[86] Orcan F. Parametric or non-parametric: Skewness to test normality for mean comparison. *International Journal of Assessment Tools in Education*. 2020 Jun 10;7(2):255-65.

[87] Wu AD, Zumbo BD. Understanding and using mediators and moderators. *Social Indicators Research*. 2008 Jul;87:367-92.

[88] Yong AG, Pearce S. A beginner's guide to factor analysis: Focusing on exploratory factor analysis. *Tutorials in quantitative methods for psychology. 2013* Oct 1;9(2):79-94.

[89] Sgier L. *Qualitative data analysis*. An Initiat. GebertRufStift. 2012 Apr 19;19:19-21.

[90] Chen CH, Härdle WK, Unwin A, editors. *Handbook of data visualization*. Springer Science & Business Media; 2007 Dec 18.

[91] Schulze T, Eicker U. Controlled natural ventilation for energy efficient buildings. *Energy and buildings*. 2013 Jan 1;56:221-32.

[92] Evola G, Gagliano A, Marletta L, Nocera F. Controlled mechanical ventilation systems in residential buildings: Primary energy balances and financial issues. *Journal of Building Engineering*. 2017 May 1;11:96-107.

[93] Schweiker M, Berger C, Day J, Mahdavi A. Fundamentals of IEQ and Occupant Needs. In *Occupant-Centric Simulation-Aided Building Design*, Routledge. 2023 May 31;10-33.

[94] Liu C, Hsu PC, Lee HW, Ye M, Zheng G, Liu N, Li W, Cui Y. Transparent air filter for high-efficiency PM2. 5 capture. *Nature communications*. 2015 Feb 16;6(1):6205.

[95] Pilechiha P, Mahdavinejad M, Rahimian FP, Carnemolla P, Seyedzadeh S. Multi-objective optimisation framework for designing office windows: quality of view, daylight and energy efficiency. *Applied Energy*. 2020 Mar 1;261:114356.

[96] Konstantzos I, Sadeghi SA, Kim M, Xiong J, Tzempelikos A. The effect of lighting environment on task performance in buildings–A review. *Energy and Buildings*. 2020 Nov 1;226:110394.

[97] Gu J, Liu H, Lu H. Can Even a Small Amount of Greenery Be Helpful in Reducing Stress? A Systematic Review. *International Journal of Environmental Research and Public Health*. 2022 Aug 9;19(16):9778.

[98] Gholamzadehmir M, Del Pero C, Buffa S, Fedrizzi R. Adaptive-predictive control strategy for HVAC systems in smart buildings–A review. *Sustainable Cities and Society*. 2020 Dec 1;63:102480.

[99] Zhong W, Schröder T, Bekkering J. Biophilic design in architecture and its contributions to health, well-being and sustainability: A critical review. *Frontiers of Architectural Research*. 2022 Feb 1;11(1):114-41.

[100] Colim A, Carneiro P, Costa N, Arezes PM, Sousa N. Ergonomic assessment and workstation design in a furniture manufacturing industry—a case study. In *Occupational and Environmental Safety and Health* 2019 Feb 28 (pp. 409-417). Cham: Springer International Publishing.

[101] Guo H, Murray F, Lee SC. The development of low volatile organic compound emission house—a case study. *Building and environment*. 2003 Dec 1;38(12):1413-22.

[102] Wang S, Ma Z. *Supervisory and optimal control of building HVAC systems: A review*. HVAC&R Research. 2008 Jan 1;14(1):3-2.

[103] Licina D, Wargocki P, Pyke C, Altomonte S. *The future of IEQ in green building certifications*.

Biographical Sketch

Sunil K. Sansaniwal

Dr. Sunil K. Sansaniwal brings extensive experience in research and academia within the energy and environment sector. His work is centered on fostering a sustainable built environment, with expertise spanning sustainable cooling, energy efficiency, clean energy adoption, indoor environmental quality and policy advocacy. Dr. Sansaniwal earned his Ph.D. with a focus on enhancing indoor environmental quality through occupants' adaptive actions in buildings. He is a qualified Mechanical Engineer and a certified Energy Professional, further solidifying his technical expertise in the field. Throughout his career, Dr. Sansaniwal has received several awards and recognitions from prestigious organizations worldwide, underscoring his contributions to the field. His exceptional science communication skills have garnered affiliations with various international journals, where he has served in multiple capacities. He has authored numerous research articles, which have accumulated significant citations, reflecting the impact and reach of his work. Dr. Sansaniwal has played a pivotal role in several high-profile research projects aimed at net-zero energy transitions, sectorial energy efficiency, power sector reforms, building energy demand reduction and sustainable cooling technologies. Currently, Dr. Sansaniwal is associated as a Consultant with NITI Aayog, Government of India. In this role, he continues to make significant contributions to the field of Energy, Green Transition and Climate Change, driving forward innovative solutions and promoting sustainable practices within the energy and environment sectors.

Julia K. Day

Dr. Julia K. Day is an expert in building science and energy-efficient design, serving as an Associate Professor in School of Design and Construction at Washington State University (WSU), Pullman (Washington). She teaches building science courses and coordinates the industry-led MEP course for construction management students. Dr. Day is the Director of WSU's Integrated Design + Construction Lab, part of a regional network of university labs focused on advancing high-performance building practices. The lab conducts applied research, provides technical assistance and supports energy efficiency outreach to improve comfort, reduce carbon impact and enhance occupant health and productivity. Her interdisciplinary Ph.D. from WSU and current research focus on occupant behavior, education and energy use in high-performance buildings. Previously, she taught and conducted research at Kansas State University, where she directed both the Energy, Behavior, and Built Environment Laboratory and the Energy Efficiency & Human Behavior Program at the Institute of Environmental Research. Professionally, Day has held roles in architectural design and energy consulting, including work with Callison Architecture in Seattle and as a project manager with Integrated Design Labs at both WSU and the University of Idaho, partnering with Idaho Power and NEEA on energy efficiency initiatives. Dr. Day holds leadership roles in several national and international organizations, including the IEA's Annex 79 (Occupant-Centric Building Design and Operation), the NSF's Sustainable Human-Building Ecosystems network, and ASHRAE, where she chairs the Education & Training subcommittee for Technical Committee on Operations & Maintenance.

Chapter 4

The Implications of Organizational Ecology on Ecological Innovation

José G. Vargas-Hernández[1,*]
Absalón J. Salmerón-Zapata[1]
and M. C. Omar C. Vargas-González[2,†]
[1]Financial Literacy Research Center, Universidad Cristóbal Colón, Veracruz, Mexico
[2]Instituto Tecnológico de México, Campus Cd. Guzmán, Jalisco, Mexico

Abstract

This study aims to analyze the implications of organizational ecology on organizational ecological innovation within organizations, from the assumption that the theoretical and conceptual framework of organizational ecology is positively associated with ecological innovation in organizations. The method employed is analytical and reflective based on the theoretical and conceptual literature review. It is concluded that major organizational ecological innovations leading to technical changes are pioneered by entrepreneurial organizations shedding light on the positive relationships between the concepts and theories of organizational ecology and the competing mechanisms proposed in the results of the organizational innovative ecology.

Keywords: ecological innovation, organizational aging, organizational ecology, patents

Introduction

The debate on organizational ecology surrounds the mechanisms underlying the effects of age on life mechanisms (Barron, West & Hannan, 1994; Hannan, 1998). There are numerous debates on the conceptual, theoretical, and methodological issues related to organizational ecology, with little effort to integrate them into an emerging research field (Wholey, & Brittain, 1986). The debates around organizational ecology regarding the mechanisms of age and their

* Corresponding Author's Email: jvargas2006@gmail.com
† Corresponding Author's Email: omar.vg@cdguzman.tecnm.mx

In: Psycho-Environmental Variables That Ensure People's Well-Being and Health …
Editors: Roberto Alonso González Lezcano and Guadalupe Cantarero García
ISBN: 979-8-89530-831-8
© 2025 Nova Science Publishers, Inc.

effects on life changes still rage (Barron, West, & Hannan, 1994; Hannan, 1998). There are many organizational ecology studies on the effects of organizational age on the life and behavior of organizations. There is a trend in applying organizational ecology in business research (Liu et al., 2022).

Organizational ecology fosters an interdisciplinary and transdisciplinary framework of sustainable development (Carayannis & Campbell, 2010) where the knowledge and innovation blend, and can be interpreted as an approach to sustainable development and social ecology (Atiku, 2020; Fields & Atiku, 2017; 2018). Organizations possess information-processing routines and technological trajectories used to facilitate incremental innovation (Tushman & Anderson, 1986; Henderson, 1993). Organizations generate, develop, and communicate socio-ecological knowledge, norms, sentiments, and innovation sensitive to the entrepreneurs and stakeholders in the scientific and technological inventories and socio-ecological projects that create a macro-effect in social and ecological dimensions.

The fundamental difference between the organizational ecological and economic approaches lies in the empirical consideration of organizational survival. There is a link between organizational survival and innovation with an indirect link between innovation and survival. Organizational survival and innovational outcomes are not always transparent. The critical differences between organizational ecological theory and organizational economic approaches are the identification of the relevance of competition and mutualism within and between environmental niches (Atiku, 2019). The indicators for voluntary environmental regulation elements are the environmental and ecological certifications, the environmental information disclosure, and the environmental supervision.

The growing gap between organizational innovative capabilities and technological frontiers presents an opportunity for new organizations to align their internal routines with technological development. It needs to be studied, as do the joint effects of age and innovation outcomes in organizational growth and mortality models. Organizational innovation becomes incremental, and process innovation increases with product innovation.

Existing research shows that organizations not only focus on improving their current performance but also try to create greater value for the business ecosystem when making strategic choices (Liu et al., 2022). This research on organizational ecology and its implications on organizational ecological innovation aims to study the assumption that the theoretical and conceptual framework of organizational ecology is positively associated with ecological innovation in organizations. To achieve this objective, it reviews the conceptual and theoretical elements of organizational ecology to explain some of the main implications in the organizational innovation. Finally, some conclusions are presented.

Background

Organizational Ecology

The concept of organizational ecology refers to an organizational field whose interrelations among the organizations compose a system, becoming the object of inquiry. The emergence of organizational ecology is traced from empirical studies in organization theory based on the institution-building tasks, in a complex and interdependent environment (Trist, 1977). In organizational ecology, firms compete in standards (David, 1985). Organizational ecology is an evolutionary theory that describes structural changes in organizations (Sisaye, 2021).

Organizational ecology studies the planning, design, and management of physical settings that affect and are affected by expectations, organizational values, and work practices (Becker, 1988). The consistent performance of leadership styles tends to stimulate the ecological innovativeness of the project supported by the inputs of ecological knowledge, information, and competence. Without the injection of knowledge, information, and competence, the performance of the leadership style does not stimulate ecological innovativeness (Bossink, 2004). Socio-ecological knowledge communication and insights contribute to changing values and attitudes, trust building, and facilitating conflict resolution to ecosystem management (Fields & Atiku, 2017).

Organizational ecology attends to the consequences of aging for organizational functioning outcomes although there is no consensus on whether the effects of aging are positive or negative on organizational functioning (Hannan, 1998). The organizational ecology aging theories distinguish between the competitive perspectives of the liability of newness (Stinchcombe, 1965; Hannan and Freeman, 1984) and the perspective of liability of senescence (Barron, West, & Hannan, 1994).

Organizational ecology combines the influences of inertia, imprinting, and environmental changes to render obsolete the core technologies of old aging organizations (Barron, West, and Hannan, 1994; Aldrich and Auster, 1986; Ranger-Moore, 1997). Time passage in organizations leads to the accumulation of knowledge and an increasing in organizational competence, paralleling the theoretical perspectives of aging in organizational ecology: liability of newness (Stinchcombe, 1965; Hannan & Freeman, 1984) and the liability of senescence (Barron, West, & Hannan, 1994). Organizational ecology infers the effects of organizational age in models failing to control the organizational size with a correlation between age and size (Barron, Hannan, & West, 1994).

Organizational ecology theories sustain an equilibrium model based on continuous change and strategic adaptation. The innovation community is a proposed framework based on organizational ecology to be used in research developing an institutional theory of technology commercialization (Lynn, Reddy, & Aram, 1996). The legal framework including the institutional arrangements and property rights is exogenous to the local voluntary collaboration socio-ecological systems (Hahn, 2000).

Organizational ecology theories sustain that at the population level, the adaptation of organizational structures occurs with the replacement of new organizations by old ones that fail to adapt. Socioecological research has firm-level variations in shaping external environments (Baum & Mezias, 1992; Lubatkin et al., 2001). In organizational ecology, competition is assumed the central mechanism via which organizations interact (Downie, 2022). Actors and organizations, underlined by the formal rules and informal social norms and conventions as institutions underlying this management, link a conceptual model of the socio-ecological dynamics to a socio-ecological system consisting of ecosystem management.

The dynamics of social responses can be assessed at different organizational levels to enhance the process of adaptive co-management and change the socio-ecosystem with the support of local self-organized steward associations and other authorities at various levels, to learn, experiment with management practices, generate socio-ecological knowledge, and collaboration (Olsson et al., 2004).

Socio-ecological systems determine resilience by ecological dynamics and the social capacity to respond and shape ecosystem changes that sustain, develop, and enhance the ecological conditions for human societies and the socio-ecological change trajectory under conditions of uncertainty (Carpenter et al., 2001, Folke et al., 2003). Socio-ecological system challenges the acceptance of uncertainty by enhancing the capacity to deal with disturbance (Berkes et al., 2003).

A resilient socio-ecological system makes use of disturbances to transform into desired states (Walker et al., 2004). A socio-ecological system that is non-resilient is vulnerable to external changes. Community transformation must adopt the socio-ecosystem approach to create a trajectory of building the resilience of the social-ecological system (Olsson et al., 2004) supported by the interactions of a social network to generate socioecological knowledge and provide memory for the management socio-ecosystem (Berkes & Folke, 1992; McIntosh et al., 2000). Building resilience in socio-ecological systems is a relevant tool to influence physical planning for land use in communities.

An ecosystem's adaptive governance is related to socio-ecological systems (Dietz et al., 2003; Eckerberg & Joas, 2004; Folke et al., 2005; Ostrom, 2005). Adaptive governance is supported by social memory of responses to ecological crises requiring social incentives and enabling legislation for collaboration (Malayang et al., 2005; Pretty, 2003). The adaptive governance of socio-ecological systems tends to reduce organizational transaction costs of collaboration and value formation providing social incentives that have lasting effects on behaviors for implementing socio-ecological projects (Pretty, 2003).

Any governance system must count on social processes, policies, and strategies to promote and sustain socio-ecosystem management, generating, developing, and communicating ecological knowledge. The socio-ecological knowledge and the levels of dynamic governance that bridge local actors are relevant dimensions of socio-ecosystem management to generate legal, financial, and political support.

Ecological knowledge can be fed into adaptive management practices characterized by continuous monitoring of adaptive responses with management plans adapted to the inherent uncertainty in complex systems (Berkes et al., 2003). The socio-ecosystem management system is based on collaboration and landscape management concerned with adaptive governance, adaptive management, eco-management, and resilience with social response resulting from self-organization at the local level and involving interaction between organizations. Collaboration resulting from an open dialogue resulting among stakeholders at local inventories is more concerned with conservation ecology, ecotourism, and cultural heritage issues.

Vertical links enable knowledge to be incorporated from other socio-ecosystems to the local socio-ecological knowledge for management planning (Olsson et al., 2004). There should be feedback and responses between the social and ecological systems and responses avoiding the creation of systemic friction in the case of actors and agents with higher access to financial resources and assets to support various projects replaced by less interested people in the socio-ecosystem management.

Adaptive approaches for socio-ecosystem management under conditions of uncertainty involve building knowledge, linking people and organizations with knowledge systems, and mobilizing resources and socio-ecosystem dynamics to reduce ecological illiteracy, detecting environmental feedback and responding to enhance the resilience of socio-ecosystem processes and functions (Folke et al., 2005; Gadgil et al., 1993; Olsson & Folke, 2001).

Organizational growth and survival are outcomes of organizational ecology used to evaluate different mechanisms (Ranger-Moore, 1997). Organizational aging has consequences and implications in organizational ecology, evolutionary, and learning theories leading to obsolescence processes in organizational innovation. Organizational obsolescence has a specific innovation trajectory (Dosi, 1982). Organizational innovation is enhanced by organizational learning as the source of competitive advantages in industrial ecology. The strategy of learning organizations achieves a corporate competitive advantage in industrial ecology (Chen, Wang, Lin & Chang, 2018). Organizational ecology has inferences drawn on the effects of organizational aging in models failing to control the size, correlates age and size (Barron, West, & Hannan, 1994). Organizational ecology takes into consideration the aging consequences for organizational outcomes, failing to reach a consensus to determine the negative and positive aging effects on organizational functioning (Hannan, 1998). The decline of organizational responsiveness leads to reduced levels of organizational innovation (Aldrich & Auster, 1986).

Ecological change in organizations can be incorporated into the organizational adaptation framed by the organizational ecological theory (Barnett, 1990). The implementation of organizational ecology among the strategic research groups of firms leads to performance differences in the organizational forms. Implementing the use of an organizational ecological model of resource has led to the findings supporting the use of an organizational ecological model of form-specific density and resource-partitioning (Carroll & Waminathan, 1992) found that the founding rates of firms increase with density and then tend to decline, mortality rates decline with density and industry concentration. The organizational ecological approach incorporated that organizational systems influence the operations of class and economic structures and lead to the regulation of social and political order. (Sisaye, 2021).

Organizational aging is a ubiquitous process that has a multifaceted influence on organizational innovation, although the relationship between organizational behavior and aging has not been resolved (Hannan, 1998). It is important to study the gap between the benefits of proactive turnaround strategies and the obstacles faced by organizations (Gotteiner et al., 2019). Organizational ecology processes are an essential element that may influence the changes in organizational populations over time. Aging has positive consequences for innovative activities on accumulated experience as in the case of older firms that tend to innovate more frequently, and these innovations are more significant.

The relationships between organizational aging and innovation improve the organizational dynamics of technological leadership in markets. A consistent negative relationship between aging and innovation is expressed in tales of displacement implying that organizations are unable to generate innovations (Abernathy & Utterback, 1978; Tushman & Anderson, 1986).

Organizational ecology sustains that the combination of imprinting, environmental changes, and inertia leads to organizational and technological innovation obsolescence of old organizations (Barron, West & Hannan, 1994; Aldrich & Auster, 1986; Ranger-Moore, 1997).

Organizational population ecology sustains that individual organizations are subject to inertial forces and have limitations to succeed in radical structural and strategic changes. The organizational ecology has implications for strategic choice as perspectives on organizational strategy are constrained by environmental conditions and industry change over time. Organizational ecology and evolutionary theories do not tend to consider the contextual factors of organizational change. Central organizational populations are considered more ecologically dominant, coordinating, and controlling the flows of resources through and into the community (Hawley, 1963; Lincoln, 1976).

Commercially owned technological firms that become organizational ecologically dominant result from technological interdependence and centrality of the network of the salient feature of technological systems displaying positive consumption externalities rather than from ownership (Katz & Shapiro, 1985: 424).

Organizational ecology gives support for the theoretical framework and operational methodology for the interdependence analysis of competition and mutualism using the model density-dependent mortality (Barnett & Carroll, 1987; Tucker et al., 1988; Carroll & Hannan, 1989; Delacroix, Swaminathan, & Solt, 1989). In the ecological framework, mutualism is considered to favor some populations over others and results from supplementary similarities and complementary differences. For Downie (2022), the organizational ecology assumes that competition is the principal form of interaction, but the same population can cooperate and are more likely to when they have a shared governance goal.

The ecological principles give perspective for the analysis from the ecological view of technological interdependence. Singh and Lumsden, (1990), review theory and research in organization and population levels of organizational ecology analysis and processes of changes in findings and mortality. Organizational mortality in which firms proliferate and fail under conditions or organizational technological change draws on the community ecology theory, which predicts when technologies are systemic and organizational technological change does not favor. The organizational ecological theory of adaptation incorporates technological change.

The organizational theory presents two different perspectives; on the one hand, there is the perspective of surviving by adapting to environmental changes, and on the other, extinction by selection in the face of environmental changes (Ozturk & Dil 2022, Hannan & Freeman 1977).

Ecological Innovation

Organizational ecology, learning, and evolutionary theories derive propositions of organizational aging as obsolescence processes related to organizational innovation. An organizational ecological framework is used to study and analyze systemic technological innovation in terms of more elemental systems (Hawley, 1950). Organizational ecology and evolutionary theories explain the dynamic relationships between organizational innovation and evolution at the industry population levels using historical data, the organizational research tends to examine the organizational adaptation process.

The approach based on ecological principles to study technological change and competition is different from the Schumpeterian approach. This approach to innovation is relevant in the history of industry because of its effects on the cost, range, and quality of service (Wasserman, 1985). Corporations undertake initiatives to address social and ecological degradation by adapting organizational design and developing new business models (Doppelt, 2003; Dunphy et al., 2003).

The Darwinist explanation of progress is simple, unorganized complexity where any change of the system is determined by the environment while the ecological explanation is a more complex modeling with new elements and activities. Ecological modernization and innovation diffusion theories based on the adoption of green supply management practices identify early adopters, followers, and laggards. The adoption affects organizational performance leading to the advancement of the theory of innovation diffusions (Zhu, Sarkis, & Lai, 2012).

The dynamic, complex, and uncertain changes in the global economy environment and industrial ecology enhance the learning organization to cope with and transform the organizational innovation processes. The environmental fit refers to the fit between the innovations and the state of the art of modern technologies. Older firms tend to build on previous innovative activities. Aging firms in elaborate innovation in old technological areas are the result of the fit between the technological environment and organizations' innovative activities that influence the technological community.

The environmental and organizational fit relates to the match between the innovations of the firm and the current state of the art, which is receptive to other producers of related modern technologies (Abernathy & Utterback, 1978; Tushman & Anderson, 1986; Rosenbloom & Christensen, 1994). Environmental developments and changes external to the organizations make it difficult to keep pace leading to organizational innovative outputs to become suited to the demands.

The analysis of the relationship between aging and the rate of production of innovations by organizations. As organizations age, they gradually refine the organizational routines and competencies underlying the production of innovations. The internal time passage processes govern organizational innovation processes. In organizational routines, the passage of time in organizations leads to incremental improvements as the result of experience-dependence in which age is associated with innovation increases. Organizations more experienced in developing innovation routines tend to move beyond past innovation activities and are more likely to experiment with local investments in technology and tend to avoid non-local. The innovative activities of the organization may become insulated from external non-domestic technological developments. An increasing gap between the technological frontier and the organizational innovation capabilities creates and develops opportunities with the alignment of internal routines with technological development.

Organizational aging is positively associated with innovation. Organizational aging is a ubiquitous organizational process that addresses the issue of nature in the organizational theory of the relationships between organizational behavior and aging, which has a multifaceted influence on organizational innovation (Hannan, 1998). There is evidence of how organizational aging alters the internal features of organizations and affects innovations. Differences across and among organizations in recruitment and turnover patterns mediate the relationships between organizational aging and innovation. Differences across organizations in the patterns of personnel recruitment and turnover time mediate the relationship between organizational aging and innovation. Elevated levels of turnover in key organizational roles dilute institutional memory.

Increasingly knowledge-based economy pinpoints the factors shaping the organizational ability to generate innovations. At the organizational level, innovation is governed by organizational search strategies and routines, which are repositories of organizational knowledge that combined, generate outputs (Cyert & March 1963; Nelson & Winter, 1982; Hannan & Freeman, 1984; March 1988). The organizational level is a determinant of innovation activity, and the aging results are due to the influence of unmeasurable variables correlated with organizational aging. Organizational knowledge is required to accumulate innovative activities and assimilate ideas in a solid base of knowledge (Cohen & Levinthal,

1990: 136; Nelson & Winter, 1982; March 1991). The organizational innovation and knowledge accumulation cycle tends to self-reinforce the knowledge base aimed to pursue innovative opportunities (Cohen & Levinthal, 1990).

Innovation at the organizational level is governed by innovation at the industry level, with time in different economic and technical contexts. Organizational innovation level processes are governed by the organization's internal lifecycle leading to several organizations facing similar constraints at the industry level and functionally responding differently according to their aging. Organizations drawn from high technology industries are affected by the organizational aging routine strategies (Cyert & March 1963; Nelson & Winter, 1982; Hannan & Freeman, 1984).

Organizational knowledge of the industry domains suggests that innovation is rapid in some of them experimenting with radical innovation and competence for destroying technological change. Radical innovation spawns' new technological fields emerging from small entrepreneurial organizations. The organizational ability of a firm to use its knowledge for innovation is dependent on knowledge distribution and communication patterns (Cohen & Levinthal, 1989; 1990). Firms engaged in the exploitation of competencies are more prone to building upon prior innovations. Organizational competence is the capacity to create and develop innovations of modern technologies and products with a broader quality and acceptance. The development of the ability to innovate high technology areas hinges on heavy investments in long-standing competence building (Abernathy & Utterback, 1978; Burgelman, 1983; Tushman & Anderson, 1986; Henderson & Clark, 1990).

The relationship between organizational innovation and aging has consequences for the fitness of the environmental demands and organizational routines that affect organizational competence. A technologically driven industry field well fitted between aging and environment tied to innovative ability is expected to experience lower failures. Microelectronics and biotechnology are among the most innovation-intensive industries in the economy, they differ in underlying technologies and development efforts in the manufacture, distribution, and marketing of their innovations (Barley, Freeman, & Hybels, 1992). The maturation of the industrial context in the analysis of the industry life cycle is related to the composition of organizational innovation.

The organizational ability to innovate requires investments in long-established competence building in specific areas as a way of adapting to technological regimes (Abernathy & Utterback, 1978; Burgelman, 1983; Tushman & Anderson, 1986; Henderson & Clark, 1990). The ability to innovate in high-technology markets requires investing in competence building in areas of technology (Abernathy & Utterback, 1978; Burgelman, 1983; Tushman & Anderson, 1986; Henderson & Clark, 1990).

Large organizations are likely to invest slack resources in innovative activities because they tend to possess market power aimed at getting the appropriate returns (Schumpeter, 1942). Large organizations tend to spend more on research and development leading to innovation to benefit from improvements (Cohen & Klepper, 1996). Organizational background knowledge reduces and impedes opportunities to capitalize on new developments to create innovations (Cohen & Levinthal, 1990). Large organizations are often less entrepreneurial and more bureaucratic than small organizations; the size of organizations harms innovation (Blau & Schoenherr, 1971; Abernathy, 1978; Aldrich & Auster, 1986).

The organizational cycle between the accumulation of knowledge and innovation is self-reinforcing. Organizations with larger knowledge bases develop more opportunities to accumulate knowledge (Cohen & Levinthal 1990). Lack of background and accumulated organizational knowledge impedes the development of the ability to generate innovations (Cohen & Levinthal, 1990).

Organizational innovative activities of older organizations are less relevant compared to the most recent technological developments as the age of firms in changing environments leads to technological obsolescence (Tushman & Anderson, 1986; Henderson, 1993; Barron, West & Hannan 1994). Technological obsolescence is the result of age affecting nature and quality of organizational innovation outcomes of developments. The obsolescent organization is the result of a specific innovation trajectory (Dosi, 1982). Organizational and technological obsolescence is the result of age affecting the nature and quality of the organizational innovative outputs.

The research and development investments of the organization increase the generation of patents in innovative domains that are new and have no impact on the patenting rates. Obsolescence as the age concomitant leads to mismatches in the innovative outputs with the environmental demands and becomes irrelevant to the innovative activities of other organizations in the technological community. Innovation and obsolescence are part of the process of establishing the scope of patents. The analysis of age on the innovativeness outputs of organizations from the impact of patents of the organizations that have been cited in subsequent inventions. The foundation age of the organizational period increases with the age of the organization. Patent data derive measures of innovation.

Organizational age increases the propensity to generate firm patents as opposed to working on innovative domains. Firms age tends to work on older areas of technology incorporating technological developments measured by the age of patents cited prior. Older organizations produce innovations and patents as the function of organizational age. Older organizations trail behind the leading age technology focusing on innovative activities in new technological domains. Obsolescence is concomitant of organizational age leading to a mismatch with innovative outputs between the environmental demands and the innovative activities in the technological community.

The organizational outputs and the environmental demands decline with organizational aging. In cases such as the innovations of older organizations are more consistent with extensions of innovative domains. The decline of innovation in older organizations is manifested in the innovative domains associated with organizational aging and patent self-citation rates.

Age-related decline in the fit between environment and organization tends to lead innovative organizations to create and develop on older technological foundations. Innovative organizations are likely to succumb to the competency traps occurring when the competency has better performance with inferior procedures (Levitt & March 1988). The organizational age increasingly generates innovation by exploiting existing competencies.

Innovative organizations must face competency traps to achieve performance with inferior procedures leading to accumulated knowledge and experiences for a superior procedure but inadequate to be rewarding to use (Levitt & March, 1988, 322). Prior organizational innovations reinforce routines and trajectories in technological frontiers to enter new fields, despite facing competency traps.

Learning organizations led to organizational innovation capabilities and enhancement of adjustments and performance behaviors (Lopez et al., 2016). An ecological organization encourages multiple learning processes to enhance team competitiveness, encourage decision-making and execution to transform into learners, promote common cooperative high learning level, and promote organizational innovation competitiveness. Organizational learning theory sustains that a set of experiences and improved routines enhance organizational competence with the accumulation of knowledge leading to technical innovations (March 1991; Cohen & Levinthal, 1990). The accumulated knowledge required for innovative activities assimilates innovative ideas (Cohen & Levinthal, 1990; Nelson & Winter, 1982; March, 1991).

An organizational ecology must transfer an integrated thinking system to encourage cooperation and trust spirit, creating and supporting a learning organization aimed at continuous enhancement of innovation, positive organizational culture, and climate through common learning and development, the capability of transformation, and adaptation to social change. However, there are some contradictory outcomes related to the organizational learning and innovation processes (March, 1991).

Organizational innovation models are based on cross-functional problem-solving leading to less integration with regulations in process innovation for economic, social, and ecological performance. Innovative organizations may succumb to competency traps occurring when an inferior procedure leads to favorable performance and accumulating more experience (Levitt & March 1988). Organizations with smaller ecological footprints can align organizational innovation models with sustainable goals. The comprehensive concept of Quintuple Helix frames knowledge and innovation in the context of the natural environment leading to sustainable development and social ecology (Carayannis et al., 2012).

There is a relationship between organizational change and innovation supported by the incremental and evolutionary view. Organizational incremental innovation consists of incremental improvements. Organizations possess processing information routines along the technological trajectories able to facilitate incremental innovation (Tushman & Anderson, 1986; Henderson, 1993). Organizational changes in evolutionary theories occur through incremental skills change in organizational routines. Organizational innovative capabilities are better suited to creating and developing incremental innovations along with the existing technological trajectories.

Innovation can be incremental and radical but neither involves competence-destroying technological change. In periods of organizational radical technical change, organizations are unable to adapt their activities to external advances and environmental demands. Incremental and radical technological change and innovation processes fall along a continuum of innovative capabilities defined by organizational aging leading to predictable changes occurring independently of the innovative context. Current innovations of aging organizations elaborate on older technological areas.

The distinction between entrant incremental or radical technological change, the innovative capabilities of organizations fall into a continuum defined by organizational aging leading to the prediction of innovative changes and activities in a broader innovative context. The innovative capabilities of an organization are better suited to generate incremental innovations in the technological trajectories.

Organizational aging is associated with increasing experience-dependent enhancements of innovation. Organizational aging affects innovation and promises to inform important theoretical debates in organizational theory. Organizational aging leads to an increase in the rigidity and ossification of structures and communication patterns, which may reduce the competence and innovations over time and lead to increased organizational structure rigidity and ossification of communication and distribution patterns resulting in the production of fewer innovations as related to their age. The organizational capability and ability to use a knowledge base for innovation depends on the communication and distribution patterns. As firms age, they become more likely to create and exploit competences to generate innovations.

High-technology organizations survive for a longer period because they have created and developed innovative competencies in their domains. This statement is confirmed by the assumptions that organizational age is positively associated with innovation, because of age the larger size is associated with elevated levels of bureaucracy and complexity (Belau & Schooner, 1971). Organizational size and innovation rates are relevant in the association with patenting behavior.

Organizational size has effects on the firm's innovation. The patents of other organizations depending on the industry sector may less or more cite the patents of large organizations. Organizational innovation is an output that has a direct impact on organizational viability and effects on economic and social change. The success of organizational innovation depends on the social capital and reputation of the organizations that sponsor innovativeness on underlying technical specifications (Tushman & Rosenkopf, 1992; Wade, 1995; Podolny & Stuart, 1995).

Organizational size has some positive effects on innovation outcomes, evident in the technological patent rate. Larger organizations tend to spend more resources on R&D toward process innovations because of their greater production to benefit the improvements (Cohen & Klepper, 1996). Organizational resources in interdependent markets are often distributed based on organizational promises and the reputation of large corporations able to attract innovators, elaborators, and adapters of technologies. Large organizations generate a large quantity of innovation (Schumpeter, 1942; Cohen, Levin, & Mowry, 1987; Cohen & Klepper, 1996).

Large firms' patents may be less cited on a per-patent basis although the innovations of large technological firms tend to be more cited by the patents of other organizations because large firms tend to be less entrepreneurial than medium and small enterprises and more bureaucratic (Blau & Schoenherr, 1971; Abernathy & Utterback 1978; Aldrich & Auster 1986).

Entrepreneurial firms support the assertion that organizational aging is a source of dynamic change often-pioneer major innovations. However, organizational size may have discrepant effects on the innovations of organizations. The patent application has negative effects on its use as the foundation for other innovations. Organizational aging affects the fit between internal competence and the environment as determinant of innovative performance. The innovations of older firms are less influential on subsequent innovative processes in the industrial and technological community. An age-related decline in the fit between the organization and the environment becomes a tendency for innovative activities of older organizations based on older technology. The fit between the innovative activities of firms and their technological environment influences the innovations in their technological community.

Organizational aging gauges the length of operational experience and the duration of the organizational exposure to environmental changes (Carroll, 1983). In a technological community, the innovations of older organizations are less influential on technology development, subject to the differences in technologies and the types of firms of the ecological population, the market dynamics, etc. Older firms are more likely to build upon previous innovative activities. Older firms with specific innovation areas are expected to harvest in their fields of established competence. Older organizations tend to exploit the established innovative domains without moving into innovative areas. Older organizations that are slow in changing due to inertia are unhurried in moving beyond prior innovation areas.

Aging has positive consequences for organizational innovation on one extreme and the other aging impedes the capability and ability to innovate. Organizational aging has positive consequences for organizational innovative activities. Based on the accumulation of experience, older organizations innovate more frequently and with greater significance. Experience outweighs the negative consequences of bureaucratization of organizations becoming more adapted in the creation of organizational innovations per their ages. The production of organizational innovation processes results from the experience of negative consequences of bureaucratization. A consistent negative relationship between innovation and aging implies that organizations can generate important innovations with age.

Independent of radical competence destroying innovative processes, the consequences of aging at organizational innovation processes and activities are generic for all the different innovative contexts. These scenarios have direct implications for organizational demography and ecology in high technology industry. High technology fields have predictive effects of firms on innovative activities.

Organizational competence refers to the capacity of firms to generate and develop innovations, regardless of the acceptance and quality of modern technologies. Relationships between organizational innovation and aging are related to the distinction from theoretical perspectives on how may affect organizational competence and the consequences for the fitting between the environmental demands and the organizational routines.

Findings of organizational aging for innovation in rudimentary dimensions and across contexts have been validated and generalizable using patent-based measures of innovation. The patent citation data enables the construction of measures of inventions, proximity of inventions to current technological developments, and inter-temporal stability in innovative activities. Patent citations have a positive association with organizational age and patents manifested in technological building relations. New patents of organizations are closely related to prior innovative activities and earlier inventions.

Highly cited patents on innovations are perceived to be the most relevant inventions in the specific technological field (Albert et al., 1991). Self-citing patents are elaborations of prior innovation activities that increase with aging and differentiate from non-self-citing. Self-citing patents are affected by the innovative activities of organizational aging. Patents in innovative domains that are new to the organizations do not have an impact on the existing work of the firm.

The organizational aging process can be explored with other measures of innovation. An innovation index that does not examine the effects of organizational aging on the commercialization of innovative technologies, is one relevant limitation for patents. Patents have limitations as an innovation index to examine the organizational age affecting the commercialization of modern technologies. Inertia is a force in high-technology firms, and patent-based measures can further the study of management practice to moderate-age innovation relationships.

Older organizations produce more innovations than younger organizations. Innovations of older organizations are less relevant than those of younger organizations. Firms incorporating recent technological developments into innovations can be measured by the age of patents. As the age of technology organizations increases, the generation of patents based on prior innovations increases. Increases in the aging of the firm´s innovative activity are due to the age of cited prior patents. Organizational aging increases the likelihood of innovation in the technological fields' trajectories (Dosi, 1982).

The age of organizations increases the period of innovation, leading older firms to innovate at a higher rate because the organization's age gradually refines the organizational competencies and routines of innovation. The organization's current period patents the age of the prior innovation cite the innovation period. Highly cited patents cover innovations in expert technological areas that are perceived as the most relevant (Albert et al., 1991).

Organizational aging is related to innovation processes to signal the dynamics of high-technology industries and organizational theory on the effects of aging on organizational functioning. Organizational aging has effects on the innovations at the time they are developed by the effects of the patent citations. The aging consequences may be contradictory for organizational innovation increases associated with the difficulties of keeping pace with external developments causing innovative inputs to avoid becoming obsolete to the environmental demands. The contradictory outcomes are interrelated and reflect inherent trade-offs in organizational innovation and learning processes (Sørensen & Stuart, 2000).

Evidence on the relationship between organizational innovation and aging enhances the understanding of the dynamics of organizational technological leadership (Anane-Simon & Atiku, 2023). Mandatory retirements, leadership replacements, and volitional departures lead to alterations in the innovative foci of the organizations. Leadership as a variable change's innovation as an expression of organizational aging. Managerial and leadership changes due to retirements and volitional departures, the replacements enable alterations in the organizational innovation-related manifestations of aging. Leadership changes do not have an impact on patent rates. Older firms are less likely than younger organizations to incorporate recent technological developments into their innovative activities, which can be evaluated by measuring the aging of the organization's current-period innovations.

The program of organizational ecological innovation research is based on the theoretical and empirical development of issues facing ecological research (Atiku & Anane-Simon, 2022; Amburgey & Rao Hayagreeva, 2017).

Research Methodology

The bibliometric analysis was limited to data retrieved from electronic literary and scientific sources providing the necessary information to conduct the study. The study was conducted using scientific search engines. The research is in English and is related to the publications and consulting reports, only articles from peer-reviewed journals were included in this study. Besides, only the publications published in journals in the fields of "business" and "management" were used as the basis for on ecological innovation, organizational aging, organizational ecology, patents, and its impact on the organizational ecology innovation. Using the Prisma Flow diagram, we identify the journals that fulfill the requirements for the bibliometric analysis.

Results and Discussion

This study analyzes the implications of organizational ecology on the ecological innovation of organizations departing from the assumption that the theoretical and conceptual framework of organizational ecology is positively associated with ecological innovation in organizations. The main conclusion is that ecological innovations leading to technical changes are pioneered by entrepreneurial organizations, highlighting the positive relationships between the concepts and theories of organizational ecology.

The work has theoretical implications by studying the ecology organization reinforced by rewards that should be created and developed as a learning organization. Organizational ecology faces challenges to become learning organizations and to cope with the needs. An analytical framework of environmental regulation contributes to the formulation, development, and implementation of strategies to cultivate green technology innovation capabilities of firms aimed at improving the ecological environment, alleviating environmental pollution, and leading to ecological governance.

The socio-ecosystem's capacity to generate valuable ecosystem services is dependent on the socio-ecological dynamics, and organizational and institutional capacity to manage. Preservation of socio-ecological values, and cultural heritage, and the use of natural resources to sustain and recreate values must be the main purpose of any socio-ecosystem management program involving all the members and stakeholders of the organization. Socio-ecology values for recreation and ecotourism require enhanced accessibility provided by institutions. Socio-ecological values emerge through socio-ecosystem inventories supported by scientific and local ecological knowledge and, the engagement of actors, agents, and other stakeholders in collaborative learning and problem-solving processes.

Major innovations leading to technical changes are pioneered by entrepreneurial organizations. Innovations in specific technological areas lead to related prior organizational innovative activities that are technologically distant from the organizational past activities. The proximity of inventions, innovations, and patents of technological developments leads to intertemporal stability in organizational innovative activities. Patenting behavior in economic analysis is relevant in controlling for organizational size in association with innovation. Old organizations are less likely to incorporate recent technological developments into previous innovative activities, by measuring the foundation organizational age.

Recommendations

There is dedicated support for the relationship between organizational aging and the organizational innovation processes in such a way that there is evidence that as organizations age, they generate more innovations. As an organization ages, it generates more innovations and patents; However, these gains may result in increasing divergence between organizational competence and current environmental demands. Organizational age affects the capacity to survive, grow, change, and innovate. The competence to generate innovations improves with organizational aging.

It is essential to conduct more studies to understand the impact of organizational ecology in different contexts. Nowadays we can find studies in recent years that examined the organizational ecology of different organizations. Research on the Path Selection of Enterprise Performance Improvement from the Perspective of Organizational Ecology (Liu et al. 2022). On the other hand, Tuncer (2022) lists the following examples of organizational ecology in case studies:

- Downie 2022 - International organizations in global energy management.
- Olvera & Sutton (2021) - Organizational ecology of small food businesses in New York City.
- Lake (2021) – Relationship between private governance organizations, intergovernmental organizations, and states together via the organizational ecology.

Future Areas of Research

More studies on the implications of organizational ecology on the ecological innovation of organizations must be done from different perspectives. It is important to start from the assumption that the theoretical and conceptual framework of organizational ecology is positively associated with ecological innovation and should be reviewed in more organizations, especially in the new paradigms of competition, cooperation, and adaptation that the world is facing.

Further research must be conducted to explore the impact of the value chain network, related to order suppliers and customers, complementors and competitors aligning organizational model with economic, financial, societal, and ecological goals.

Conclusion and Limitations

The relationships between organizational age and innovation highlights the competing mechanisms proposed in organizational ecology theories, despite the scarce empirical evidence of organizational aging and its effects on the associated behavioral changes. The relationship between organizational age and organizational innovation sheds light on the competing mechanisms posited in ecological theories. Its contribution is scarce to the debates over organizational aging leading to behavioral changes. Aged organizations tend to exploit their innovative domains in specific innovation areas that have repeated successfully without moving into new fields of organizational and technologically innovative activities, McQuillan (2019) defines that size and chronological age are not factors in organizational aging.

It has been suggested that most organizations face a decline in their performance at some time during their existence (Gotteiner et al., 2019) which is why it is important to explore the organizational aging processes with other innovation measures. The existing empirical research on the effects of organizational aging in organizational ecology and technical change and innovation leads to the conclusion that there are contradictory consequences for organizational innovation.

Institutional and ecological research converges on issues such as the effects of institutional variables on vital rates, the role of legitimacy in population dynamics, and challenges identified for future research.

References

Abernathy, W. J. (1978). *The Productivity Dilemma.* Baltimore, MD: Johns Hopkins University Press.

Abernathy, W. J., & Utterback, J. M. (1978). Patterns of industrial innovation. *Technology Review* June/July: 41-47.

Albert, M. D., D. Avery, F. Narin, and R McAllister (1991). Direct validation of citation counts as indicators of industrially important patents. *Research Policy*, 20: 251-259.

Aldrich, H., and Auster, E. R. (1986). Even dwarfs started small: Liabilities of age and size and their strategic implications. *Research in Organizational Behavior* 8: 165-198.

Amburgey, T. L. & Rao, Hayagreeva (2017). Organizational ecology: past, present, and future directions. *Academy of Management Journal 39*, 5 https://doi.org/10.5465/256999.

Anane-Simon, R., & Atiku, S. O. (2023). Inclusive leadership for sustainable development in times of change. *Routledge Open Research*, *2*(16), 16.

Atiku, S. O. & Anane-Simon, R. (2022). Stimulating Creativity and Innovation Through Apt Educational Policy. In Z. Fields (Ed.), *Achieving Sustainability Using Creativity, Innovation, and Education: A Multidisciplinary Approach* (pp. 113-133). IGI Global. https://doi.org/10.4018/978-1-7998-7963-3.ch006.

Atiku, S. O. (2019). Institutionalizing Social Responsibility Through Workplace Green Behavior. In S. Atiku (Ed.), *Contemporary Multicultural Orientations and Practices for Global Leadership* (pp. 183-199). IGI Global. https://doi.org/10.4018/978-1-5225-6286-3.ch010.

Atiku, S. O. (2020). Knowledge Management for the Circular Economy. In N. Baporikar (Ed.), *Handbook of Research on Entrepreneurship Development and Opportunities in Circular Economy* (pp. 520-537). IGI Global. https://doi.org/10.4018/978-1-7998-5116-5.ch027.

Barley, S. R., Freeman, J. and Hybels, R. C. (1992) Strategic alliances in commercial biotechnology. In Nitin Nohria and Robert Eccles (eds.), *Networks and Organizations: Structure, Form and Action.* Boston, MA: Harvard Business School Press.

Barnett, W. P. (1990). The Organizational Ecology of a Technological System. *Administrative Science Quarterly*, March., 1990, Vol. 35, No. 1, Special Issue: Technology, Organizations, and Innovation (March, 1990), pp. 31-60. https://www.jstor.org/stable/2393550.

Barnett, W. P., and Carroll, G. R. (1987). Competition and mutualism among early telephone companies. *Administrative Science Quarterly*, 32: 400-421.

Barron, D. N., West, E. and Hannan, M. T. (1994). A time to grow and a time to die: Growth and mortality of credit unions in New York City, 1914-1990. *American Journal of Sociology* 100: 381-421.

Baum, J. A. C., Mezias, S. J. (1992). Localized competition and organizational failure in the Manhattan hotel industry, 1898-1990. *Administrative Science Quarterly*, 37 (4): 580-604.

Becker, F. D. (1988). Chapter 52 - Technological Innovation and Organizational Ecology, Editor Martin Helander, *Handbook of Human-Computer Interaction,* North-Holland, Pages 1107-1117, https://doi.org/10.1016/B978-0-444-70536-5.50057-9.

Berkes, F., and Folke, C. (1992). A Systems Perspective on the Interrelations between Natural, Human-made and Cultural Capital. *Ecological Economics* 5: 1–8.

Berkes, F., Folke, C., and Colding, J. (eds.) (2003). *Navigating Social-Ecological Systems: Building Resilience for Complexity and Change*, Cambridge University Press.

Blau, P. M., and Schoenherr, R. A. (1971). *The Structure of Organizations*. New York: Basic Books.

Bossink, B. A. G. (2004), Effectiveness of innovation leadership styles: a manager's influence on ecological innovation in construction projects, *Construction Innovation*, 4, 4, pp. 211-228. https://doi.org/10.1108/14714170410815105.

Burgelman, R. A. (1983). A Process Model of Internal Corporate Venturing in the Diversified Major Firm. *Administrative Science Quarterly* 28: 223-244.

Carayannis, E. G., & Campbell, D. F. (2010). Triple Helix, Quadruple Helix, and Quintuple Helix and how do knowledge, innovation and the environment relate to each other? A proposed framework for a trans-disciplinary analysis of sustainable development and social ecology. *International Journal of Social Ecology and Sustainable Development, 1*(1), 41–69.

Carayannis, E. G., & Wang, V. W. L. (2012). Competitiveness model—A double diamond. *Journal of the Knowledge Economy, 3*(3), 280–293.

Carpenter, S. R., Walker, B., Anderies, J. M., & Abel, N. (2001). From Metaphor to Measurement: Resilience of What to What? *Ecosystems* 4: 765–781.

Carroll, G. R. & Waminathan, S. (1992). The Organizational ecology of strategic groups in the American brewing industry from 1975 to 1990, *Industrial and Corporate Change*, 1, 1, 1992, Pages 65–97, https://doi.org/10.1093/icc/1.1.65.

Carroll, G. R. (1983). A stochastic model of organizational mortality: Review and reanalysis. *Social Science Research* 12: 303-329.

Carroll, G. R. (1984). Organizational ecology. Annual Review of Sociology. Vol. 10:71- 93 https://doi.org/10.1146/annurev.so.10.080184.000443

Carroll, G. R., and Hannan, M. T. (1989). Density dependence in the evolution of populations of newspaper organizations. *American Sociological Review*, 54: 524-541

Chen, K. H., Wang, J. S., Lin, M. H., & Chang, W. Y. (2018). The Influence of Learning Organization on Organizational Innovation and Organizational Performance Relationship: The Case of Ecology Industry. Ekoloji, 2018, Issue 106, Pages: 329-335, Article No: e106080

Cohen, W. M & Levinthal, D. A. (1990). Absorptive Capacity: A New Perspective on Learning and Innovation. *Administrative Science Quarterly*, 35:123-138.

Cohen, W. M. & Levinthal, R. C. (1989). Empirical studies of innovation and market structure. Pp. 1060-1107 in R. Schmalensee and R. D. Willig (eds.), *Handbook of Industrial Organization*, vol. III. Elsevier Science Publishers

Cohen, W. M., and Klepper, S. (1996). Firm size and the nature of innovation within industries: The case of process and product R&D. *The Review of Economics and Statistics* 78:323-243.

Cohen, W. M., R. C. Levin, and D. C. Mowrey, (1987). Firm size and R&D intensity: A re-examination. *Journal of Industrial Economics*, 35: 543-565.

Cyert, R. M., and March, J. G. (1963). *A Behavioral Theory of the Firm*. Prentice-Hall.

David, P. A. (1985) Clio and the economics of QWERTY. *American Economic Review*, 75: 332-337.

Delacroix, J., Swaminathan, A. and Solt, M. E. (1989) Density dependence versus population dynamics: An ecological study of failings in the California wine industry. *American Sociological Review*, 54: 245-262.

Dietz, T., Ostrom, E., and Stern, P. L. (2003). The Struggle to Govern the Commons. *Science* 302: 1907–1912.

Doppelt, B. (2003). *Leading change toward sustainability: A change-management guide for business, government, and civil society* (p. 296). Sheffield, UK: Greenleaf.

Dosi, G. (1982). Technological paradigms and technological trajectories. *Research Policy*, 11: 147-162.

Downie, C. (2022). Competition, cooperation, and adaptation: The organizational ecology of international organizations in global energy governance. *Review of International Studies, 48*(2), 364-384. https://doi.org/10.1017/S0260210521000267.

Dunphy, D. C., Griffiths, A., & Benn, S. (2003). *Organizational change for corporate sustainability: A guide for leaders and change agents of the future*. London: Routledge.

Eckerberg, K., and Joas, M. (2004). Multi-level Environmental Governance: A Concept under Stress? *Local Environment* 9(5): 405–412.

Fields, Z. & Atiku, S. O. (2017). Collective Green Creativity and Eco-Innovation as Key Drivers of Sustainable Business Solutions in Organizations. In Z. Fields (Ed.), *Collective Creativity for Responsible and Sustainable Business Practice* (pp. 1-25). IGI Global. https://doi.org/10.4018/978-1-5225-1823-5.ch001.

Fields, Z. & Atiku, S. O. (2018). Collaborative Approaches for Communities of Practice Activities Enrichment. In N. Baporikar (Ed.), *Knowledge Integration Strategies for Entrepreneurship and Sustainability* (pp. 304-333). IGI Global. https://doi.org/10.4018/978-1-5225-5115-7.ch015.

Folke, C., Colding, J., & Berkes, F. (2003). Synthesis: Building resilience and adaptive capacity in social-ecological systems. In Berkes, F., Folke, C., and Colding, J. (eds.), *Navigating Social-ecological Systems: Building Resilience for Complexity and Change*, Cambridge University Press, Cambridge, pp. 352–387.

Folke, C., Hahn, T., Olsson, P., and Norberg, J. (2005). Adaptive Governance of Social-ecological Systems. *Annual Review of Environment and Resources.*

Gadgil, M., Berkes, F., and Folke, C. (1993). Indigenous Knowledge for Biodiversity Conservation. *Ambio* 22: 151–156.

Gotteiner, S., Mas-Machuca, M., Marimon, F. (2019). Fighting organizational decline: a.

Hahn, T. (2000). *Property Rights, Ethics, And Conflict Resolution: Foundations of the Sami Economy in Sweden*, Doctoral dissertation, Agraria 258, SLU, Dept of Economics, Uppsala.

Hannan, M. T. (1998). Rethinking age dependence in organizational mortality: Logical formalizations. *American Journal of Sociology*, 104:126-164.

Hannan, M. T., and J. Freeman (1984). Structural inertia and organizational change. *American Journal of Sociology*, 49: 149-164.

Hawley, A. H. (1950) *Human Ecology: A Theory of Community Structure*. New York: Ronald Press.

Hawley, A. H. (1963). Community power and urban renewal success. *American Journal of Sociology,* 68: 422-431.

Henderson, R. M. (1993). Underinvestment and incompetence as responses to radical innovation: Evidence from the photolithographic alignment equipment industry. RAND *Journal of Economics*, 24: 248-270.

Henderson, R. M., and Clark, K. M. (1990). Architectural innovation: The reconfiguration of existing product technology and the failure of established firms. *Administrative Science Quarterly* 35: 9-31. https://doi.org/10.1146/annurev.so.16.080190.001113.

Katz, M. L., & Shapiro, C. (1985). Network externalities, competition, and compatibility. *American Economic Review*, 75: 424-440.

Lake, D. A. (2021). The organizational ecology of global governance. European Journal of International Relations, 27 (2), 345–368. doi: 10.1177/1354066120959407.

Levitt, B., & March, J. G. (1988). Organizational learning. *Annual Review of Sociology* 14: 319-340.

Lincoln, J. R. (1976). Power and mobilization in the urban community: Reconsidering the ecological approach. *American Sociological Review*, 41: 1-15.

Liu, X., Yu, H., Lai, G., Wang, S., Xie, Y. (2022). Imitation or Innovation? Research on the Path of Enterprise Performance Improvement from the Perspective of Organizational Ecology. *Sustainability, 14*, 7223. https://doi.org/10.3390/su14127223.

Lopez, I. F., Amaku, M., Coutinho, F. A., Quam, M., & Burattini, M. N. (2016) Modeling Importations and Exportations of Infectious Diseases via Travelers. *Bull. Math. Biol*, 78: 185-209. https://doi.org/10.1007/s11538-015-0135-z.

Lubatkin, M., Schulze, W. S., Mainkar, A., & Cotterill, R. W. (2001). Ecological investigation of firm effects in horizontal mergers. *Strategic Management Journal*, 22(4): 335–357.

Lynn, L. H., Reddy, N. M., Aram, J. D. (1996). Linking technology and institutions: the innovation community framework, *Research Policy*, 25, 1, Pages 91-106, https://doi.org/10.1016/0048-7333(94)00817-5.

Malayang III, B. S., Hahn, T., and Kumar, P. (2005). Responses to ecosystem change and to their impacts on human well-being. In *Millennium Ecosystem Assessment, Findings of the Sub-global Assessments Working Group*, chapter 9. Island, http://www.maweb.org.

March, J. G. (1988). *Decisions in Organizations*. New York: Blackwell.

March, J. G. (1991). Exploration and exploitation in organizational learning. *Organization Science* 2: 71-87.

McIntosh, R., Tainter, J., and McIntosh, S. (2000). *The Way the Wind Blows: Climate, History, and Human Action*, Columbia University Press, New York.

McQuillan, J. (2019). Is your organization aging? Journey Consulting. https://www.journeyconsult.com/post/is-your-organization-aging.

Nelson, R. & Winter, S. (1982). *An Evolutionary Theory of Economic Change.* Cambridge: Harvard University Press.

Olsson P., and Folke, C. (2001). Local Ecological Knowledge and Institutional Dynamics for Ecosystem Management: A Study of Lake Racken Watershed, Sweden. *Ecosystems* 4: 85–104.

Olsson, P., Folke, C., and Hahn, T. (2004b). Social-ecological Transformation for Ecosystem Management: The Development of Adaptive Comanagement of a Wetland Landscape in Southern Sweden. *Ecology and Society* 9(4): 2. [Online] URL: http://www.ecologyandsociety.org/vol9/iss4/art2/print.pdf.

Olvera, J., Sutton, S. A. (2021). An organizational ecology approach to new food marts in New York City neighborhoods. International Journal of Urban Sciences, 25 (2), 252–271. doi: 10.1080/12265934.2020.1804988.

Ostrom, E. (2005). Understanding Institutional Diversity, Princeton University Press, Princeton New Jersey, USA. Ovesson, P. (2003). *Markhävdkartering 2002, Hävdtillståndet på betesmarker och slåtterängar inom Nedre Helgeåns våtmarksområde i Kristianstads Vattenrike. Länsstyrelsen i Skåne län, Kristianstads kommun, Högskolan i Kristianstad.*

Ozturk, O., & Dil, E. (2022). Bibliometric Analysis of Organizational Ecology Theory (OET): To Review Past for Directing the Future of the Field. *Ege Akademik Bakis, 22*(2), 195-212. https://doi.org/10.21121/eab.980638.

Podolny, J. M., & Stuart, T. E. (1995). A role-based ecology of technological change. *American Journal of Sociology* 100:1224-1260.

Pretty, J. (1995). Participatory Learning for Sustainable Agriculture. *World Development* 23: 1247–1263.

Pretty, J. (2003). Social Capital and the Collective Management of Resources. *Science* 302: 1912–1914.

Ranger-Moore, J. (1997). Bigger may be better, but is older wiser? Organizational age and size in the New York life insurance industry. *American Sociological Review*, 62: 903-921.

risk-based approach to organizational anti-aging. *Management Research Review*, Vol. 42, Issue 11, pp. 1259-1277, doi 10.1108/MRR-09-2018-0367

Rosenbloom, R. S., and C. M. Christensen (1994). Technological discontinuities, organizational capabilities, and strategic commitments. *Industrial and Corporate Change*, 3: 655-685.

Schumpeter, J. A. (1942) *Capitalism, Socialism and Democracy*. Harper.

Singh, J. V., Lumsden, Ch. J. (1990). Theory and Research in Organizational *Ecology Annual Review of Sociology*. Vol. 16:161-195 (Volume publication date August 1990).

Sisaye, S. (2021). The organizational ecological resource framework of sustainability reporting: implications for corporate social reporting (CSR). *Journal of Business and Socioeconomic Development* Vol. 2 No. 2, pp. 99-116. doi 10.1108/JBSED-05-2021-006..

Sørensen, J. B. & Stuart, T. E. (2000). Aging, Obsolescence, and Organizational Innovation. *Administrative Science Quarterly*, Vol. 45, No. 1, pp. 81-112 http://www.jstor.org/stable/2666980.

Stinchcombe, A. L. (1965). Social structure and organizations. Pp. 142-193 in James G. March (ed.), *Handbook of Organizations*. Chicago: Rand McNally.

Trist E. A. (1977). Concept of Organizational Ecology. *Australian Journal of Management*. 2(2):161-175. doi:10.1177/031289627700200205.

Tucker, D. J., Singh, J., Meinhard, A. G., & House, R. J. (1988). Ecological and institutional sources of change in organizational populations. In Glenn R. Carroll (ed.), *Ecological Models of Organizations*: 7-31. Ballinger.

Tuncer, M., Akbulut, N., Turhan, M. S., & Ari, Y. (2022). Time-Varying Network Connectedness between the Organizational Ecology of Transportation and Storage Firms and Macroeconomic Variables. Folia Oeconomica Stetinensia, 22(2), 209-223. https://doi.org/10.2478/foli-2022-002.

Tushman, M. L., & Anderson, P. (1986) Technological discontinuities and organizational environments. *Administrative Science Quarterly* 31: 439-465.

Tushman, M. L., & Rosenkopf, L. (1992). Organizational determinants of technological change: Toward a sociology of technological evolution. *Research in Organizational Behavior* 14: 311-347.

Wade, J. (1995). Dynamics of organizational communities and technological bandwagons: An empirical investigation of community evolution in the microprocessor market. *Strategic Management Journal* 16: 111-133.

Walker, B., Holling, C. S., Carpenter, S. R., & Kinzig, A. (2004). Resilience, Adaptability, and Transformability in Social-ecological Systems. *Ecology and Society* 9(2): 5. [Online] URL: http://www.ecologyandsociety.org/vol9/iss2/art5/.

Wasserman, N. (1985). *From Invention to Innovation: Long Distance Telephone Transmission at the Turn of the Century*. Johns Hopkins University Press.

Wholey, D. R. & Brittain, J. W. (1986). Organizational Ecology: Findings and Implications. Academy of Management ReviewVol. 11, No. 3. https://doi.org/10.5465/amr.1986.57140723.

Zhu, Q., Sarkis, J., & Lai, K. (2012). Green supply chain management innovation diffusion and its relationship to organizational improvement: An ecological modernization perspective, *Journal of Engineering and Technology Management*, 29, 1, Pages 168-185, https://doi.org/10.1016/j.jengtecman.2011.09.012.

Biographical Sketches

José G. Vargas-Hernández

José G. Vargas-Hernandez is currently a research professor at Financial Literacy Research Center, Universidad Cristóbal Colón, at National technological Institute of México, ITS Fresnillo and a research professor at Broward International University (Miami). He is a member of the National System of Researchers of Mexico. He has been a researcher at Budapest Centre for Long-term Sustainability (BC4LS), University Center for Economic and Managerial Sciences, Universidad de Guadalajara and at University Center for Social research, Universidad de Colima, a visiting scholar at Carleton University Canada, University of California Berkeley and Laurentian University, Canada. Professor Vargas-Hernandez holds a PhD. in Economics from Keele University and a PhD. in Public Administration from Columbia University. He has published nine books and more than 600 papers in international journals and reviews, as well as more than 300 essays in national journals and reviews. His main research is in organizational economics and strategic management. He teaches for several doctoral programs and has won 17 international awards. His main research focuses on the organizational economics and green economy in sustainable green urban planning for urban green innovation areas.

Absalón J. Salmerón-Zapata

Absalón J. Salmerón-Zapata holds a PhD in Administrative Sciences from the Cristóbal Colón University, where he currently works as a research professor. He has a Master's degree in Administration and a Bachelor's degree in Psychology from the same university. He is a theologian from the Pontifical Gregorian University. He directs the DCM Program, an analysis model based on labor competencies, at the Cristóbal Colón University and is the Vice-Rector General of the same university. His line of research is on human talent optimization and organizational development. Among his most recent publications are: Conceptual, Theoretical-Methodological, and Empirical Approaches on the Multidimensional Relationship Between Human Talent Management and Organization.

Omar C. Vargas-Gonzàlez

Professor, research assistant and former Head of Computer Systems Department at Tecnológico Nacional de México Campus Ciudad Guzmán, professor at Telematic Engineering at Centro Universitario del Sur Universidad de Guadalajara with a master's degree in Computer Systems. Has been trained in Innovation and Multidisciplinary Entrepreneurship at Arizona State University (2018) and a Generation of Ecosystems of Innovation, Entrepreneurship and Sustainability for Jalisco course by Harvard University T. H. Chan School of Health. At present conduct research on diverse fields such as Entrepreneurship, Economy, Statistics, Mathematics and Information and Computer Sciences. Has collaborated in the publication of many scientific articles and conducted diverse Innovation and Technological Development projects.

Chapter 5

An Investigation of Physical Environmental Design Requirements for Individuals with Dementia

Gökçen Firdevs Yücel Caymaz*
and Nigar Zeynalova
İstanbul Aydın University, Istanbul, Turkey

Abstract

The aim of the present study is to investigate the design parameters intended to improve the comfort of use in the built environment of patients with dementia. Accordingly, the parameters suggested by previous studies were reviewed, and subsequently, an up-to-date checklist was developed. The list was reviewed on the basis of videos, photos, and information available on the Internet digital database about four different dementia villages, which are limited in numbers across the world. As a result of the analyses conducted in this study it was concluded that use of handrails and sign boards were required similar to children's playground designs.

Keywords: age-friendly design, exterior environment, design for dementia, elderly-nature connection, dementia villa Ges, design elements

Introduction

The Madrid International Plan of Action, which was adopted at the Second World Assembly on Ageing held in Madrid, in 2002, underscored "ensuring enabling and supportive environments" among the three priority areas (United Nations, 2002). Older individuals need space for development and recreation, and therefore, streets should be envisaged to serve as an extension of home and allow playfulness for all ages, including the old age (Spencer et al., 2013). Wu et al. (2019) suggested that individuals with dementia required spaces, where they are understood, respected, supported, and trusted for their contribution to society. Environments for older individuals may include private and public planting spaces, legible

* Corresponding Author's Email: gokcenfyucel@aydin.edu.tr

In: Psycho-Environmental Variables That Ensure People's Well-Being and Health …
Editors: Roberto Alonso González Lezcano and Guadalupe Cantarero García
ISBN: 979-8-89530-831-8
© 2025 Nova Science Publishers, Inc.

gardens that appeal to the senses of smell, touch, sight, taste, and hearing, comfortable and easily distinguishable exterior seating, access to public transportation means, integrated library and reading clubs, nearby medical facilities, religious buildings, shopping centers, and memory centers containing the spatial components of the past and future, properly marked spaces, non-disturbing public parking lots, good street lighting, clear signage, and use of color (Halsall and MacDonald, 2015). Difficult access, high and steep steps, level alterations, damaged sidewalks, heavy-traffic streets with few crossing points, isolated dark bus stops, lack of adequate urban furniture, and lack of public toilets would prevent the older individuals from using the city centers (Hanson, 2002).

More than 55 different diseases may induce dementia (Cotter, 2007). According to Alzheimer's Disease International (2003), approximately 47 million people worldwide had dementia in 2015, and this number was projected to exceed 131 million by 2050. Environmental design would play an important role in improving the daily living comfort of older individuals with dementia. Cleanliness, visual appeal, fresh clean air, and reducing noise and traffic congestion may encourage older individuals to use public spaces (World Health Organization, 2007). Strong evidence suggested that person-oriented approaches might improve behavior. Moderate evidence was supportive of noise regulation, environmental design, unobtrusive visual barriers, and environmental relocation strategies to reduce problematic behaviors (Jensen and Padilla, 2017).

Environment design for patients with neurodegenerative disease should be aligned with behavioral patterns and focus on reducing stress (Goto et al., 2014). As Beckwith and Gilster (2014) suggested in their work, each garden should meet the unique environmental, social and physical needs of each population throughout the progression of dementia (Cohen-Mansfield and Werner, 1998). The basic proposition of the model as suggested by Lawton in the 1970s is that an environment that places high demands on its inhabitants (i.e., 'environmental pressure') has a negative impact, particularly on older individuals (Lawton and Nahemow, 1973). The results of Mooney and Nicell's study (1992) were indicative of the fact that utilization of exterior spaces reduced the aggressive behavior of patients with dementia and significantly contributed to the risk management program. People with dementia are often very active and generally find it frustrating to be in an environment with constraints. Patients with dementia frequently lose their sense of time, their perception of days and seasons. Access to nature and the exteriors may help mitigate that symptom by exposing residents to natural sunlight and darkness, which helps with keeping an individual's internal clock synchronous with real time. Ulrich (1984) suggested that natural views would be effective in the recovery of patients compared to building views. The availability of water and vegetation might attract interest and attention, reduce sentiments of fear and anxiety by blocking stressful thoughts (Mooney and Nicell, 1992).

Environmental perception issues, including color, taste, smell, touch, acoustics, and microclimate; location of the garden; design issues associated with garden entrance, pedestrian paths, pavements, railings, navigation, water elements, activity areas, and urban furniture; planting and maintenance issues should be taken into consideration for the design of quality and comfortable exterior spaces for patients with dementia.

Environmental Perceptions

A calming environment reduces wandering behavior and anxiety, whereas highly elevated sund variations or an interesting environment may result in increased wandering. Philips et al. (2013) suggested that an appropriate sound level, poor signage, confusing spaces, and poor flooring would create barriers for the older individuals in new environments, and that the presence of landmarks and distinctive structures in unfamiliar areas would prove to be important. Exterior freedom is associated with the extent the exteriors are accessible to the residents. Residents should know that the garden exists and should be able to readily find the way thereto. They should also be able to make active or passive use of the garden (Ulrich, 1999). Lee et al. (2021) suggested stated that an appropriate sound level or familiar music would help create a positive stimulus for individuals with dementia. Colors and patterns, including strong contrasts, can impact residents. However, patterns and dark lines can be confusing and even lead to falls. (McAdam, 2017).

Location

The exterior space should be located on the southeastern side of a building with an aim to provide a monolithic building shadow (Randall et al., 1990). In case the exterior spaces are close to activity and living areas, residents would tend to visit them. Incontinence is a prevalent condition in care settings, and therefore, toilet facilities should be located as close to the exterior spaces as possible.

Design Elements

Orientation, privacy, autonomy, sensory comprehension, range of movement, encounters, and activities are considered key factors for individuals with dementia (Nillesen and Opitz, 2014). Memory care and dementia gardens are often enclosed to ensure a sense of security. They contain wide, plain paths or labyrinths, non-glare surfaces, social areas, and seating units for patients to rest (Figure 1). Familiar features, including wind chimes, clotheslines, and bird baths are also frequently introduced in such places.

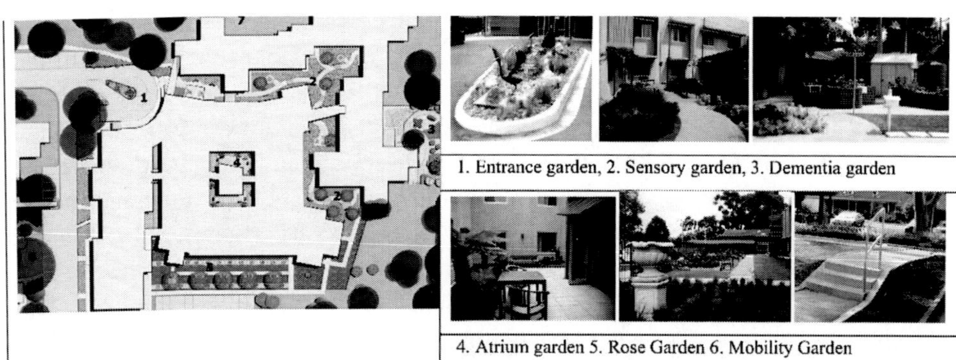

Figure 1. Resthaven Paradise, 61 Silkes Road, Paradise, SA, 2011 (Graham-Cochrane, 2010).

For patients with dementia, spatial appearance and views are important not only to improve the spatial attraction, but also to reassure them that the space is warm and safe. It was reported that patients with dementia could make decisions more easily in buildings with well-articulated entrances and signs (Barnes and Design in Caring Environments Study Group, 2002). A single entrance and/or exit door to the garden with a simple road system should be envisaged to help patients in consideration of spatial perception problems (Şahin and Erbek, 2018). In case of multiple doors, the main door should be more prominent compared to the other(s).

Studies on ageing indicated that older individuals moved more slowly and took smaller steps to adapt to physical changes (Zeisel and Tyson, 1999). Creating a continuous route may ensure that 'users' easily navigate around and search for different impulses. Pollock (2007) suggested that a simple return path system-based circulation (loop, circular, figure eight, loop divided into two), minimal selection points to minimize confusion, and no dead ends were imperative. Exterior walkability should be facilitated by means of a loop with a maximum total length of 500 meters (Marcus, 2005).

The color of pavement materials can help separate pathway from seating area. Road fabric or materials can also help navigate along with color contrast. Open ground helps define the roadside thanks to the contrast created against the grass surface and vegetation. People living with dementia may forget where they have gone and where they have come from. This could prove to be restrictive and hinder their exterior mobility. Landmarks, doorways, change in ground surface, and open signage can help them gain a sense of control and self-confidence in the garden, setting (McBride, 1999). Colors, lighting, furnishings, and pictorial signs are viable cues to help navigation of individuals with dementia (Phillips et al., 2013). Brawley (2007) recommended oval-shaped and large flat surface handrails to provide a better gripping surface. Zeisel and Tyson (1999) suggested that the door to return inside the building was a vital landmark in a garden setting designed for people with dementia. McBride (1999) asserted that fountains acted as centers, which facilitated orientation and wayfinding. Natural sounds are the best for mood and meditation and a fountain can also serve to mask other unpleasant sounds in the environment. They also promote visual, auditory, kinesthetic, and tactile stimulation. There is limited research available on the specific effects of water elements. Nevertheless, in a study of 12 elderly patients with dementia, average systolic blood pressure ratios decreased from 127 to 123 in the presence of water elements (HDC, 2008).

The space is shaped upon the building's relationship therewith; thus, a good garden design starts at the building scale. The building orientation should be aligned to allow sunlight and air into both the gardens, and the spaces. In this case, height is also very important (Michon, 2016). Cohen and Weisman (1991) suggested that exterior views from indoor common areas would reduce the feeling of confinement and provide residents with valuable stimuli and information. Access to privacy or socializing areas should be provided. Perceived privacy adds to the comfort of the residents and provides a peaceful atmosphere and a calm environment. Socializing areas may be designed so as to accommodate an intimate setting for two persons or provide a setting, where small or large groups can come together. Socialization can be improved by safeguarded, comfortable seating that would promote eye contact (Sommer, 1970). Falls are associated with serious fractures in older individuals. Therefore, street furniture and signage are crucial in design for patients with dementia. Patients with dementia would benefit the most from light-colored furniture with a dark background (Singh and Tiwari, 2020). Seating areas placed closer to the entry points would allow the use of garden also in rainy weather (Cobley, 2003). Arbors, flower or vine-covered trellises, plants, and groups of plants surrounding a bench can all be used to create exterior private spaces (Brawley, 2002). Sturdy seats with backrests and armrests are comfortable and help people with mobility issues and weak muscles to more easily lift themselves from the sitting position (Zeisel and Tyson, 1999). Dementia may have an adverse effect on eyesight (Rauch, 2022). People with dementia Disease need high levels of lighting with even distribution. Too much light reflection or darker areas are not helpful for older individuals with likely vision problems. Road lighting with motion sensors can be used to aid walking in the night and to inconspicuously monitor the residents (Marquardt et al., 2014). Well-lit transition areas would increase usage preferences (Algase et al., 2010). Adequate lighting during the night not only contributes to the security perception but also allows users to see each other and provides an informal monitoring system (McBride, 1999).

Planting

Trees, hedges, shrubs, and scattered vegetation help define borders, pedestrian circulation areas, views, and spaces. Evolving gardens within a garden (vegetable patches, flowers for cutting, herb garden, potted plants and raised container gardens) that would evolve over time and change with the seasons (Zeisel and Tyson, 1999). Flowering plants would provide the opportunity to feel the changing times of the year. A 2002 study suggested that patients with dementia, who participated in activities, including plant growing and harvesting, regained their old skills and learned new ones (Jarrott and Gigliotti, 2004). Horticultural activities, including planting, planning, or maintenance may serve as a therapeutic tool that could improve participation and strengthen identity through communication and the expression of feelings and experiences (Katz, 2010). Sensory garden elements, including sunlight, colors, smells, nature sounds, and touching plants in the open air would prove to be beneficial for patients with dementia (Suznjevic, 2013). Patients with dementia would likely pick leaves, flowers, and fruit from plants and may eat them without realizing the consequences on their health. Therefore, non-toxic plants should be used in gardens (Zeisel and Tyson, 1999). Memories can be alluded by traditional garden plants, including roses and lilies. Furthermore, an associative garden activity featuring daisy chains, dandelion clocks, conkers, may be a part of conversation spanning from extraordinary recipes from the days of war to ancient natural reliefs.

Maintenance

Maintenance is defined as keeping structural and plant design and furniture in a well-maintained status and allowing access for assistance in cases of emergency. Individuals with dementia frequently experience memory impairment, impulsiveness, distraction, and restlessness, and thus, require 24-hour surveillance to ensure their personal safety in advanced stages of the disease.

Gardens and exterior environments in safe dementia care homes provide access and exposure to nature that is known to be beneficial to health and provide space for exercise and rest (a basic human right). Therefore, they are considered a necessity rather than optional amenity (Ministry of Health, 2016). The present study aimed to investigate how to increase the quality of physical space in order to improve the comfort of daily living of patients with

Dementia's under the topics of environmental perceptions, selection of location, design elements, planting and maintenance.

Method

The study methodology is based on two stages. The first stage included a literature review to understand the basics of a successful exterior dementia landscape followed by development of a check list. The checklist was tested against 4 different dementia villages. The Dementia villages were selected on the grounds that there was only a limited number of studies in the aforementioned areas. The main criteria in the checklist were adopted as the research questions. A three-level scale based on the project performance was developed for each layer in order to standardize the scores for each domain in question. Performance: 1- Poor, 2 - Moderate, 3 - Good. A detailed and repeated scan of the videos, images, and articles available on the Internet was conducted with an aim to improve the assessment reliability.

Research Questions

Main question: What are the criteria of an exterior design intended for the older individuals?

Sub-questions:

1. Which design criteria related to environmental perceptions should be taken into consideration in outdoor landscape designs for individuals with dementia?
2. Which design criteria should be considered in outdoor landscape designs for dementia patients in choosing the location for the garden?
3. Which structural design criteria should be considered in outdoor landscape designs for dementia patients?
4. Which planting design criteria should be considered in outdoor landscape designs for dementia patients?
5. Which maintenance criteria should be considered in outdoor landscape designs for dementia patients?

Sample Areas

Nursing home residents in the Netherlands go out for a period of 96 seconds as an average per day and 60% thereof *never* receives visitors. 35% of patients with dementia leave their homes, whether it is their residence for years or an assisted living/memory care community, *only once a week, where 10% only once a month* in the USA. Villages chosen in the scope of the study offered small-scale living spaces as an alternative to nursing homes. In the dementia villages, the healthcare providers, caregivers and other workers engage in coordinated efforts to support individuals with dementia to participate in 'village life' (Dyer, 2020). These care facilities are designed so as to serve like a regular village. Residents of those centers maintain access to restaurants, shops, hairdressers, and other amenities, including theaters and courtyards. Four dementia villages located in different countries were selected for the purposes of the present study; and numbered as DV1, DV2, DV3, and DV4 (Table 1).

Table 1. General Information on Villages

NAME	DV1	DV2	DV3	DV4
Plan	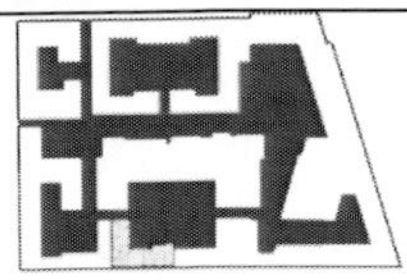	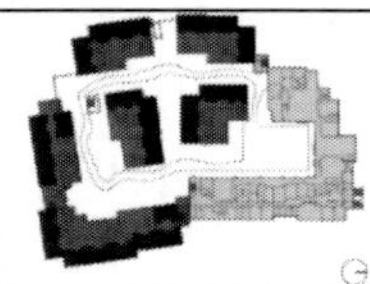	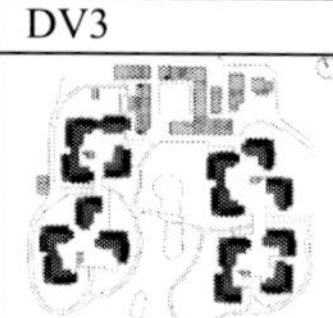	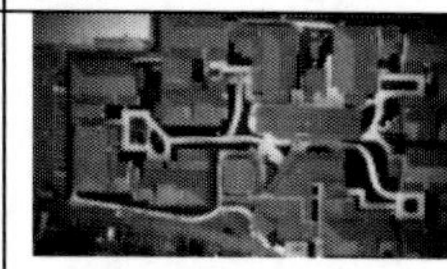
Architect	Molenaar & Bol & Van Dillen	Nordic Office of Architecture	Champagnat & Grègoire Architects, Nord Architects	Stephen Geason, Cykel Architecture in collaboration with Thomson Adsett.
Landscape Architect	Niek Roozen		Sarl Cauros	Papworth Davies
City/Town	Weesp		Dax	Glenorchy
State/Provence	Amsterdam	Bærum	Landes	Tasmania
Country	The Netherlands	Norway	France	Australia
Year	2008	2016-2020	2018	2021
Project Size:	11.500 m^2	18.000 m^2	10.700 m^2	
Houses	27 houses (6 or 7 residents per house)	136 communal housing units, 22 high-care dementia units	120 rooms	12 cottages
Activity Venues	Cafe, restaurant, shared courtyard places, barber shop beauty saloon, healthcare center, supermarket, grocery store, theater-cultural center, movie theater			
Fitness		√		
Carpentry		√		
Post office	√			√
Auditorium	√		√	
Cycling	√			√

Study Results

The use of color in DV2 and DV4 was better compared to the other villages; DV2 was better in taste, smell and touch, and acoustics criteria, where DV4 provided better advantages in terms of microclimate. There was no issue associated with location in all the four villages, where there was no defined parking lot in DV1.

The designs of the entry points in all the four villages were considered adequate. Varying route length was insufficient in DV1 and DV2; DV2 lacked sufficient roads for the passage of the disabled; and there were dead ends in DV4.

DV2 was not adequately designed as regards creating consistent colors on paths and avoiding dark lines and patterns and featuring non-glare paved surfaces (tinted concrete, colored); and furthermore, the ratio of green area to hard ground was less than 70:30 in DV2 and DV4. Although the use of stairs was avoided in garden designs in all the four villages; there were stairs at the entrance in DV2.

Table 2. An Analysis of the Physical Environment of Dementia Villages (analyzed and developed by authors)

VILLAGES	DV1	DV2	DV3	DV4
ENVIRONMENTAL PERCEPTIONS				
Color				
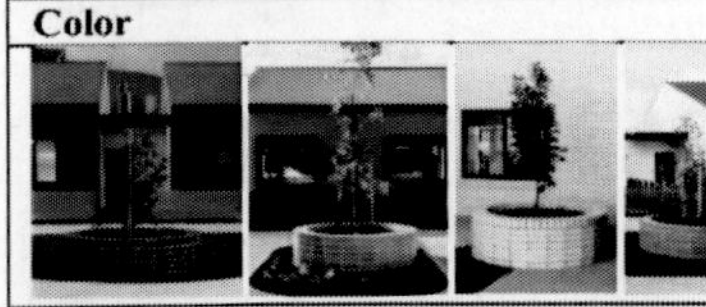 DV4	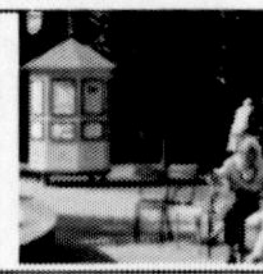	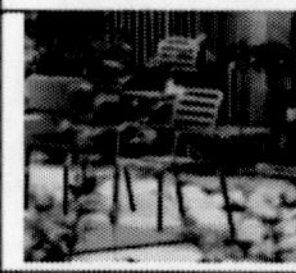	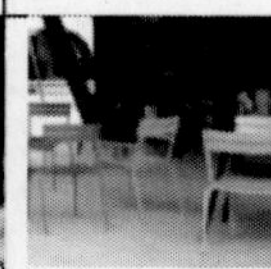	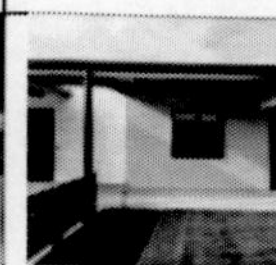
Surfaces, planes, and objects with respect to each other	2	3	2	3
Provision of strong light-dark, textural and color contrasts	2	3	2	3
Color-coded floors and areas	2	3	2	3
More redder colors of the spectrum	3	2	3	3
Incorporation of certain bright accents to a sense of excitement and youth	2	2	2	3
Taste, Smell and Touch				
Opportunity to touch and smell plants, herbs, and flowers	2	3	2	2
Provision of pleasant auditory experiences	1	3	3	2
Acoustics				
Pleasant auditory stimuli, such as the sound of wind in the trees or leaves	2	2	2	1
Acoustic barriers, such as planting and fencing, intended for minimizing background noise	2	3	2	2
Microclimate				
Garden is exposed to sun at least half a day	3	2	2	3
	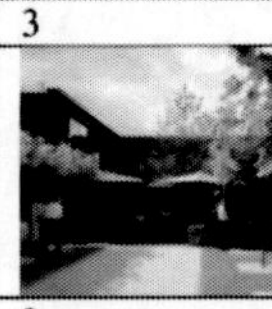	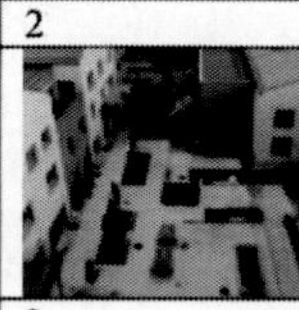	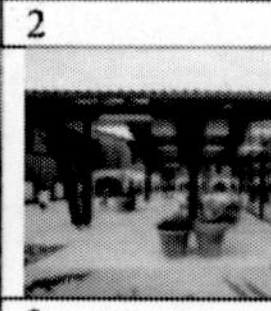	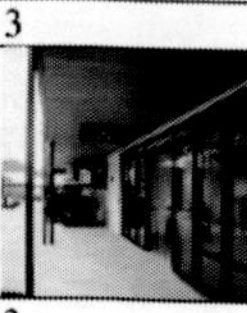
Availability of shade (Provision of Arbores, tables with umbrella, shaded swings)	2	2	3	3
Protection from glare	2	2	2	2
Adaptation to seasonal changes in temperature	2	2	2	2
LOCATION				
Domestic scale	3	3	2	3
Located far from any industrial area	3	3	3	3
Accessible for neighbors	3	2	2	3
	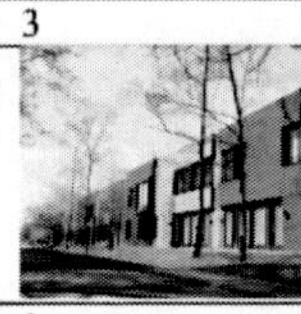	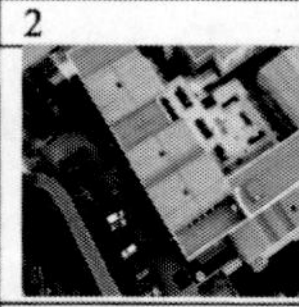	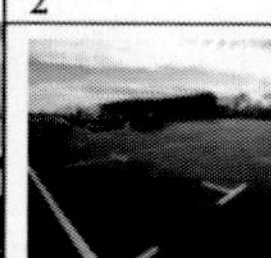	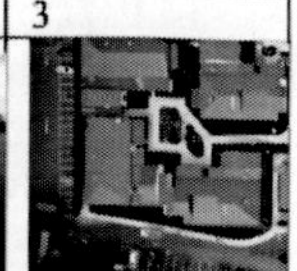
Parking area located outside the main landscape area	2	3	3	3
Garden should be easily accessible from within the residence	3	2	2	2
Garden space at the southeast of the facility building is recommended	2	3	3	3
Easily accessible toilets	3	3	3	3
DESIGN ELEMENTS				
Enclosing Walls				
Fenced-off spaces	3	3	2	2
Exit Control				

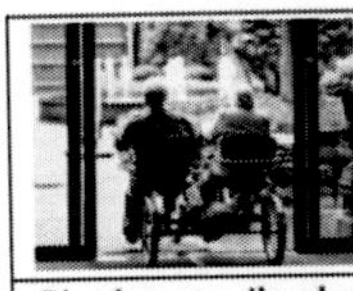 DV1 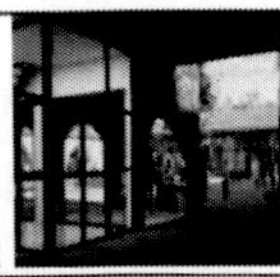 DV3	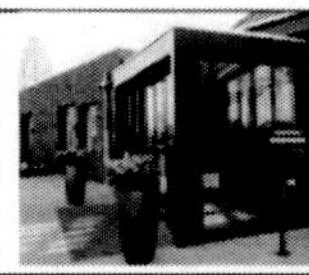	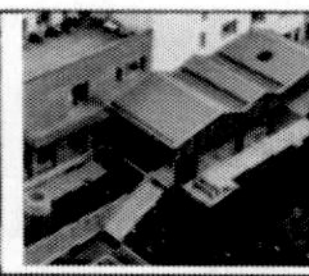	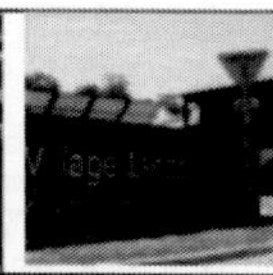	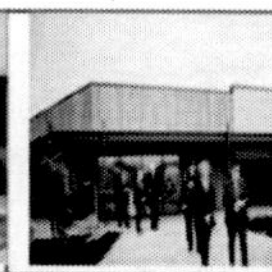
Single entry 'landsmark' door	2	2	2	2
Clear Gateways (Contrasting door surroundings)	2	2	2	2
Automated door	3	2	3	3
Usually unlocked	3	3	2	3
Visible from inside	3	3	3	3
Shaded entry	3	3	3	3
Seating available	3	3	3	3
Walking Path				
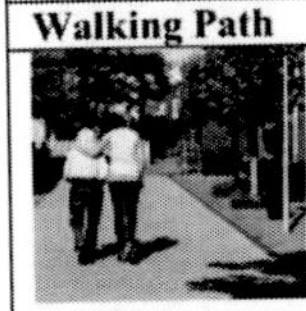 DV1 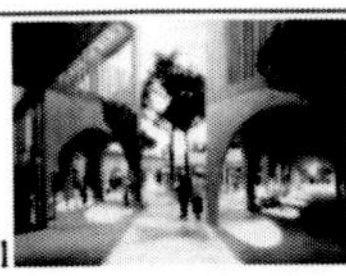 DV3	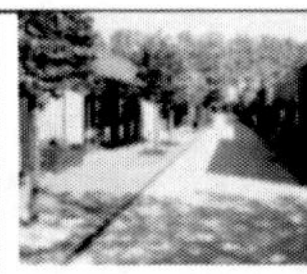	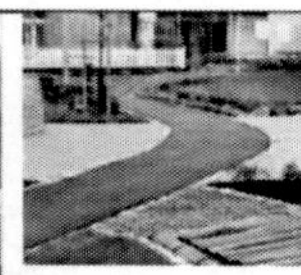	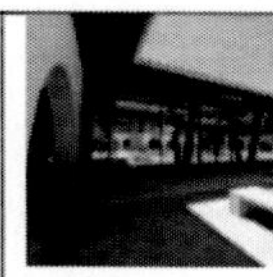	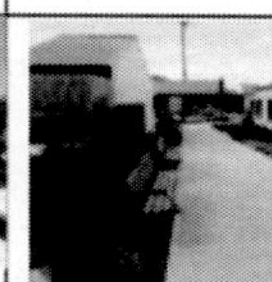
Varying route lengths	1	1	3	2
Paths wide enough for 2 wheelchairs	3	1	2	
Corridors and common spaces lead towards a particular direction	2	2	3	2
Continuous circulation loops with destination points	3	3	2	2
No dead ends to reduce cognitive demand and panic	2	3	3	1
Social area or hearth at the end of the roads such as the entrance to a garden	2	3	2	2
Avoided raised edges posing tripping hazards	3	3	3	2
Minimal crossroads	2	2	2	2
Paving				
Materials contrast between space and building	2	3	2	3
Creates consistent colors on paths and avoid dark lines and patterns.	3	1	3	2
Defines texture changes on path edges.	2	3	3	2
Fine texture	2	3	2	2
High ratio of green to hard surfaces - 70:30	2	1	3	1
Granular materials, textured concrete or asphalt are acceptable options	3	3	3	2
Features non-glare paved surfaces (tinted concrete, colored)	3	1	3	2
Features non-slip paved surfaces	3	2	3	3
Steps and Ramps				
Avoids steps	3	2	3	3
If necessary, should have clearly visible alternatives - lifts or ramps	-	1	-	-
Handrails				
Implements handrails	1	1	1	1
Prevent patients from interacting with the vegetation	2	2	1	1
Comfortable to hold	3	2	1	1
Oval shape a broad flat surface	3	2	2	1
Wayfinding				
Signage				
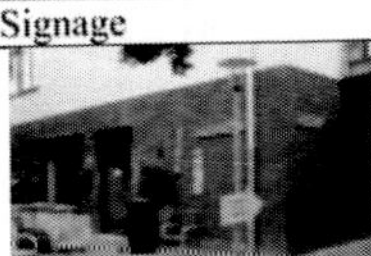 DV1 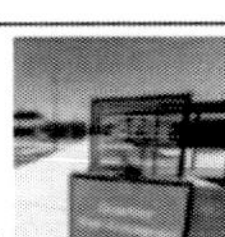 DV3 *Image by Debbie Selsalvage.* H	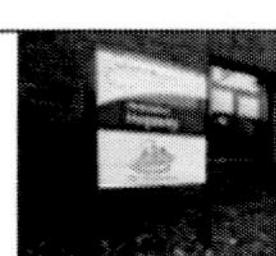	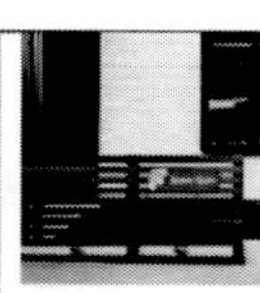	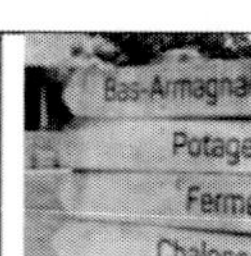	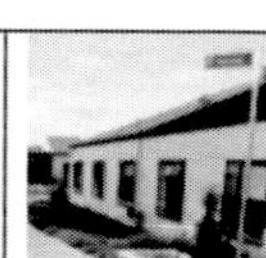
Design features that trigger memory	3	3	2	3
Consistents colors on paths	1	3	3	2

Table 2. (Continued)

Combined text & signs	1	1	2	1
Positions signs lower than normal	2	2	2	2
Minimal signs giving simple information at decision points	3	3	2	3
Directional signs on single pointers	1	2	1	3
Locational signs for primary services positioned perpendicular to the wall	3	2	2	3
Signs with larger graphics and symbols in color contrast to the background	3	2	2	2
Signs with non-glare lighting and non-reflective coverings	3	2	1	1
Visual access to landmarks & orientation points	3	3	1	3
Visual barrier	2	2	2	2
Water				
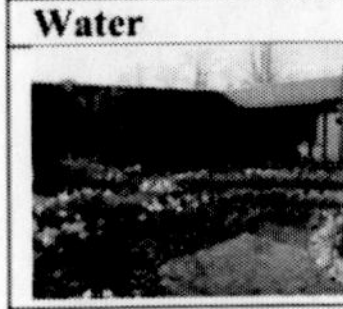 DV1 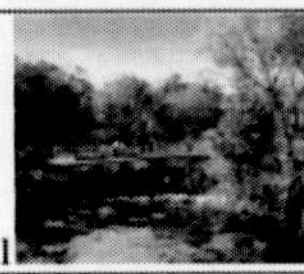 DV3	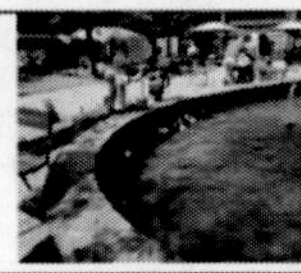	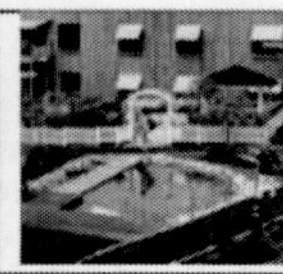	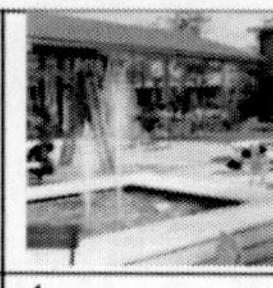	X
Drinking water	1	1	1	3
Slowly water	2	3	3	1
Bubbling fountain	3	1	3	1
Mount or Hill				
Subtle, with a low gradient, and as different configurations of space	2	2	3	2
Place				
	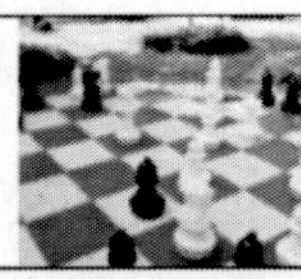	X	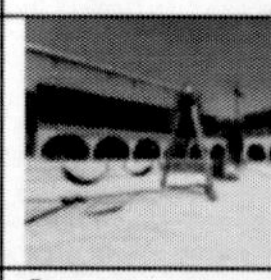	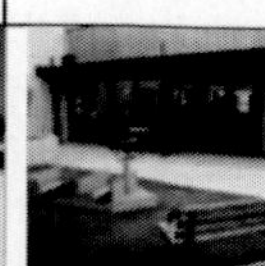
Playground	1	1	2	1
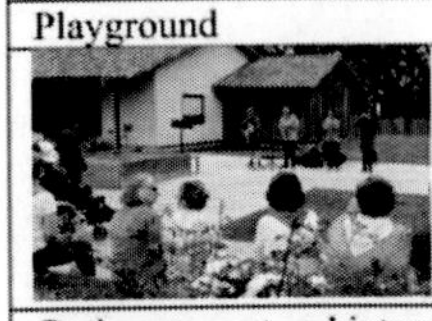 DV1	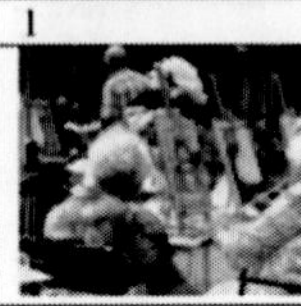	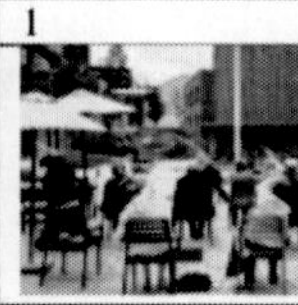	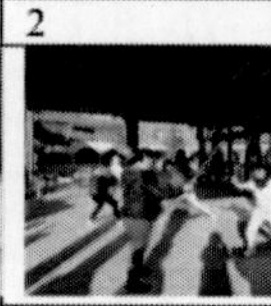	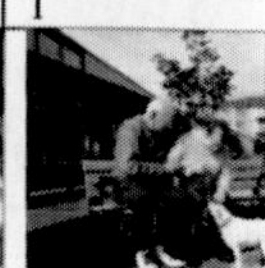
Options to rest and interact	3	3	3	2
Two or more common places	3	2	2	2
Clusters of tables and chairs	2	2	2	2
Possible nodes	3	2	2	2
To view or interact with birds and other animals	3	1	3	3
Toilets along loop	1	1	1	3
Sitting Areas	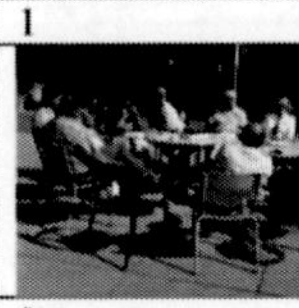	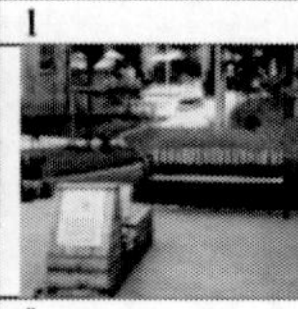	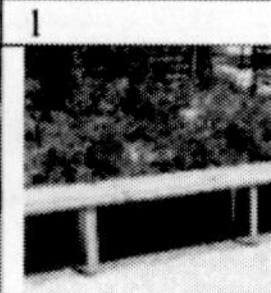	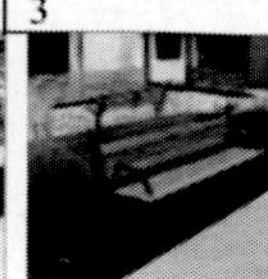
Seating for groups	3	3	3	3
Appropriate seating design (with back and arms)	2	3	2	2
Comfort seating material (wood, fabric, or hard plastic)	3	3	3	2
Seating opportunities in both sunny and shaded locations	3	2	2	2
Seating spaced every 4.5m	3	2	2	3
Features fixed heavy seating	3	2	2	3
45cm seating height	3	3	3	3
Alternative types of seating	3	2	2	2
Situated in on the way out from the building	2	2	2	2

into the garden				
Situated around the activities	3	2	2	2
On patients' routes	2	2	1	2
	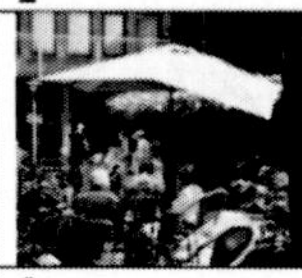	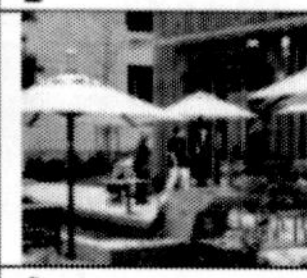	X	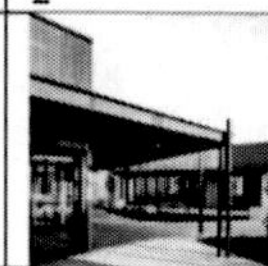
Using adjustable umbrellas	2	2	1	2
Moveable seating available	3	2	2	2
Artwork				
Recognizable Artwork	3	2	3	2
Lighting				
Adequate lighting	3	3	2	3
Waste	3	2	1	2
PLANTING				
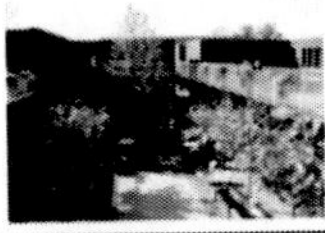 DV1 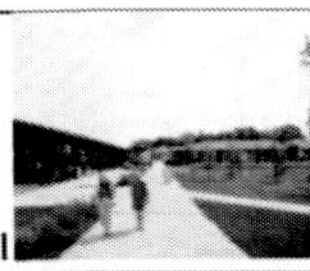 DV4	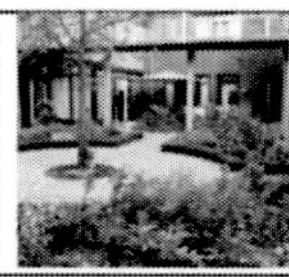	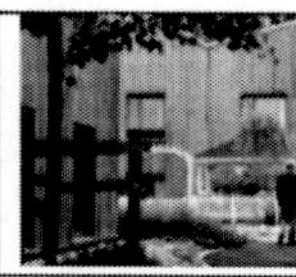	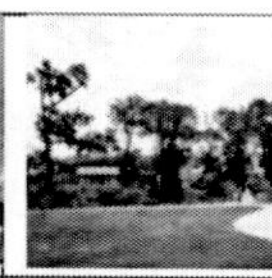	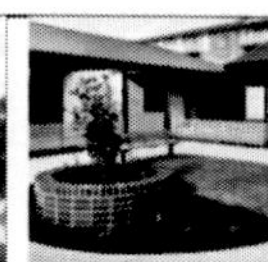
Vegetable gardens (mini farm)	3	2	3	2
Locate groups of strongly scented or colorful plants as navigational markers	2	2	2	2
Avoidance of trees whose fruit or leaves	2	2	3	2
	X	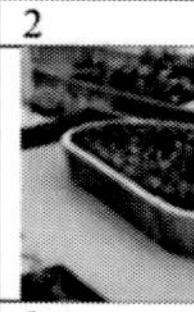	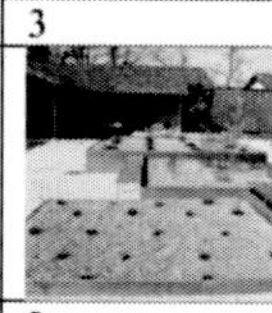	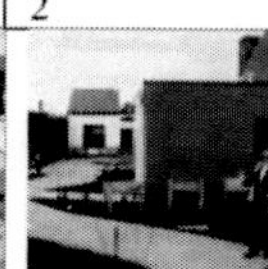
Raised planters	1	2	2	3
Provision of a large enough flat lawn area	2	2	3	2
Non-deciduous plants	2	3	3	2
No thorns or spines	3	3	3	2
	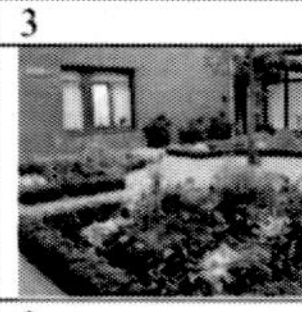	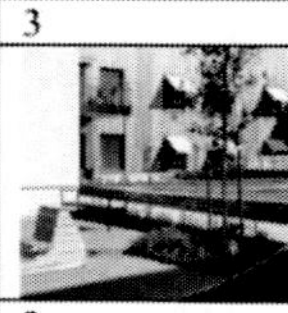	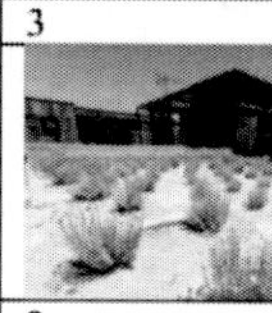	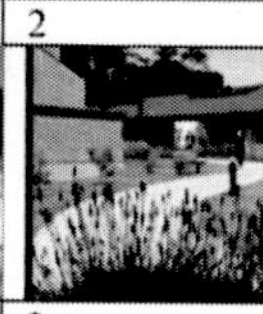
Flowering plants	3	2	2	2
Featuring herbs, vegetables, and traditional flowers	2	2	3	1
Avoidance of messy trees	2	2	3	2
Non-toxic plants are used	3	3	3	2
Scented plants	2	2	2	2
Healing garden available (horticulture programs)	3	2	3	3
Fine textures and darker colors in background	3	2	3	2
Bolder textures and lighter colors in foreground	2	2	3	2
MAINTENANCE				
Furniture	3	3	2	3
Plant health	3	3	2	3
Maintenance quality of litter pick-up	3	3	2	3
Availability of telephone or communication devices for emergency purposes	2	1	1	1
Provision of a specific exterior smoking area	1	1	1	1
Storage facility for maintenance staff	1	1	2	1

1. Poor, 2. Moderate, 3. Good (Calking, 1988; Lovering, 1990; Randall et al., 1990; Passini, 2000; Brawley, 2001; Dixon, 2002; Mitchell et al., 2003; Ziesel, 2003; Marcus, 2005; Blackman, 2007; Chalfont, 2007; Hasselkus and Murray, 2007; Hernandez, 2007; Rappe and Topo, 2007; Brawley, 2009; Marquardt and Schmieg, 2009; Raske, 2010; Marquardt, 2011; Mitchell and Burton, 2012; MacKerron and Mourato, 2013; Feddersen and Lüdtke, 2014; Pallasmaa, 2015; Moyle et al., 2016; Muir-Hunter and Montero-Odasso, 2017; Prolo and Sassi, 2017; Kuş and Erbek, 2018; Liao, et al., 2018; Garrett, 2019; Motealleh et al., 2019; Olson and Albensi, 2021 and Tierney, 2022).

Handrail usage was inadequate in all the four villages; design features intended to trigger memory was insufficient in DV3 compared to other villages; and there was no choice of consistent colors on the paths in DV1. Furthermore, combined text and graphic expression in the markings was not in use in all the four villages and the positions of the signposts were generally not lower than normal; and that the directional signs were inadequate in DV1 and DV3. Visual access to landmarks and orientation points were insufficient in the cases of DV3 and DV4. There was no drinking water fountain available in the villages; there was no bubbling fountain in DV2 and DV4. Except for DV3, playground spaces were insufficient; DV2 did not offer opportunities to view or interact with birds and other animals; and that access to the toilet was not easy except for DV4. DV4 failed to provide options to rest and interact compared to other villages; and there were more gathering points in DV1 vis-a-vis other villages. DV3 featured less seating units around roads compared to other villages in question; there were insufficient trash cans and umbrellas for shade.

There was no vegetable garden in DV2 (other than greenhouse) and DV4; there was no elevated planting in DV1; DV4 provided insufficient herbs, vegetables, and traditional flowers; DV2 had inadequate healing garden (horticulture programs) facilities.

All the four villages lacked sufficient telephone or communication devices for emergencies, a specific exterior smoking area, and storage facility of maintenance staff (Table 2).

Discussion

Zeisel (2003) suggested that people with dementia would need to live in safe and carefully planned environments, because they might have great difficulty remembering the places they visited and locating those environments, among other problems related to the dementia. As Brawley (2001) suggested exteriors would expand the residents' opportunities to use all their remaining senses and physical abilities. It is important to provide a safe, enabling, and vibrant physical environment for individuals with dementia (Mitchell and Burton, 2006; Tierney 2007). Exterior space design is envisaged as an extension of indoor space (Feddersen and Lüdtke, 2014). The view of or access to the garden may reduce the level of agitation and make a positive contribution to the building's environment and the wider visual environment, as well as greatly improving self-confidence and dignity of a person with dementia (Chalfont, 2007 and Hernandez, 2007; Mitchell and Burton, 2012; Motealleh et al., 2019 and Olson and Albensi, 2021). Therefore, they are necessary amenities rather than merely being optional.

People with dementia may have difficulty seeing color shades or tonal differences (Brawley, 2009). It is important to define spaces in environmental designs and to use contrasting colors on surfaces for patients with dementia. Environmental perception for people with dementia can be improved by stimulation based on color, smell, and wildlife sounds. There is now available a range of environmental manipulation to aid individuals in way finding, including the use of pattern and colors (Lovering 1990; McAdam, 2017 and Kuş and Erbek, 2018). Each building cluster in DV4 had a planting area with clored brick materials with a different tree at the entrance. The entrance of each house had its own unique color and hydro wood covered verandas at the building entrances. Thus, residents were able to better remember their homes. DV2 also featured bricks as the main material in all the facades, with two color shade variations that gave a bright and consistent impression. In other villages, improvements can be made as regards the perception of exterior spaces, especially with the use of more colors. Untreated wood cladding and wooden arrows of ore pine were in use as a secondary material to create variety and give a homely character. Additions can be made for the use of color in DV1 and DV3, especially incorporating a color-coding system. Hearing, smelling, and touching senses would reinforce the impaired visual abilities over age. Therefore, elements that would appeal to those senses is necessary in any environment intended for older individuals. There is a strong correlation between high noise levels and undesirable behaviors (including wandering, agitation), while pleasant sounds are positively stimulating. Sound therapy is associated with improved symptoms of dementia (Moyle et al., 2018). In order to stimulate the auditory stimuli, the use of leafy trees in the DV4 and the use of moving water elements in all the four villages could be improved. Additions to other villages except for DV2 would help increase the comfort of use. Microclimate is another important issue for older individuals. Further efforts would improve the microclimate in all the four villages.

There were no issues in all the four villages regarding location. It is important to provide an adequate parking lot to access the villages. For DV1, it seems that a more defined parking lot is required instead of lots provided around the building perimeters. Considering the entry points to the villages, there was an undesired use of stairs in DV2 was, and use of a ramp is required in parallel. Residents in the advanced stages of dementia would not need a higher fence to keep them from leaving. If a garden gate is required (depending on fire regulations and maintenance needs), it should be of the same material as the rest of the fence to help hide it.

Safe, circular pathways, exterior lighting during nighttime, seating units, water elements, and gardens would encourage residents to be active and spend time exterior. Mitchell et al. (2003) suggested that services and facilities featuring adequate seating, lighting, shelter, and well-maintained, smooth, level, plain paving within walking distance would help improve attending problems of physical frailty. Circular or eight-shaped paths are a particularly important design element as they would allow individuals with dementia to return to their starting point without assistance. In all the four villages in question, those conditions were provided (except for the dead-end streets in DV4). In DV1, the exterior landscape provides a route for residents, ensuring a navigable and legible experience. The landmarks, including ponds and fountains, which were occupied by ducks in springtime, seemed to provide the residents with familiarity with their surroundings. In DV3, the width of the secondary paths could be increased.

In DV1, varied tiling, materials, planting, greenery, and trees found use in support of orientation criterion along with multiple sensorial experiences as linked to temporal and seasonal changes. Slatted roofs should be avoided, because the shadows of the slats on the pavement could feel depressive and therefore confusing, just as the juxtaposition of dark and light-colored pavements would have the same effect. As for the road color tiling in DV2, it had the potential to have an adverse impact on its users. Although the use of stairs was avoided in garden designs in all the four villages in question; there were stairs at the entrance of DV2. A clearly visible ramp should be provided nearby when there are steps.

The elements that would help find direction in spaces are important due to cognitive deficits, including memory loss and sensory problems in patients with dementia (Marquardt, 2011; Marquardt and Schmieg, 2009 and Passini et al., 2000). Although there was no serious issue of orientation in the villages, visual access to landmarks and orientation points were insufficient in DV3. The number of landmarks and signboards can be increased in the villages.

Furthermore, secondary landmarks, including furniture, plants, land surface, and even framed landscapes could be improved as suggested by Zeisel and Tyson (1999). It is necessary to reduce the height of the signs in DV2 and increase the signage elements in DV1 and DV3. It is disruptive for the comfort of the users that there were crossroads with 3 or 4 options in DV1, where some of the roads were dead ends. Blackman, Van Schaik, Martyr (2007) pointed out the significance of combined use of graphics and texts in signage. This was not considered in the villages in question.

Water is an important element in a sensory garden, because it provides a sense of movement and sound (Prolo and Sassi, 2017; Garrett et al, 2019 and Motealleh et al., 2019). McBride (1999) suggested that fountains may serve as focal points to assist in orientation and wayfinding. The results of a study by Prolo and Sassini (2017) were indicative of the fact that the patients liked the presence of fountains and running water. Especially bubbling fountains were recommended. Bubbling fountains may be incorporated to DV2 and DV4. Considering that the families would visit the residents in environments intended for the older individuals, the presence of playgrounds and equipment for children would be favorable and encourage the use thereof by the visiting families. The insufficient number of playgrounds except for DV3 indicates that this should be revised for all four villages.

Meeting areas would provide the opportunity for the older individuals to participate in formal or informal group activities (Zeisel and Tyson, 1999). Previous studies reported that such activities supported sense of belonging and closeness between people (Hasselkus and Murray, 2007; Muir-Hunter and Montero-Odasso, 2017). Options to rest and interact should be improved in DV4. Adequate shade is very important, as patients with dementia may have a hard time recognizing that they are too hot and barely think of wearing a hat or protecting themselves against the sun. As an integral part of street furniture, seats may prove to be confusing. Seats should have a look of seats. It is important to provide plenty of seating for different types (fixed, movable, glider or swing seat) in different locations and with a choice of sun or shade. In DV3, the number of seats around the roads, the use of trash cans and umbrellas for shade can be increased. Persons with dementia need high levels of evenly distributed lighting and transition space illumination. Gradual light level changes should be included in all designs (Dixon, 2002). There were no issues regarding lighting in all the four villages.

It is important to design green spaces and gardens for the older individuals, which stimulate the senses, reveal their memories, and encourage them to walk and spend time outside (Rappe Topo, 2007; Liao et al., 2018 and Raske, 2010). Although DV1 offers different views across all the four seasons, it may have a negative visual effect in winter due to the abundance of deciduous species. All the villages reserved space for green areas. Notwithstanding the above, it is also important to offer different alternatives such as healing gardens and vegetable gardens, especially for the older individuals. Additional horticulture programs should be incorporated in DV2 and DV4. Again, the issue of elevated plantation is particularly important in terms of wheelchair use. Elevated plantation areas should be considered in DV1 and DV2.

Furthermore, emergency telephone or communication devices, specific exterior smoking areas, and storage facilities for maintenance staff should be considered in all the four villages.

Conclusion

Understanding the human-nature relationship is essential to ensure that built environments meet the needs of their inhabitants. (Pallasmaa, 2015). Sensitive environmental modifications may increase an individual's ability to function by reducing their cognitive demand to navigate their environment (Calkins, 1988). Access to the exteriors provides individuals with dementia with a certain level of potential autonomy (Rodiek, Schwarz, 2007) and an opportunity to experience the design of the physical environment and enjoy nature with an aim to meet the needs of people living with dementia for ready access to open space and gardens. Form, function, interiors, and exteriors should be designed simultaneously so that exteriors can positively impact the well-being of individuals with dementia. Here, although the general design rules for older individuals do not differ much, the present study primarily focuses on exterior design principles.

As a result of the study; the villages in the scope of the study generally met basic design requirements; DV4 had environmental acoustics and paths with dead ends; DV2 had dark lines and patterns; DV2 and DV4 failed to meet the standards for the relationship between green space and hard ground; Directional signage was insufficient in DV1; landmarks and bins were lacking in DV3; and there was no accessible drinking f ountain except in DV4; and elevated plantation was insufficient in DV1 and DV3. It was concluded in the light of the above analysis that future designs should consider the use of handrails and sign boards, and playgrounds for children.

References

Abbott, P. S. (Ed.). (2009). *Re-creating neighborhoods for successful ageing*. Health Professions Press.

Alheimer' s Disease International (2023). https://www.alzint.org/.

Algase, D. L., Beattie, E. R., Antonakos, C., Beel-Bates, C. A., & Yao, L. (2010). Wandering and the physical environment. *American Journal of Alzheimer's Disease & Other Dementias®*, *25*(4), 340-346.

ArcDaily (2023). Alzheimers Village / NORD Architects, https://www.archdaily.com/973948/alzheimers-villa-nord-architects.

Barnes, S., & Design in Caring Environments Study Group. (2002). The design of caring environments and the quality of life of older people. *Ageing & Society*, *22*(6), 775-789.

Beavis, L. (2020). Inside the Tasmanian village where everyone will be living with dementia, https://www.abc.net.au/news/2020-07-10/inside-hobart-dementia-village/12434416.

Beckwith, M. E., & Gilster, S. D. (2014). The paradise garden: A model garden design for those with Alzheimer's disease. In *Horticultural therapy and the older adult population* (pp. 3-16). Routledge.

Bissell, K. (2010). *Designing for those with Dementia using the principle of Wayfinding* (Doctoral dissertation).

Blackman, T., Van Schaik, P., & Martyr, A. (2007). Outdoor environments for individuals with dementia: An exploratory study using virtual reality. *Ageing & Society*, *27*(6), 811-825.

Brawley, E. C. (2009). Enriching lighting design. *NeuroRehabilitation*, *25*(3), 189-199.

Brawley, E. C. (2007). Designing successful gardens and outdoor spaces for individuals with Alzheimer's disease. *Journal of Housing for the Elderly*, *21*(3-4), 265-283.

Brawley, E. C. (2002). Therapeutic gardens for individuals with Alzheimer's disease. *Alzheimer's Care Today*, *3*(1), 7-11.

Brawley, E. C. (2001). Environmental design for Alzheimer's disease: a quality of life issue. *Aging & Mental Health*, *5*(sup1), 79-83.

Bruce, H. (2014). Gardening activities can help enrich the quality of life for those with Alzheimer's, and their caregivers.

Calkins, M. (1988). Design for dementia: Planning ideas for the elderly and confused.

Carpe Diem Dementia Village/Nordic Office of Architecture (2021). ArchDaily. https://www.archdaily.com/955466/carpe-diem-dementia-village-nordic-office-of-architecture, ISSN 0719-8884.

Chalfont, G. (2007). *Design for nature in dementia care.* Jessica Kingsley Publishers.

CLPNA Think Tank (2014). A vision and the outcome: De Hogeweyk, https://www.clpna.com/wp-content/uploads/2014/12/CLPNA-2014-Think-Tank-Eloy-van-Hal.pdf.

Cobley, M. (2003). Designing a garden for individuals with dementia sets out principles for designing a garden to be used by individuals with dementia. *Journal of Dementia Care*, *11*(5), 22-23.

Cohen, U., & Weisman, G. D. (1991). Holding on to home: Designing environments for individuals with dementia (pp. 61-63). Baltimore, MD: Johns Hopkins University Press.

Cohen-Mansfield, J., & Werner, P. (1998). The effects of an enhanced environment on nursing home residents who pace. *The Gerontologist*, *38*(2), 199-208.

Cotter, V. T. (2007). The burden of dementia. *American Journal of managed care*, *13*(8), S193.

Davey, J. A. (2017). Age-friendly Cities and Communities World experience and pointers for New Zealand. Ministry of Social Development: Wellington, New Zealand.

Dementia Villages Associates (2023). DVA De Hogeweyk, https://www.dementiavillage.com/projects/dva-de-hogeweyk/.

Département des Landes (2023). Visitez le Village Landais Alzheimer [version longue], https://villagealzheimer.landes.fr/en/.

Dixon, C. J. M. (2002). A return to the garden: design criteria for therapeutic exterior environments for people with Alzheimer Disease. (Master's thesis).

Dyer, S., van den Berg, M., Brown, A., Johnstone, G., Laver, K., Lowthian, J., ... & Winsall, M. (2020). *Review of innovative models of aged care* (No. Research paper 3). Royal Commission into Aged Care Quality and Safety.

Feddersen, E., & Lüdtke, I. (Eds.). (2014). *Lost in space: architecture and dementia.* Birkhäuser.

Halsall, B., & MacDonald, R. (2015). Design for Dementia–A Guide with helpful guidance in the design of exterior and interior environments. *Liverp. Halsall Lloyd Partnersh; The Halsall Lloyd Partnership: Liverpool, UK.*

Garrett, J. K., White, M. P., Huang, J., Ng, S., Hui, Z., Leung, C., ... & Wong, M. C. (2019). Urban blue space and health and wellbeing in Hong Kong: Results from a survey of older adults. *Health & place*, *55*, 100-110.

Glenview Community Services (2023). Korongee Advancing dementia care, https://glenview.org.au/korongee/

Goto, S., Kamal, N., Puzio, H., Kobylarz, F., & Herrup, K. (2014). Differential responses of individuals with late-stage dementia to two novel environments: A multimedia room and an interior garden. *Journal of Alzheimer's Disease*, *42*(3), 985-998.

Graham-Cochrane T. (2010). *Gardens that care: Planning outdoor environments for individuals with dementia.* Alzheimer's Australia SA. http://www.enablingenvironments.com.au/uploads/5/0/4/5/50459523/gardens_that_care.planning_outdoor_environments_for_people_with_dementia.pdf.

Grozdanic, L. (2014). Self-Contained Dementia Village Protects People Suffering from

Dementia and Alzheimer's, https://inhabitat.com/self-contained-dementia-village-protects-people-suffering-from-dementia-and-alzheimers-from-themselves/.

Hanson, J. (2002). The inclusive city, what active ageing might mean for urban design.

Harris, C. W., & Dines, N. T. (1988). Time-saver standards for landscape architecture: design and construction data.

HDC (2008). The effects of a waterfall on the systolic blood pressure of individuals with dementia. https://healthcaredesignmagazine.com/architecture/effects-waterfall-systolic-blood-pressure-individuals-dementia/.

Jarrott, S. E., & Gigliotti, C. (2004). From the garden to the table: Evaluation of a dementia-specific HT program. *Acta Horticulturae*, 139-144.

Jensen, L., & Padilla, R. (2017). Effectiveness of environment-based interventions that address behavior, perception, and falls in people with Alzheimer's disease and related major neurocognitive disorders: A systematic review. *The American Journal of Occupational Therapy*, *71*(5), 7105180030p1-7105180030p10.

Hasselkus, B. R., & Murray, B. J. (2007). Everyday occupation, well-being, and identity: The experience of caregivers in families with dementia. *The American Journal of Occupational Therapy*, *61*(1), 9-20.

Hernandez, R. O. (2007). Effects of therapeutic gardens in special care units for individuals with dementia: Two case studies. *Journal of Housing for the Elderly*, *21*(1-2), 117-152.

Katz, J. (2010). Katherine Froggatt, Sue Davies and Julienne Meyer (eds), Understanding Care Homes: A Research and Development Perspective, Jessica Kingsley Publishers, London, 2008, 264 pp., pbk£ 19.99, ISBN 13: 978 1 84310 553 4. *Ageing & Society*, *30*(5), 914-916.

Kus Sahin, C., Erbek M. (2018). Evaluating Therapeutic Landscapes: An Approach To Designing Healing Garden For Alzheimer's Patients In Antalya, Turkıye, *World Journal of Pharmaceutical Research, 8* (1), 1301-1313. https://wjpr.s3.ap-south-1.amazonaws.com/article_issue/1546318552.pdf.

Lawton, M. P., & Nahemow, L. (1973). Ecology and the ageing process. In C. Eisdorfer & M. P. Lawton (Eds.), *The psychology of adult development and ageing* (pp. 619–674). American Psychological Association. https://doi.org/10.1037/10044-020.

Lee, S. Y., Hung, L., Chaudhury, H., & Morelli, A. (2021). Staff perspectives on the role of physical environment in long-term care facilities on dementia care in Canada and Sweden. *Dementia*, *20*(7), 2558-2572.

Liao, M. L., Ou, S. J., Heng Hsieh, C., Li, Z., & Ko, C. C. (2020). Effects of garden visits on individuals with dementia: A pilot study. *Dementia*, *19*(4), 1009-1028.

Lovering, M. J. (1990). Alzheimer's disease and outdoor space: Issues in environmental design. *American Journal of Alzheimer's Care and Related Disorders & Research*, *5*(3), 33-40.

MacKerron, G., & Mourato, S. (2013). Happiness is greater in natural environments. *Global environmental change*, *23*(5), 992-1000.

Marcus, C. C. (2007). Alzheimer's garden audit tool. *Journal of Housing for the Elderly*, *21*(1-2), 179-191.

Cooper Marcus, C. (2005). No ordinary garden. Alzheimer's and other patients find refuge in a Michigan dementia-care facility. *Landscape Architecture*, *95*(3), 26-39.

Marquardt, G. (2011). Wayfinding for individuals with dementia: a review of the role of architectural design. *HERD: Health Environments Research & Design Journal*, *4*(2), 75-90.

Marquardt, G., Bueter, K., & Motzek, T. (2014). Impact of the design of the built environment on individuals with dementia: An evidence-based review. *HERD: Health Environments Research & Design Journal*, *8*(1), 127-157.

Marquardt, G., & Schmieg, P. (2009). Dementia-friendly architecture: environments that facilitate wayfinding in nursing homes. *American Journal of Alzheimer's Disease & Other Dementias®*, *24*(4), 333-340.

McAdam, K. (2017). *Dementia friendly design features for walking paths: A focused practice question.* Region of Peel Public Health.

McBride, D. (1999). Nursing home gardens. *Healing Gardens: Therapeutic Benefits and Design Recommendations. Wiley, New York*, 385-436.

Mitchell, L., & Burton, E. J. (2012). Dementia-friendly neighbourhoods–a step in the right direction.

Michon, M. (2016). Dementiekliniek als integraal onderdeel van de stad.

Ministry of Health (2016). Secure Dementia Care Home Design: Information Resource. Wellington: Ministry of Health. https://www.health.govt.nz/system/files/documents/publications/secure-dementia-care-home-design-information-resource.pdf.

Mitchell, L., & Burton, E. (2006). Neighbourhoods for life: Designing dementia-friendly outdoor environments. *Quality in Ageing and Older Adults*, *7*(1), 26-33.

Mitchell, L., Burton, E., Raman, S., Blackman, T., Jenks, M., & Williams, K. (2003). Making the outside world dementia-friendly: design issues and considerations. *Environment and Planning B: Planning and Design*, *30*(4), 605-632.

Mooney, P., & Nicell, P. L. (1992, July). The importance of exterior environment for Alzheimer residents: Effective care and risk management. In *Healthcare management forum* (Vol. 5, No. 2, pp. 23-29). Sage CA: Los Angeles, CA: SAGE Publications.

Motealleh, P., Moyle, W., Jones, C., & Dupre, K. (2019). Creating a dementia-friendly environment through the use of outdoor natural landscape design intervention in long-term care facilities: a narrative review. *Health & Place*, *58*, 102148.

Moyle, W., Jones, C., Dwan, T., & Petrovich, T. (2018). Effectiveness of a virtual reality forest on individuals with dementia: A mixed methods pilot study. *The Gerontologist*, *58*(3), 478-487.

Muir-Hunter, S. W., & Montero-Odasso, M. (2017). The attentional demands of ambulating with an assistive device in older adults with Alzheimer's disease. *Gait & Posture*, *54*, 202-208.

Nicelocal (2023). The Hogeweyk — Dementia Village | Be Advice, https://en.nicelocal.co.nl/north-holland/shops/the_hogeweyk_-_dementia_village_be_advice/.

Nillesen, J., & Opitz, S. (2014). Dimensie voor dementie. *Denkbeeld*, *26*(2), 4–4. https:// doi.org/10.1007/s12428-014-0026-3

Del Nord, R. (Ed.). (2003). *Architecture for Alzheimer disease*. Alinea Editrice.

Olson, N. L., & Albensi, B. C. (2021). Dementia-friendly "design": Impact on COVID-19 death rates in long-term care facilities around the world. *Journal of Alzheimer's Disease*, *81*(2), 427-450.

Open House Oslo (2003). Carpe Diem Dementia Village Main programme OSLO, https://www.openhouseworldwide.org/films/carpe-diem.

Pallasmaa, J. (2015). Body, mind, and imagination: the mental essence of architecture. *Mind in architecture: Neuroscience, embodiment, and the future of design*, 51-74.

Passini, R., Pigot, H., Rainville, C., & Tétreault, M. H. (2000). Wayfinding in a nursing home for advanced dementia of the Alzheimer's type. *Environment and Behavior*, *32*(5), 684-710.

Phillips, J., Walford, N., Hockey, A., Foreman, N., & Lewis, M. (2013). Older people and outdoor environments: Pedestrian anxieties and barriers in the use of familiar and unfamiliar spaces. *Geoforum*, *47*, 113-124.

Pollock, A. (2007). *Designing Gardens for People with Dementia*. Sterling: University of Sterling press.

Prolo, P., & Sassi, E. (2017). A sensory garden in dementia care: from design to practice Balerna Diurnal Therapeutic Centre. *Alzheimers Dement Cogn Neurol*.

Randall, P., Burkhardt, S. S., & Kutcher, J. (1990). Exterior space for patients with Alzheimer's disease and related disorders. *American Journal of Alzheimer's Care and Related Disorders & Research*, *5*(4), 31-37.

Rauch, K. (2022). Alzheimer's Disease, Dementia and the Eye. https://www.aao.org/eye-health/diseases/alzheimers-disease-dementia-eye.

Rappe, E., & Topo, P. (2007). Contact with outdoor greenery can support competence among individuals with dementia. *Journal of Housing for the Elderly*, *21*(3-4), 229-248.

Raske, M. (2010). Nursing home quality of life: Study of an enabling garden. *Journal of Gerontological Social Work*, *53*(4), 336-351.

Samzun, M. (2019). Au village Alzheimer des Pays-Bas. https://www.solidarum.org/sante/au-village-alzheimer-des-pays-bas.

Rodiek, S., & Schwarz, B. (Eds.). (2007). Outdoor Environments for People with Dementia (1st ed.). Routledge. https://doi.org/10.4324/9780203726310.

Singh, A., & Tiwari, S. (2020). Studies in Habitat with Academic Alliance in Planning Environment and Design (SHAAPED), https://www.researchgate.net/publication/344627842_Designing_healing_outdoor_spaces_for_Alzheimer's_patients_in_India.

Sirivastava, A. (2022). Dementia Villages – Experimenting with Universal Design Treatment, https://sites.dartmouth.edu/dujs/2022/09/29/dementia-villages-experimenting-with-universal-design-treatment/

Sommer, R. (1970). Small group ecology in institutions for the elderly. *Spatial behavior of older people*, 25-39.

Spencer, B., Williams, K., Mahdjoubi, L., & Sara, R. (2013). Third places for the third age: the contribution of playable space to the well-being of older people. In *Landscape, well-being and environment* (pp. 123-142). Routledge.

Street Furniture (2021). Korongee Dementia Village, https://streetfurniture.com/projects/korongee-dementia-village/.

Struthers, K. (2017). Interite Healthcare's Inspirational Design Tour of De Hogeweyk Aged Care Concept Weesp Netherlands, https://www.linkedin.com/pulse/interite-healthcares-inspirational-design-tour-de-aged-kim-struthers/.

Suznjevic, A. A (2013). Fantasy and reality: design for dementia, Controlled Multi-Sensory Environment, https://www.semanticscholar.org/paper/Fantasy-and-reality-%3A-design-fordementia-Suznjevic/4ed3282df34d3285a634fe9781af0129533dda41?p2df.

THW Design (2023). 5 Considerations for Memory Gardens. https://www.thw.com/blog/15-5-considerations-of-membory-gardens.

Tierney, L., Doherty, K., Breen, J., & Courtney-Pratt, H. (2022). Community expectations of a village for people living with dementia. *Health & Social Care in the Community*, *30*(6), e5875-e5884.

Ulrich, R. S. (1999). Theory and Research. *Healing gardens: Therapeutic benefits and design recommendations*, *4*, 27.

Ulrich, R. S. (1984). View through a window may influence recovery from surgery. *science*, *224*(4647), 420-421.

Ulrich, R. S., Bogren, L., & Lundin, S. (2012). Towards a design theory for reducing aggression in psychiatric facilities. In *ARCH12 Conference: International Conference ARCH12 and Forum Vårdbyggnad Nordic Conference 2012*. Chalmers Institute of Technology.

United Nations (2002). Madrid international plan of action on ageing, 2002. https://www.un.org/development/desa/ageing/madrid-plan-of-action-and-its-implementation.html.

Wells, S. (2014). *Horticultural therapy and the older adult population*. Routledge.

World Health Organization. (2007). *Global age-friendly cities: A guide*. World Health Organization.

Wright, J. (2014). Garden therapy for those with special needs. Retrieved June 2015, http://www.thegardener.co.za/kb/article.php?id=996.

Wu, S. M., Huang, H. L., Chiu, Y. C., Tang, L. Y., Yang, P. S., Hsu, J. L., ... & Shyu, Y. I. L. (2019). Dementia-friendly community indicators from the perspectives of people living with dementia and dementia-family caregivers. *Journal of Advanced Nursing*, *75*(11), 2878-2889.

Volicer, L., & Bloom-Charette, L. (2013). *Enhancing the quality of life in advanced dementia*. Routledge.

Zeisel, J. (2003). Marketing therapeutic environments for Alzheimer's care. *Journal of architectural and planning research*, 75-86.

Zeisel J, Tyson M (1999) Alzheimer's treatment gardens. InHealing Gardens: Therapeutic Benefits and Design Recom-mendations, Cooper Marcus C, Barnes M, eds. John Wiley &Sons, New York, pp. 437-504 *(PDF) Healing gardens: Recommendations and criteria for design.* Available from: https://www.researchgate.net/publication/231214688_Healing_gardens_Recommendations_and_criteria_for_design.

Biographical Sketch

Gökçen Firdevs Yücel Caymaz

Affiliation:
Istanbul Aydın University, Architecture and Design Faculty, Industrial Design Program

Education:

- 1998-2006 Graduated from İstanbul Technical Univerity Landscape Planning Doctory Program
- 1995-1998 Graduated from İstanbul Technical Univerity Landscape Planning Master Program
- 1991-1995, İstanbul University, Landscape Architecture

Business Address:
Beşyol, İnönü Cd. No:38, 34295 Küçükçekmece, İstanbul, Türkiye

Research and Professional Experience:
Full senior research fellow position at İstanbul Aydın University since 2012.

Publications from the Last 3 Years:

https://scholar.google.com/scholar?as_ylo=2019&q=street+furniture+g%C3%B6k%C3%A7en++caymaz&hl=tr&as_sdt=0,5.

Chapter 6

Leveraging AI in Telehealth and Telepharma: A Transformative Approach for the Healthcare System

Miguel Ángel de Miguel Paraíso[1,*]
Daniel Arranz Paraíso[2]
and Sandra Arranz Paraíso[3]
[1]Rey Juan Carlos University, Madrid, Spain
[2]R&D Development Manager at Pinisan SL. C/Gran Canaria, Madrid, Spain
[3]Complutense University of Madrid, Madrid, Spain

Abstract

In the last decade, the field of Artificial Intelligence (AI) has undergone a remarkable revolution, transforming various industries and aspects of our daily lives. From advanced Machine Learning (ML) algorithms to Natural Language Processing (NLP) and computer vision techniques, AI is nowadays revolutionizing a wide range of activities.

In healthcare, alongside traditional on-site medicine attention, one of the areas where these modern technologies could lead to significant transformation is the emerging field of telehealth and telepharma.

One of the primary advantages of integrating AI into telehealth is the ability to enhance patient care through intelligent decision support systems. AI-powered chatbots and virtual assistants using state-of-the-art NLP models, can offer tailored patient attention, medication reminders and queries, and triage services to contact the appropriate specialist, enhancing the patient experience.

Moreover, AI algorithms can analyze vast amounts of patient data, enabling accurate diagnosis, personalized treatment recommendations, and proactive monitoring of chronic conditions, serving as a support to the responsible doctor in charge of the telemedicine service, assisting in providing more accurate and fast diagnosis and treatment.

In addition to patient-centric applications, AI can also improve telepharma services. AI-powered medication management systems can ensure medication adherence, detect adverse drug interactions, and assist with medication reconciliation, improving medication safety and reducing errors. In addition, intelligent inventory management systems can optimize pharmaceutical supply chains, reducing stock-outs and wastage while ensuring timely availability of medicines.

* Corresponding Author's Email: miguelangel.demiguel@urjc.es

In: Psycho-Environmental Variables That Ensure People's Well-Being and Health …
Editors: Roberto Alonso González Lezcano and Guadalupe Cantarero García
ISBN: 979-8-89530-831-8

© 2025 Nova Science Publishers, Inc.

To summarize, the integration of AI in telehealth and telepharma has the potential to significantly impact the healthcare landscape. However, ensuring the responsible and ethical use of AI requires a robust regulatory framework, careful consideration of privacy and security, and close interdisciplinary collaboration. These factors are critical to harnessing the transformative power of AI to revolutionize and improve healthcare.

Keywords: telehealth, telepharma, artificial intelligence, machine learning, medicine*

Introduction

In the rapidly evolving landscape of healthcare, the convergence of Artificial Intelligence (AI) and telecommunication technologies has ushered in a new era of possibilities. This synergy has given rise to innovative solutions that transcend traditional healthcare boundaries, leading us into an era where patient-centric care is achievable. This chapter explores the transformative intersection of AI, telehealth, and telepharma, offering a comprehensive insight into the revolutionary changes these technologies are bringing to the healthcare system.

Here we delve into the intricacies of how AI algorithms are reshaping the healthcare paradigm. We will unravel the potential of AI-driven telehealth platforms to enhance accessibility, improve diagnostic accuracy, and personalize treatment plans, thus fostering a more inclusive and effective healthcare system.

Additionally, we will explore the transformative impact of AI in pharmaceuticals, where telepharma is emerging as a key player in streamlining medication management, ensuring adherence, and improving safety. By leveraging the power of AI, telepharma is not only facilitating remote consultations but also revolutionizing the way medications are prescribed, monitored, and delivered.

As we embark on this exploration, it is crucial to acknowledge the ethical, regulatory, and security challenges that accompany the integration of AI into healthcare systems. The potential benefits are vast, but so too are the responsibilities. This chapter will address these considerations, providing a balanced perspective on the risks and rewards of adopting AI in telehealth and telepharma.

This chapter provides a review of different state-of-the-art AI methods applied in the field of telehealth (section 0) and telepharma (section 0), as well as their limitations and considerations from an ethical and social point of view (section 0), followed by an analysis of the current situation of new AI-based technologies applied to the healthcare field, as well as the steps to be taken for their widespread implementation in the future (section 0). Additionally, the following section will provide a brief description of the most relevant technologies that will be referred to throughout this chapter.

AI Technologies Background

To provide context for the following sections of this chapter, the following paragraphs provide a brief overview of relevant technologies related to the application of AI in the fields of medicine and pharmacy.

Among these technologies, the most notable is Machine Learning (ML), a subset of AI that empowers computers to learn from data and improve their performance on specific tasks without being explicitly programmed. It leverages a variety of algorithms and techniques to enable systems to discern patterns, make predictions, and derive insights from vast and complex datasets. In the context of telemedicine and telepharmacy, ML plays a pivotal role in augmenting healthcare services and facilitating remote patient care. This technology encompasses several key techniques, including supervised learning, computer vision, and Natural Language Processing (NLP), which together empower healthcare providers to enhance diagnosis, treatment, and patient interactions, advancing the capabilities and accessibility of telemedicine and telepharmacy. The following sections delve into these ML techniques and their applications in critical healthcare domains.

Supervised Learning

Supervised learning is a paradigm in machine learning where a model is trained from labeled training data to make predictions or decisions. This approach involves extracting general characteristics from observed examples composed of labeled data through a process called training where a model "learns" those characteristics. These observed examples consist of input-output data pairs that can be of any kind and are usually generated manually or with human supervision (Bzdok, Krzywinski, and Altman 2018, 5). Supervised learning is well understood and widely used in various domains, such economics, robotics, and medicine among many others (Kanavati et al. 2021, 15330338211027901; Sahu et al. 2023), especially in scenarios where there is a requirement for precise classification models, as it yields classification models that can predict the label of previously unseen data (Lu and Cukic 2012, 79-88; Van Engelen and Hoos 2020, 373-440).

Computer Vision

Computer vision is a multidisciplinary field that allows computers to interpret and understand the visual world, revolutionizing various industries (Hashimoto et al. 2019). It plays a pivotal role in enhancing our ability to comprehend, analyze, and extract meaningful information from visual data, opening new frontiers for innovation and automation (Jopling, Pridgen, and Yeung 2021). Traditional computer vision techniques, such as image processing and feature extraction, have been enhanced and improved through the integration of AI methods, particularly deep learning and convolutional neural networks (CNNs) (Chartrand et al. 2017). The integration of AI methods in computer vision has not only improved the performance of traditional techniques but has also opened new frontiers for innovation and automation. The ability of AI-powered computer vision algorithms to automatically learn complex hierarchical features from visual data has led to superior performance in tasks such as image classification, object detection, and image generation (Chartrand et al. 2017). Furthermore, the application of AI in computer vision has facilitated the development of novel approaches for triaging medical images, inspecting critical infrastructure, and analyzing complex visual data, thereby transforming various industries and domains (Habib et al. 2022; Zakaria, Karaaslan, and Catbas 2022).

Natural Language Processing (NLP)

NLP is a field of AI that focuses on enabling computers to understand, interpret, and generate human language in a valuable and meaningful way (Al 2019). NLP involves the use of computational techniques to analyze and synthesize natural language data, enabling machines to comprehend human language and derive meaning from it (Tilton and Arnold 2019). This field has a wide range of applications across various domains, including finance, healthcare, information retrieval, and sentiment analysis (Lee, J. et al. 2023). The application of NLP tools for fraud detection, sentiment analysis, and financial market prediction has gained significant attention in recent years (Lee, J. et al. 2023; Goel et al. 2010). NLP has also been utilized in healthcare for tasks such as automated detection of radiology reports that require follow-up imaging, demonstrating its potential to improve healthcare processes (Lou et al. 2019).

The benefits of NLP are multifaceted. By leveraging NLP, organizations can automate repetitive tasks such as information extraction, classification, and summarization, leading to increased efficiency and productivity (Al 2019). Furthermore, NLP enables the extraction of valuable insights from large volumes of unstructured textual data, which can be utilized for decision-making and trend analysis (Badal, Kundrotas, and Vakser 2018). In the financial sector, NLP has been employed to decode Federal Reserve communications, providing valuable insights for macroeconomics (Lee, J. et al. 2021). Additionally, NLP has the potential to enhance the interpretability of language models, contributing to improved performance in various NLP tasks (Lee, H. 2023).

Overall, NLP plays a crucial role in enabling machines to understand and process human language, with applications in areas as diverse as finance, healthcare, and information retrieval. Benefits of NLP include automating tasks, extracting valuable insights from textual data, and improving the interpretability of language models, contributing to improved decision making and efficiency.

Telehealth

Telehealth, as a subset of eHealth, involves the use of telecommunication technologies to provide remote healthcare services, such as virtual consultations and remote monitoring. It requires the digitization of all data, including voice consultations, audiovisual material, and medical results, to be transported between the patient and the healthcare provider (Rodriguez et al. 2021).

The use of AI in telehealth has the potential to improve aspects such as time, diagnostic accuracy, and service, by leveraging ML and AI computer vision technologies. Taking advantage of all this digitized data, AI has the potential to improve different telehealth aspects such as time, diagnostic accuracy, and service, by leveraging different ML technologies (Mahtta et al. 2021).

The following sections will describe with more detail NLP, ML, and computer vision-based healthcare systems, which are highlighted as technologies that can lead to a major revolution in the telehealth sector.

Chatbots with NLP

Chatbots for medical support have been in use for the past decades. However, their implementation and expansion has been slow due to a several issues:

They are perceived to lack quality and accountability compared to face-to-face interactions with human doctors (Palanica et al. 2019) as they are usually based on pre-defined guidelines, which limits their adaptability and responsiveness to user queries (Kohnke, Moorhouse, and Zou 2023). Moreover, traditional chatbots lack the ability to establish smart and responsive communication with users, predict user problems or diseases, and understand and respond to the emotional state of patients (Parviainen and Rantala 2021). These limitations hinder their capacity to provide comprehensive and empathetic care to patients, which is essential in healthcare settings.

However, in recent years, language processing and generation technologies such as New NLP models have significantly improved chatbots in medicine by enhancing their capabilities in various aspects. The latest generation of NLP models leverages deep-learning Large Language Models (LLMs) built on Transformer architectures, along with techniques like Reinforcement Learning, resulting in emergent properties not seen in earlier generations of chatbots (Yeung et al. 2023). These advancements have enabled chatbots to understand and interpret user queries and responses in a more human-like manner, leading to more effective communication between patients and healthcare providers, ultimately improving diagnosis and treatment (Palanica et al. 2019). Furthermore, NLP algorithms have enhanced the ability of chatbots to generate natural language responses that are easily understood by users, thereby improving the overall user experience and making interactions with chatbots more seamless and intuitive (Palanica et al. 2019).

NLP algorithms have also been utilized for sentiment analysis, allowing chatbots to understand and respond to the emotional state of patients, which is particularly useful in providing emotional support and guidance for individuals dealing with mental health issues (Palanica et al. 2019).

However, despite all the benefits described above, modern chatbots cannot fully replace the caregiver, but can only adopt a coaching approach and support the doctor's activity. Further studies are needed to validate these conversational interfaces through experiments in real-world contexts (Valtolina, Barricelli, and Di Gaetano 2020, 108-132).

ML Analysis of Patient Data

ML algorithms have been widely utilized in the medical field to predict and diagnose various diseases by analyzing large sets of medical data and identifying patterns and correlations (Erickson et al. 2017). These algorithms are trained on labeled datasets, incorporating diverse features related to the disease, such as symptoms, medical history, and test results, to produce accurate diagnoses or predictions (Jiang et al. 2017). ML methods, such as the reviewed in this chapter, have been popularly employed for structured data analysis in healthcare, demonstrating their effectiveness in disease prediction and diagnosis (Cao et al. 2022).

The application of ML methods in disease prediction and diagnosis across various medical specialties has shown significant potential as can be seen in the following examples shown below:

In ophthalmology, deep learning algorithms have been developed to detect diabetic retinopathy in retinal fundus photographs, demonstrating the potential of ML in diagnosing diabetic eye diseases (Gulshan et al. 2016). In medical imaging, ML has been extensively utilized for MRI analysis, particularly in the domain of neurology and radiology, offering significant advancements in medical image processing and analysis (Lundervold and Lundervold 2019). Additionally, in pulmonology, quantitative computerized tomography (CT) analysis has been applied to diagnose various lung diseases, including obstructive, infiltrative, and restrictive pulmonary conditions such as emphysema, cystic fibrosis, and idiopathic pulmonary fibrosis (Chen, A. et al. 2020). In gastroenterology, AI has been increasingly employed for endoscopic ultrasonography, demonstrating high performance and becoming an essential technique for medical diagnosis (Kuwahara et al. 2020). In the cardiovascular domain, ML methods have been utilized for predicting cardiovascular events, providing insights into subclinical disease markers without a priori assumptions of causality, thereby enhancing prognostic capabilities (Ambale-Venkatesh et al. 2017). Furthermore, in the context of infectious diseases, ML techniques have been applied in the diagnosis and prediction of diseases such as dengue fever, allowing for accurate analysis based on clinical and laboratory symptoms (Mello-Román et al. 2019). Additionally, in oncology, ML has been instrumental in the early diagnosis of gastric cancer, showcasing its applicability in diverse medical fields, including cardiology, hematology, and surgery (Mortezagholi et al. 2019). Furthermore, the application of ML in neurology has extended to Alzheimer's disease classification using deep convolutional neural networks based on MRI and fMRI data, highlighting its potential in medical image analysis and disease prediction (Sarraf et al. 2016). Lastly, in the context of chronic kidney disease, both supervised ML and neural network approaches have been effectively utilized for early prediction and diagnosis of the condition (Nag and Jammula 2021).

Despite these positive results, the use of AI in medicine for disease prediction and diagnosis presents challenges related to confidence. Authors in (Zhou et al. 2020) highlighted challenges in developing AI tools, including data heterogeneity, low data quality, insufficient data sharing, and concerns about the security and interpretability of the models.

One of the reasons for that is that they are often treated as a 'black box', i.e., they provide an answer, but it is difficult to know how and why they arrived at that conclusion, which can make it difficult for practitioners to trust them. However, work such as (Ahmad, Eckert, and Teredesai 2018, 559-560) based on interpretable ML models (a type of ML model that can provide explanations for its predictions or decisions) can help healthcare professionals understand why a particular diagnosis or treatment recommendation was made. This can help improve confidence in the model and increase the likelihood that the recommendation will be followed. In addition, interpretable ML models can help identify which features or factors are most important in making a prediction, which can help healthcare professionals better understand the underlying mechanisms of a disease or condition.

However, the evolution of AI applied to medicine is indeed promising, with numerous studies indicating its transformative potential in healthcare. The application of AI in medicine is expected to become an integral part of medical attention in the future. The work of (Guo et al. 2020) demonstrated the exponential growth of health care–related AI research publications, signifying the continued expansion of AI applications in healthcare. Authors in (Maassen et al. 2021) highlighted that AI in medical practice is expected to meet higher expectations of medical treatment, increase the efficiency of clinical care, and accelerate the growth of personalized medicine. Similarly (Shu, Ren, and Song 2021) emphasized that AI is regarded as a revolutionary frontier technology in the field of medicine, particularly in cardiovascular medicine. Bajwa et al. (Bajwa et al. 2021) outlined recent breakthroughs in the application of AI in healthcare, describing a roadmap to building effective, reliable, and safe AI systems, further supporting the notion that AI will play a significant role in shaping the future of medical practice.

Computer Vision in Imagery Analysis

Computer vision has become an integral part of medical diagnosis and treatment, leveraging advanced algorithms to analyze medical imagery. The application of computer-aided diagnosis (CAD) in medical imaging has become a major research subject, offering significant assistance to medical professionals in disease diagnosis (Doi 2007). ML techniques have shown success in image-based diagnosis, disease detection, and prognosis (Kaur, Singh, and Kaur 2018; OLABI, Yilmaz, and Aslan 2020). The integration of various cues and modalities can enhance the performance of image or vision-based analysis, contributing to more accurate and efficient medical diagnosis (Rahman Ahad, Kobashi, and R. Tavares 2018). Additionally, computer-aided diagnosis can provide considerable assistance for pathologists, revolutionizing clinical research and diagnosis (Kang et al. 2021). The use of non-invasive biomarkers facilitated by innovation in biomedical imaging can lead to improved patient outcomes through better therapy prediction and monitoring (Anonymous2019).

Computer vision's main application is to analyze medical images and videos to assist with diagnosis and treatment planning in different specialties. These include cardiology, pathology, dermatology, and ophthalmology, among others. In cardiology, AI can assist with diagnosis and screening using imaging modalities such as echocardiography, CT, and magnetic resonance imaging MRI. In pathology, deep learning can help with the analysis of tissue samples for cancer diagnosis and treatment planning. In dermatology, deep learning can assist with the diagnosis of skin conditions using images of skin lesions. In ophthalmology, deep learning can help with the diagnosis and monitoring of eye diseases such as diabetic retinopathy and age-related macular degeneration. These applications have the potential to improve the accuracy and efficiency of medical diagnosis and treatment planning, leading to better patient outcomes (Gao et al. 2018).

Additionally, clinical workflows can integrate computer vision to enhance patient care. We can find several examples of medical video applications that can benefit from computer vision, such as monitoring patient movements and detecting falls in hospitals and nursing homes.

However, there exist different challenges and hurdles for real-world clinical deployment of computer vision. These include issues related to data quality, model limitations, community participation, and trust building. Data quality is a key factor in determining model quality, and identifying and addressing inequities in the data can lead to more equitable healthcare. Planning for model limitations, community participation, and trust building are also important considerations for successful deployment of these technologies in healthcare (Gao et al. 2018).

Moreover, computer vision techniques have been demonstrated to achieve a higher classification rate than previous works, indicating their potential to enhance the accuracy of medical diagnoses (Civit-Masot et al. 2020). These advancements in computer vision have the potential to significantly impact medical diagnosis and treatment by providing accurate and efficient analysis of medical imagery. The use of deep learning in medical imaging has shown potential to outperform humans in visual recognition tasks, offering significant applications in medicine and healthcare. Overall, the application of computer vision in medical imagery analysis holds great promise for improving the accuracy and efficiency of medical diagnosis and treatment.

Telepharmacy

Telepharmacy, is a form of pharmaceutical care that utilizes information and communication technology (ICT) facilities to enable remote interactions between pharmacists and patients, which has gained significant attention in recent years. The evidence supporting the potential benefits of telepharmacy and the implementation of this technology in providing access to healthcare services in remote communities is well documented (Baldoni, Amenta, and Ricci 2019, 327).

As an example, it can offer wide coverage of pharmaceutical services, especially in economically or geographically challenged areas, and can help counter pharmacist shortages while reducing pharmacy service costs (Elnaem et al. 2022, 9; Baldoni, Amenta, and Ricci 2019, 327). Additionally, telepharmacy can alleviate the burden of travel time and costs for patients, particularly the elderly, who are more vulnerable in these aspects (Baldoni, Amenta, and Ricci 2019, 327). It is important to highlight that the quality of the technology provided, reliable internet connections, and optimal utilization of the technology have been identified as factors that could influence telepharmacy services positively (Elnaem et al. 2022, 9), therefore, a good technological infrastructure is essential for this technology.

Although this service has many positive aspects, there is a need for more rigorous evidence on the reliability, safety, and effectiveness of telepharmacy in comparison to the traditional face-to-face healthcare delivery model (Rabbani et al. 2023, 30). As an example, situations such as acute care setting (including both intensive care units (ICUs) and non-ICUs) where , the application of telepharmacy is not clear due to differing patient needs, monitoring parameters, and medication use, as well as a greater risk of medication-related events (Strnad et al. 2018, 1250-1258).

However, preliminary studies have indicated that telepharmacy services can improve safety in drug dispensing and reduce the burden on healthcare infrastructure (Hefti, Wei, and Engelen 2022, 1324-1331). The following sections will describe these two telepharmacy applications in more detail.

Medication Prescription

In the field of medication prescription, there is also considerable evidence showing that novel AI algorithms can improve in several domains of this area.

Regarding the decision of the most appropriate drug and dosage, ML algorithms have been widely used in healthcare to predict the correct medication dosage for patients and to identify individuals at risk of adverse drug effects or interactions (Ryu, Kim, and Lee 2018). These algorithms leverage various input variables such as age, weight, sex, and medical history to make more informed decisions about medication therapy and adapt the therapeutic setting accordingly (Don Jayatilake and Ganegoda 2021).

By analyzing vast quantities of data, ML algorithms can identify patterns and trends that may not be immediately apparent to healthcare professionals. This can help healthcare professionals make more informed decisions about medication therapy and adapt the therapeutic setting accordingly (Iancu et al. 2023, 105241).

Similarly, AI methods can also improve the accuracy and reliability of prescription checks in a hospital setting, and can help healthcare professionals make more informed decisions about medication therapy, reduce the risk of prescribing errors and adverse drug effects, and improve patient safety (Corny et al. 2020, 1688-1694).

However, in spite of all the advantages and applications of AI in this field, the accuracy and reliability of ML systems in performing healthcare decision tasks should be evaluated through well-designed empirical studies prior to a more generalized implementation (London 2019).

Inventory Management

When managing the inventory of medicines, two main aspects should be addressed:

On the one hand, it is essential to provide a good service to the patients, having the necessary medicine available and ensuring an appropriate use of these medicines. On the other hand, it is also important to reduce costs by avoiding storing a larger quantity of medicines than necessary, which can end up deteriorating over time.

For the first problem, AI has the potential to significantly impact inventory management in pharmacy and medicine. AI can aid in minimizing drug inventory costs through simulation optimization, ensuring optimal inventory levels to prevent drug shortages, and improving the performance of pharmacies through the use of Accounting Information Systems (AIS) without compromising patient services (Chen, C. et al. 2022, 556; Abu Zwaida, Pham, and Beauregard 2021, 2726; Shrivastava 2019, 8). Additionally, by integrating AI with pharmacology, the efficiency of drug repurposing can significantly improve, leading to cost reductions and better resource allocation (Mohanty et al. 2020, 1027-1031).

Moreover, AI can contribute to targeted drug delivery systems, enhancing localized drug delivery and potentially reducing the misuse of pharmaceutical drugs (Das 2023, 1067144). Pharmacists, who play a crucial role in preventing and reducing drug abuse, can benefit from AI in inventory and supply chain management, leading to improved pharmacy performance (Chiappini et al. 2020). Additionally, AI can aid in the development of evidence-based actions to detect, understand, and prevent drug diversion activities and the adverse effects of drug misuse (Chiappini et al. 2020; Mason 2020, 216).

Ethical, Privacy and Security Considerations

When integrating AI into healthcare, it is crucial to consider various ethical aspects to ensure responsible and ethical use of AI technologies. The literature emphasizes the importance of transparency, fairness, responsibility, privacy, and security in the development and deployment of AI systems in healthcare (Jha et al. 2022; Smallman 2022; Pasricha 2023). These considerations are essential to uphold ethical standards, safeguard patient rights and well-being.

Transparency and trust in AI systems are critical components in the context of AI-enabled medical care. The potential barriers and facilitators to trustworthy and ethical AI-enabled medical care should be carefully examined to ensure the responsible and effective use of AI technologies in healthcare (Mooghali 2023). Transparency has the potential to improve the efficacy, safety, and quality of clinical research by allowing agencies, regulators, researchers, and companies to learn from the successes and failures of devices, reflecting the ethical responsibility of regulators and manufacturers (Muehlematter, Daniore, and Vokinger 2021).

Furthermore, the ethical implications of AI in healthcare extend to the impact on clinical decision-making, patient safety, and the potential for AI-induced medical errors. Addressing issues of accountability, responsibility, and the potential for AI-induced medical errors is crucial, emphasizing the importance of human involvement in the implementation of AI in clinical pathways (Bartlett 2023; Hill et al. 2023).

Moreover, the global health context, particularly in low- and middle-income countries (LMICs), presents unique ethical challenges that need to be addressed. It is essential to consider the ethics of AI in global health and ensure inclusiveness and equity of access to AI technology in healthcare (Murphy et al. 2021; Wang, Y. and Liu 2023).

Furthermore, privacy considerations in the application of these modern technologies are crucial for ensuring ethical and secure use of AI technologies. There is a universal recognition of the importance of privacy in the context of AI in healthcare (Smallman 2022). The government's role in ensuring the ethical and transparent use of AI solutions and protecting patient privacy is crucial, emphasizing the need for regulatory frameworks that prioritize privacy protection in the context of AI-assisted healthcare (Saeed, Saeed, and AlAhmri 2023). The future regulation of AI systems in healthcare services and medical research in the European Union underscores the importance of data protection laws and regulations, particularly the purpose limitation principle, in safeguarding patient privacy and ensuring responsible data processing in healthcare (Meszaros, Minari, and Huys 2022).

Concerning the safety of integrating telemedicine and AI into the healthcare system, several security aspects need to be carefully considered to ensure the responsible and secure use of AI technologies. Cybersecurity breaches, including the theft of health information and ransomware attacks on hospitals, pose significant threats to the integrity and confidentiality of healthcare data (Coventry and Branley 2018). Additionally, privacy, security, and confidentiality issues, as well as the security of healthcare databases and applications, are key ethical concerns that must be addressed to mitigate the risk of patient harm and ensure the responsible use of AI-enabled medical care (Mooghali 2023; Wang, C. et al. 2022; Kumar, Dwivedi, and Anand 2021; Gupta, Kamboj, and Bag 2021). Furthermore, the use of AI-based cybersecurity can play a crucial role in ensuring secure data transmission and storage in digital health communication, emphasizing the importance of leveraging AI technologies to enhance cybersecurity measures in healthcare (Tyagi 2023).

Discussion and Conclusion

This chapter has explored the transformative impact of AI on the healthcare industry, particularly in the areas of telehealth and telepharma. The main findings and contributions of the document include:

- AI-powered chatbots and virtual assistants can enhance patient care in telehealth by providing personalized support and guidance, improving patient engagement and satisfaction, and reducing the burden on healthcare providers.
- AI algorithms can analyze vast amounts of patient data to provide accurate diagnosis and personalized treatment recommendations, improving the efficiency and effectiveness of healthcare delivery.
- AI-powered medication management systems can improve telepharma services by ensuring medication adherence and detecting adverse drug interactions, reducing the risk of medication errors, and improving patient outcomes.

However, all these advances and advantages, while promising, should not be considered as a technology that will replace the current healthcare system. The methods discussed in this chapter, although showing very promising results, have not been sufficiently evaluated and have not shown good enough results to replace a professional expert in the field.

Therefore, the logical evolution of healthcare involves using these technologies as tools to accelerate or enhance processes, as a complementary consultation source, or even to automate specific tasks. For this reason, it is currently essential to have a professional who supervises the actions or decisions of these modern technologies and who is ultimately responsible for the final decisions taken.

Furthermore, prior to a widespread deployment of these technologies, there are numerous aspects that need further investigation, which have been described in the previous sections. These issues are not only limited to achieving better accuracy and recall results in deployed AI technologies, but also extend to different areas that have little or nothing to do with AI, such as legal, ethical, social and privacy concerns.

To conclude, this chapter has provided a state-of-the-art revision of AI technologies applied to the field of telehealth and telepharmacy, emphasizing the different fields of these disciplines in which they can be applied, and which can greatly benefit from them. Although, as mentioned above, significant research is still needed to improve various aspects and analyze their ethical and social repercussions, the benefits they offer justify continued development efforts.

References

"Strategic Research Agenda for Biomedical Imaging." 2019. *Insights into Imaging*. doi:10.1186/s13244-019-0684-z.

Abu Zwaida, Tarek, Chuan Pham, and Yvan Beauregard. 2021. "Optimization of Inventory Management to Prevent Drug Shortages in the Hospital Supply Chain." *Applied Sciences* 11 (6): 2726.

Ahmad, Muhammad Aurangzeb, Carly Eckert, and Ankur Teredesai. 2018. "Interpretable Machine Learning in Healthcare."

Al, Umut. 2019. "Natural Language Processing Applications in Library and Information Science." *Online Information Review*. doi:10.1108/oir-07-2018-0217.

Ambale-Venkatesh, Bharath, Xinmi Yang, Colin O. Wu, Kiang Liu, W. Gregory Hundley, Robyn L. McClelland, Antoinette S. Gomes, et al. 2017. "Cardiovascular Event Prediction by Machine Learning." *Circulation Research*. doi:10.1161/circresaha.117.311312.

Badal, Varsha D., Petras J. Kundrotas, and Ilya A. Vakser. 2018. "Natural Language Processing in Text Mining for Structural Modeling of Protein Complexes." *BMC Bioinformatics*. doi:10.1186/s12859-018-2079-4.

Bajwa, Junaid, Usman Munir, Aditya V. Nori, and Bryan Williams. 2021. "Artificial Intelligence in Healthcare: Transforming the Practice of Medicine." *Future Healthcare Journal*. doi:10.7861/fhj.2021-0095.

Baldoni, Simone, Francesco Amenta, and Giovanna Ricci. 2019. "Telepharmacy Services: Present Status and Future Perspectives: A Review." *Medicina* 55 (7): 327.

Bartlett, Benjamin. 2023. "The Possibility of AI-Induced Medical Manslaughter: Unexplainable Decisions, Epistemic Vices, and a New Dimension of Moral Luck." *Medical Law International*. doi:10.1177/09685332231193944.

Bzdok, Danilo, Martin Krzywinski, and Naomi Altman. 2018. "Machine Learning: Supervised Methods." *Nature Methods* 15 (1): 5.

Cao, Ji, Lixiang Zhang, Liang Ma, Xiaojuan Zhou, Baofeng Yang, and Wenjing Wang. 2022. "Study on the Risk of Coronary Heart Disease in Middle-Aged and Young People Based on Machine Learning Methods: A Retrospective Cohort Study." *Peerj*. doi:10.7717/peerj.14078.

Chartrand, Gabriel, Phillip M. Cheng, Eugene Vorontsov, Michal Drozdzal, Simon Turcotte, Christopher Pal, Samuel Kadoury, and An Tang. 2017. "Deep Learning: A Primer for Radiologists." *Radiographics*. doi:10.1148/rg.2017170077.

Chen, Alicia, Ronald A. Karwoski, David S. Gierada, Brian J. Bartholmai, and Chi Wan Koo. 2020. "Quantitative CT Analysis of Diffuse Lung Disease." *Radiographics*. doi:10.1148/rg.2020190099.

Chen, Chia-Nan, Chin-Hui Lai, Guan-Wei Lu, Ching-Chun Huang, Le-Jean Wu, Hui-Chuan Lin, and Ping-Shun Chen. 2022. "Applying Simulation Optimization to Minimize Drug Inventory Costs: A Study of a Case Outpatient Pharmacy."MDPI.

Chiappini, Stefania, Amira Guirguis, John Corkery, and Fabrizio Schifano. 2020. "Misuse of Prescription and Over-the-Counter Drugs to Obtain Illicit Highs: How Pharmacists can Prevent Abuse." *The Pharmaceutical Journal*.

Civit-Masot, Javier, Manuel Domínguez-Morales, Saturnino Vicente-Díaz, and A. Balcells. 2020. "Dual Machine-Learning System to Aid Glaucoma Diagnosis using Disc and Cup Feature Extraction." *Ieee Access*. doi:10.1109/access.2020.3008539.

Corny, Jennifer, Asok Rajkumar, Olivier Martin, Xavier Dode, Jean-Patrick Lajonchère, Olivier Billuart, Yvonnick Bézie, and Anne Buronfosse. 2020. "A Machine Learning–based Clinical Decision Support System to Identify Prescriptions with a High Risk of Medication Error." *Journal of the American Medical Informatics Association* 27 (11): 1688-1694.

Coventry, Lynne and Dawn Beverley Branley. 2018. "Cybersecurity in Healthcare: A Narrative Review of Trends, Threats and Ways Forward." *Maturitas*. doi:10.1016/j.maturitas.2018.04.008.

Das, Kaushik Pratim. 2023. "Nanoparticles and Convergence of Artificial Intelligence for Targeted Drug Delivery for Cancer Therapy: Current Progress and Challenges." *Frontiers in Medical Technology* 4: 1067144.

Doi, Kunio. 2007. "Computer-Aided Diagnosis in Medical Imaging: Historical Review, Current Status and Future Potential." *Computerized Medical Imaging and Graphics*. doi:10.1016/j.compmedimag.2007.02.002.

Don Jayatilake, Senerath Mudalige and Gamage Upeksha Ganegoda. 2021. "Involvement of Machine Learning Tools in Healthcare Decision Making." *Journal of Healthcare Engineering*. doi:10.1155/2021/6679512.

Elnaem, Mohamed Hassan, Muhammad Eid Akkawi, Abdul Kareem Al-Shami, and Ramadan Elkalmi. 2022. "Telepharmacy Knowledge, Perceptions, and Readiness among Future Malaysian Pharmacists Amid the COVID-19 Pandemic." *Ind J Pharm Educ Res* 56 (1): 9.

Erickson, Bradley J., Panagiotis Korfiatis, Zeynettin Akkus, and Timothy L. Kline. 2017. "Machine Learning for Medical Imaging." *Radiographics*. doi:10.1148/rg.2017160130.

Gao, Junfeng, Yong Yang, Pan Lin, and Dong Sun Park. 2018. "Computer Vision in Healthcare Applications." *Journal of Healthcare Engineering* 2018.

Goel, Sunita, Jagdish Gangolly, Sue R. Faerman, and Özlem Uzuner. 2010. "Can Linguistic Predictors Detect Fraudulent Financial Filings?" *Journal of Emerging Technologies in Accounting.* doi:10.2308/jeta.2010.7.1.25.

Gulshan, Varun, Lily Peng, Marc Coram, Martin C. Stumpe, Daniel Wu, Arunachalam Narayanaswamy, Subhashini Venugopalan, et al. 2016. "Development and Validation of a Deep Learning Algorithm for Detection of Diabetic Retinopathy in Retinal Fundus Photographs." *Jama.* doi:10.1001/jama.2016.17216.

Guo, Yuqi, Zhichao Hao, Shichong Zhao, Jiaqi Gong, and Fan Yang. 2020. "Artificial Intelligence in Health Care: Bibliometric Analysis." *Journal of Medical Internet Research.* doi:10.2196/18228.

Gupta, Shivam, Shampy Kamboj, and Surajit Bag. 2021. "Role of Risks in the Development of Responsible Artificial Intelligence in the Digital Healthcare Domain." *Information Systems Frontiers.* doi:10.1007/s10796-021-10174-0.

Habib, Al-Rahim, Graeme Crossland, Hemi Patel, Eugene Wong, Kelvin Kong, Hasantha Gunasekera, Brent Richards, et al. 2022. "An Artificial Intelligence Computer-Vision Algorithm to Triage Otoscopic Images from Australian Aboriginal and Torres Strait Islander Children." *Otology \& Neurotology.* doi:10.1097/mao.0000000000003484.

Hashimoto, Daniel A., Guy Rosman, Elan R. Witkowski, Caitlin Stafford, Allison J. Navarette-Welton, David W. Rattner, Keith D. Lillemoe, Daniela Rus, and Ozanan R. Meireles. 2019. "Computer Vision Analysis of Intraoperative Video." *Annals of Surgery.* doi:10.1097/sla.0000000000003460.

Hefti, Erik, Benjamin Wei, and Kristen Engelen. 2022. "Access to Telepharmacy Services may Reduce Hospital Admissions in Outpatient Populations during the COVID-19 Pandemic." *Telemedicine and E-Health* 28 (9): 1324-1331.

Hill, Elizabeth Redrup, Colin Mitchell, Tanya Brigden, and Alison Hall. 2023. "Ethical and Legal Considerations Influencing Human Involvement in the Implementation of Artificial Intelligence in a Clinical Pathway: A Multi-Stakeholder Perspective." *Frontiers in Digital Health.* doi:10.3389/fdgth. 2023.1139210.

Iancu, Alexa, Ines Leb, Hans-Ulrich Prokosch, and Wolfgang Rödle. 2023. "Machine Learning in Medication Prescription: A Systematic Review." *International Journal of Medical Informatics*: 105241.

Jha, Nisha, Pathiyil Ravi Shankar, Mohammed Azmi Al-Betar, Rupesh Mukhia, Kabita Hada, and Subish Palaian. 2022. "Undergraduate Medical Students' and Interns' Knowledge and Perception of Artificial Intelligence in Medicine." *Advances in Medical Education and Practice.* doi:10.2147/amep.s368519.

Jiang, Fei, Yong Jiang, Hui Zhi, Yi Dong, Hao Li, Sufeng Ma, Yilong Wang, Qiang Dong, Haipeng Shen, and Yongjun Wang. 2017. "Artificial Intelligence in Healthcare: Past, Present and Future." *Stroke and Vascular Neurology.* doi:10.1136/svn-2017-000101.

Jopling, Jeffrey, Brian C. Pridgen, and Serena Yeung. 2021. "Setting Assessment Standards for Artificial Intelligence Computer Vision Wound Annotations." *Jama Network Open.* doi:10.1001/jamanetworkopen. 2021.7851.

Kanavati, Fahdi, Shin Ichihara, Michael Rambeau, Osamu Iizuka, Koji Arihiro, and Masayuki Tsuneki. 2021. "Deep Learning Models for Gastric Signet Ring Cell Carcinoma Classification in Whole Slide Images." *Technology in Cancer Research & Treatment* 20: 15330338211027901.

Kang, X., Xingbo Liu, Xiushan Nie, and Yilong Yin. 2021. "Learning Binary Semantic Embedding for Breast Histology Image Classification and Retrieval." . doi:10.1109/icassp39728.2021.9415036.

Kaur, Prabhpreet, Gurvinder Singh, and Parmeet Kaur. 2018. "A Review of Denoising Medical Images using Machine Learning Approaches." *Current Medical Imaging Formerly Current Medical Imaging Reviews.* doi:10.2174/1573405613666170428154156.

Kohnke, Lucas, Benjamin Luke Moorhouse, and Di Zou. 2023. "ChatGPT for Language Teaching and Learning." *Relc Journal.* doi:10.1177/00336882231162868.

Kumar, Pradeep, Yogesh K. Dwivedi, and Ambuj Anand. 2021. "Responsible Artificial Intelligence (AI) for Value Formation and Market Performance in Healthcare: The Mediating Role of Patient's Cognitive Engagement." *Information Systems Frontiers.* doi:10.1007/s10796-021-10136-6.

Kuwahara, Takamichi, Kazuo Hara, Nobumasa Mizuno, Shin Haba, Nozomi Okuno, Hiroki Koda, Akira Miyano, and Daiki Fumihara. 2020. "Current Status of Artificial Intelligence Analysis for Endoscopic Ultrasonography." *Digestive Endoscopy*. doi:10.1111/den.13880.

Lee, Heungmin. 2023. "Application of Pretrained Language Models in Modern Financial Research." . doi:10.31219/osf.io/5s3nw.

Lee, Jean, Hoyoul Luis Youn, Josiah Poon, and Soyeon Caren Han. 2023. "StockEmotions: Discover Investor Emotions for Financial Sentiment Analysis and Multivariate Time Series." . doi:10.48550/arxiv.2301.09279.

Lee, Jean, Hoyoul Luis Youn, Nicholas Stevens, Josiah Poon, and Soyeon Caren Han. 2021. "FedNLP: An Interpretable NLP System to Decode Federal Reserve Communications." . doi:10.1145/3404835.3462785.

London, Alex John. 2019. "Artificial Intelligence and Black-Box Medical Decisions: *Accuracy Versus Explainability*." *The Hastings Center Report*. doi:10.1002/hast.973.

Lou, Robert, Darco Lalevic, Charles M. Chambers, Hanna M. Zafar, and Tessa S. Cook. 2019. "Automated Detection of Radiology Reports that Require Follow-Up Imaging using Natural Language Processing Feature Engineering and Machine Learning Classification." *Journal of Digital Imaging*. doi:10.1007/s10278-019-00271-7.

Lu, Huihua and Bojan Cukic. 2012. "An Adaptive Approach with Active Learning in Software Fault Prediction.".

Lundervold, Alexander Selvikvåg and Arvid Lundervold. 2019. "An Overview of Deep Learning in Medical Imaging Focusing on MRI." *Zeitschrift Für Medizinische Physik*. doi:10.1016/j.zemedi.2018.11.002.

Maassen, Oliver, Sebastian Fritsch, Julia Palm, Saskia Deffge, J. Kunze, Gernot Marx, Morris Riedel, Andreas Schuppert, and Johannes Bickenbach. 2021. "Future Medical Artificial Intelligence Application Requirements and Expectations of Physicians in German University Hospitals: Web-Based Survey." *Journal of Medical Internet Research*. doi:10.2196/26646.

Mahtta, Dhruv, Marilyne Daher, Michelle Lee, Saleem Sayani, Mehdi H. Shishehbor, and Salim S. Virani. 2021. "Promise and Perils of Telehealth in the Current Era." *Current Cardiology Reports*. doi:10.1007/s11886-021-01544-w.

Mason, Andrew N. 2020. "Pharmacy Internal Controls: A Call for Greater Vigilance during the COVID-19 Pandemic." *Pharmacy* 8 (4): 216.

Mello-Román, Jorge Daniel, Julio César Mello Román, Santiago Gómez-Guerrero, and Miguel García-Torres. 2019. "Predictive Models for the Medical Diagnosis of Dengue: A Case Study in Paraguay." *Computational and Mathematical Methods in Medicine*. doi:10.1155/2019/7307803.

Meszaros, Janos, Jusaku Minari, and Isabelle Huys. 2022. "The Future Regulation of Artificial Intelligence Systems in Healthcare Services and Medical Research in the European Union." *Frontiers in Genetics*. doi:10.3389/fgene.2022.927721.

Mohanty, Sweta, Md Harun Ai Rashid, Mayank Mridul, Chandana Mohanty, and Swati Swayamsiddha. 2020. "Application of Artificial Intelligence in COVID-19 Drug Repurposing." *Diabetes & Metabolic Syndrome: Clinical Research & Reviews* 14 (5): 1027-1031.

Mooghali, Maryam. 2023. "Barriers and Facilitators to Trustworthy and Ethical AI-Enabled Medical Care from Patient's and Healthcare Provider's Perspectives: A Literature Review." . doi:10.1101/2023.10.02.23296447.

Mortezagholi, Asghar, Omid Khosravizadeh, Mohammad Bagher Menhaj, Younes Shafigh, and Rohollah Kalhor. 2019. "Make Intelligent of Gastric Cancer Diagnosis Error in Qazvin's Medical Centers: Using Data Mining Method." *Asian Pacific Journal of Cancer Prevention*. doi:10.31557/apjcp.2019.20.9.2607.

Muehlematter, Urs J., Paola Daniore, and Kerstin Noëlle Vokinger. 2021. "Approval of Artificial Intelligence and Machine Learning-Based Medical Devices in the USA and Europe (2015–20): A Comparative Analysis." *The Lancet Digital Health*. doi:10.1016/s2589-7500(20)30292-2.

Murphy, Kathleen, Erica Di Ruggiero, Ross Upshur, Donald J. Willison, Neha Malhotra, Jia Cai, Nakul Malhotra, Vincci Lui, and Jennifer L. Gibson. 2021. "Artificial Intelligence for Good Health: A Scoping Review of the Ethics Literature." *BMC Medical Ethics*. doi:10.1186/s12910-021-00577-8.

Nag, Shreya and Nimitha Jammula. 2021. "Comparison of Neural Network and Machine Learning Approaches in Prediction of Chronic Kidney Disease." *Journal of Student Research*. doi:10.47611/jsrhs.v10i3.1570.

OLABI, Nur, A. Yilmaz, and Zafer Aslan. 2020. "Automated Detection of Alzheimer's Disease using Wavelet Transform with Convolutional Neural Networks." *Euras Journal of Health*. doi:10.17932/ejoh.2020.022/ejoh.

Palanica, Adam, Peter Flaschner, Anirudh Thommandram, Michael H. Li, and Yan Fossat. 2019. "Physicians' Perceptions of Chatbots in Health Care: Cross-Sectional Web-Based Survey." *Journal of Medical Internet Research*. doi:10.2196/12887.

Parviainen, Jaana and Juho Rantala. 2021. "Chatbot Breakthrough in the 2020s? an Ethical Reflection on the Trend of Automated Consultations in Health Care." *Medicine Health Care and Philosophy*. doi:10.1007/s11019-021-10049-w.

Pasricha, Sudeep. 2023. "AI Ethics in Smart Healthcare." *Ieee Consumer Electronics Magazine*. doi:10.1109/mce.2022.3220001.

Rabbani, Syed Arman, Shrestha Sharma, Asiya Mahtab, Faheem Hyder Pottoo, and Sathvik B. Sridhar. 2023. "A Systematic Scoping Review of Implementation of Telepharmacy during COVID-19." *Journal of Applied Pharmaceutical Science* 13 (4): 30.

Rahman Ahad, Md Atiqur, Syoji Kobashi, and João Manuel R. Tavares. 2018. "Advancements of Image Processing and Vision in Healthcare." *Journal of Healthcare Engineering*. doi:10.1155/2018/8458024.

Rodriguez, Jorge A., Altaf Saadi, Lee H. Schwamm, David W. Bates, and Lipika Samal. 2021. "Disparities in Telehealth use among California Patients with Limited English Proficiency." *Health Affairs*. doi:10.1377/hlthaff.2020.00823.

Ryu, Jae Yong, Hyun Uk Kim, and Sang Yup Lee. 2018. "Deep Learning Improves Prediction of Drug–drug and Drug–food Interactions." *Proceedings of the National Academy of Sciences*. doi:10.1073/pnas.1803294115.

Saeed, Abdullah, Abdulrahman Bin Saeed, and Foton A. AlAhmri. 2023. "Saudi Arabia Health Systems Challenging and Future Transformation with Artificial Intelligence." *Cureus*. doi:10.7759/cureus.37826.

Sahu, Purnendra Kumar, P. Priyadarshini, Smritiratan Tripathy, and Suvendu Pradhan. 2023. "Machine Learning Strategies for Malaria Risk Prediction Based on Text-Based Clinical Information." . doi:10.21203/rs.3.rs-2938711/v1.

Sarraf, Saman, DeSouza Dd, John A. E. Anderson, and Ghassem Tofighi. 2016. "DeepAD: Alzheimer's Disease Classification Via Deep Convolutional Neural Networks using MRI and fMRI." . doi:10.1101/070441.

Shrivastava, Sudhir. 2019. "Analysis of Inventory Level Optimization using Artificial Intelligence Approach." *Smart Moves Journal Ijosthe* 6 (2): 8.

Shu, Songren, Ji-Hua Ren, and Jiangping Song. 2021. "Clinical Application of Machine Learning-Based Artificial Intelligence in the Diagnosis, Prediction, and Classification of Cardiovascular Diseases." *Circulation Journal*. doi:10.1253/circj.cj-20-1121.

Smallman, Melanie. 2022. "Multi Scale Ethics—Why we Need to Consider the Ethics of AI in Healthcare at Different Scales." *Science and Engineering Ethics*. doi:10.1007/s11948-022-00396-z.

Strnad, Kyle, Bethany R. Shoulders, Pamela L. Smithburger, and Sandra L. Kane-Gill. 2018. "A Systematic Review of ICU and Non-ICU Clinical Pharmacy Services using Telepharmacy." *Annals of Pharmacotherapy* 52 (12): 1250-1258.

Tilton, Lauren and Taylor Arnold. 2019. "An Introduction Natural Language Processing." *Rmc*. doi:10.46632/rmc/1/1/014.

Tyagi, Amit Kumar. 2023. "Digital Health Communication with Artificial Intelligence-Based Cyber Security." . doi:10.4018/978-1-6684-8938-3.ch009.

Valtolina, Stefano, Barbara Rita Barricelli, and Serena Di Gaetano. 2020. "Communicability of Traditional Interfaces VS Chatbots in Healthcare and Smart Home Domains." *Behaviour & Information Technology* 39 (1): 108-132.

Van Engelen, Jesper E. and Holger H. Hoos. 2020. "A Survey on Semi-Supervised Learning." *Machine Learning* 109 (2): 373-440.

Wang, Chao, Jieyu Zhang, Nicholas Lassi, and Xiaohan Zhang. 2022. "Privacy Protection in using Artificial Intelligence for Healthcare: Chinese Regulation in Comparative Perspective." *Healthcare*. doi:10.3390/healthcare10101878.

Wang, Yin and Xiang Michelle Liu. 2023. "Navigating the Ethical Landscape of AI in Healthcare: Insights from a Content Analysis." . doi:10.36227/techrxiv.22294513.v2.

Yeung, Joshua Au, Zeljko Kraljevic, Akish Luintel, Alfred Balston, Esther Idowu, Richard Dobson, and James Teo. 2023. "AI Chatbots Not Yet Ready for Clinical Use." doi:10.1101/2023.03.02.23286705.

Zakaria, Mahta, Enes Karaaslan, and F. Necati Catbas. 2022. "Advanced Bridge Visual Inspection using Real-Time Machine Learning in Edge Devices." *Advances in Bridge Engineering*. doi:10.1186/s43251-022-00073-y.

Zhou, Yadi, Fei Wang, Jian Tang, Ruth Nussinov, and Feixiong Cheng. 2020. "Artificial Intelligence in COVID-19 Drug Repurposing." *The Lancet Digital Health*. doi:10.1016/s2589-7500(20)30192-8.

Biographical Sketches

Miguel Ángel de Miguel Paraíso

Affiliation:
Rey Juan Carlos University, Fuenlabrada School of Engineering

Education:
2015 Graduated with honors in the degree of Industrial Electronics and Automation Engineering. 2017 MD in Industrial Engineering. 2022 PhD in Electrical, Electronic and Automation Engineering cum laude from Universidad Carlos III de Madrid.

Business Address:
Departamental III, Cam. del Molino, 5, 28942 Fuenlabrada, Madrid, Spain

Research and Professional Experience:
Assistant Professor at Rey Juan Carlos University. Researcher in the robotics group Intelligent Robots Lab. Participation in different research projects collaborating with national and international companies.

Professional Appointments:
Associate editor of the Journal Sensors MDPI. Author of a book chapter on international book.

Publications from the Last 3 Years:

1. De Miguel, M. Á., J. M. Armingol, and F. García. (2022). Vehicles trajectory prediction using recurrent VAE network. *IEEE Access*, 10, 32742–32749.
2. De Miguel, M. A., C. Guindel, A. Al-Kaff, and F. García. (2023). High-accuracy patternless calibration of multiple 3-d lidars for autonomous vehicles. *IEEE Sensors Journal*, 23(11), 12200–12208.
3. Madridano, A., S. Campos, J. M. Perez, A. Valle, D. Martín, R. A. Lattarulo, M. Á. de Miguel, C. Sierra, J. Del Olmo, C. O. Chacón, et al. (2023). Evolution of bus shuttle service in Madrid towards autonomous operation, a practical use case. In *2023 IEEE 26th International Conference on Intelligent Transportation Systems (ITSC)* (pp. 2698–2704). IEEE.

4. Madridano, A., S. Campos, J. M. Perez, A. Valle, D. Martín, R. A. Lattarulo, M. Á. de Miguel, C. Sierra, J. Del Olmo, C. O. Chacón, et al. (2023). Evolution of bus shuttle service in Madrid towards autonomous operation, a practical use case. In *2023 IEEE 26th International Conference on Intelligent Transportation Systems (ITSC)* (pp. 2698–2704). IEEE.

Daniel Arranz Paraíso

Affiliation:
Innovation Manager at Pinisan SL; Collaborating Doctor Professor at Universidad CEU San Pablo; Centro de Tecnología Biomédica

Education:

- 2013: Pharmacy degree (7.44/10), Universidad Complutense de Madrid
- 2015: Master's in Pharmacy and Pharmaceutical Technology (9.85/10, Cum Laude), Universidad Complutense de Madrid
- 2015: Doctorate in Pharmacy (Cum Laude), Universidad Complutense de Madrid

Business Address:
Pinisan SL, C. de Gran Canaria, 33, 28970 Humanes de Madrid, Madrid

Research and Professional Experience:

Daniel Arranz Paraiso has extensive experience in pharmaceutical technology, focusing on galenic development, quality control, and innovative health solutions. His research includes high-impact publications in areas such as mitochondria and infrared radiation, blue light filters, and vitamin C monitoring in mice. He is currently involved in a project at the Centro de Tecnología Biomédica studying compounds for brain cancer and holds two patents for drug delivery systems.

Daniel's teaching experience includes serving as a Collaborating Doctor Professor at Universidad CEU San Pablo, where he taught Pharmaceutical Technology and Dermopharmacy, and mentored undergraduate theses. He also has professional experience in the industry, developing over 300 formulations and working as an external advisor for various pharmaceutical companies.

Professional Appointments:

Innovation Manager at Pinisan SL (2023–present)

Collaborating Doctor Professor at Universidad CEU San Pablo (2017–2018, 2021–2023)

External Advisor for Carlos Langa Pharmacy and RZero Infection Prevention & Control (2019–present)

Publications from the Last 3 Years:

1. Arranz, D., et al. (2023). Mitochondria and infrared radiation: Impact on cellular functions. *Journal of Pharmaceutical Research.*
2. Arranz-Paraíso, D., Sola, Y., Baeza-Moyano, D., Benitez-Martinez, M., Melero-Tur, S., & González-Lezcano, R. A. (2023). Mitochondria and light: An overview of the pathways triggered in skin and retina with incident infrared radiation. *Journal of Photochemistry and Photobiology B: Biology*, *238*, 112614.
3. Arranz, D., et al. (2024). The role of blue light filters in dermatological treatments. *Journal of Pharmaceutical Sciences*.
4. Arranz, D., et al. (2024). Vitamin C monitoring in mice: A review. *Toxins* (under review).

Sandra Arranz Paraíso

Affiliation:
Universidad Autónoma de Madrid, Facultad de Psicología, Departamento de Psicología Básica

Education:
2016 Graduated with honors in the degree of Psychology. 2018 MD in Methodology of Behavioural and Health Sciences. 2023 PhD in Experimental Psychology (Visual Perception) cum laude from Universidad Complutense de Madrid.

Business Address:
C. Iván Pavlov, 6, Fuencarral-El Pardo, 28049, Madrid, Spain

Research and Professional Experience:
Assistant Professor at Universidad Autónoma de Madrid. Researcher in the Cognition, Attention and Learning Lab. Participation in different research projects collaborating with national and international companies.

Professional Appointments:
Author of three book chapters on international books.

Publications from the Last 3 Years:

1. Arranz-Paraíso, S. A. (2023). *Inhibitory mechanisms in visual motion perception* (Doctoral dissertation, Universidad Complutense de Madrid).
2. Arranz-Paraiso, D., & Arranz-Paraíso, S. (2024). Filters and Life: A Glimpse Into the Future for the Generation of Healthier Homes and Architectural Constructions. In *Design Strategies for Efficient and Sustainable Building Facilities* (pp. 200-221). IGI Global.
3. Arranz-Paraíso, S., & Arranz-Paraíso, D. (2024). Artificial Intelligence, Virtual Reality, and Augmented Reality to Enhance Visual Quality and Accessibility in

Sustainable Built Environments. In *Design Strategies for Efficient and Sustainable Building Facilities* (pp. 179-199). IGI Global.

4. Serrano Pedraza, I., López Bascuas, L. E., Arranz Paraíso, S., Bachtoula González, O., Llamas Cornejo, I., & Sierra Vázquez, V. (2023). Librerías Matlab para la realización de prácticas sensoriales y perceptivas dentro y fuera del aula.
5. Bachtoula, O., Arranz-Paraíso, S., Luna, R., & Serrano-Pedraza, I. (2023). Visual motion discrimination experiments reveal small differences between males and females. *Vision research*, *208*, 108222.
6. Arranz-Paraíso, S., & Arranz-Paraíso, D. (2023). The Extent of New Technologies in Urban Environments: Virtual Reality, Lighting, and Accessibility. In *Intersecting Health, Livability, and Human Behavior in Urban Environments* (pp. 251-272). Igi Global.

Chapter 7

Organizational Anthropology and Ethnography

José G. Vargas-Hernández[1,*]
María F. Higuera-Cota[2]
M. C. Omar C. Vargas-González[3]
and Absalón J. Salmerón-Zapata[4]

[1]Financial Literacy Research Center, Universidad Cristóbal Colón, Veracruz, Mexico
[2]Universidad Autónoma de Sinaloa, Mexico
[3]Instituto Tecnológico de México, Campus Cd. Guzmán, Jalisco, Mexico
[4] Universidad Cristóbal Colón, Veracruz, Mexico

Abstract

The study aims to deepen the analysis of the theoretical, conceptual and methodological implications arising from the relationship between organizational anthropology and ethnography. The research is based on the premise that both ethnographic analysis and interpretive research in organizational anthropology are fundamental tools to understand the social processes that occur in organizations, without preconceived notions and with categories defined by organizational actors. To achieve this objective, we employ an analytical and descriptive approach based on an exhaustive review of the theoretical and empirical literature available in organizational anthropology and ethnography. The combination of both perspectives has allowed a thoughtful and detailed analysis of the theoretical, conceptual and methodological implications that arise from the interaction between both disciplines.

The results of this study indicate that the ethnographic methodology is especially relevant for the analysis of the interactions between organizational anthropology and ethnography, since it allows a deeper and contextualized approach to the social processes that occur in organizations. In this sense, the ethnographic methodology is essential for the development of organizational anthropology as a new specialty within organizational studies.

In summary, this study highlights the importance of ethnographic methodology for organizational anthropology and underlines the need to deepen the relationship between both disciplines. Likewise, it offers an analytical and reflective perspective that contributes to the development of new research in the field of organizational anthropology and ethnography.

* Corresponding Author's Email: jvargas2006@gmail.com

In: Psycho-Environmental Variables That Ensure People's Well-Being and Health …
Editors: Roberto Alonso González Lezcano and Guadalupe Cantarero García
ISBN: 979-8-89530-831-8
© 2025 Nova Science Publishers, Inc.

Keywords: organizational anthropology, ethnography, interpretive research, ethnographic methodology and social processes in organizations

Introduction

The origin and establishment of organizational anthropology responds to situations, conditions, different but articulated anthropological visions that lead to diverse perspectives and approaches. Organizations are conceived as legitimate research laboratories in fields such as organizational anthropology, psychology, and sociology.

That is why organizational anthropology studies have become relevant to contribute to the organizational and administrative school of thought and provide complementarity to sociology, psychology, biology and history.

Organizational anthropology is an inclusive administrative discipline of knowledge processes in the management of organizations to increase efficiency. Anthropology, along with ethology, ethnology, sociology, and psychology in organizational and managerial studies, is relevant for analyzing administrative relations such as production-consumption management.

Various contexts in a diverse socioeconomic world demand new anthropologically oriented organizational forms as specific responses for survival and adaptability. In the words of Gonnet (2012), the organizational space from an emic perspective of its own members is in charge of nurturing anthropology and organizational theory.

Problem Statement

The relationship between the academic and professional fields of anthropology contribute to the theoretical framework supported to contribute to organizational psychology. In this regard, Fotaki, et al. (2020) point out that the reference to the discipline of anthropology is still conspicuously absent in organizational studies.

Although organizational anthropology is inherently interdisciplinary—drawing from industrial psychology, social anthropology, ethnology, and sociology—further studies are needed not only to enhance human knowledge but also to contribute to organizational development and foster dialogue in organizational studies. Even though the organizational issues mark the interdisciplinary of organizational anthropology, cultivating learning that addresses behavioral problems at work in organizations.

The term Anthropology comes from the Greek ἄνθρωπος, ánthrópos, which means man or human being, and λόγος, logos, which means word, treaty, knowledge, study. Anthropology is a science with a holistic approach to study humanity as a human being, people, human groups in terms of values, norms, lifestyles, patterns, etc. of homosocialis and culture. The study of the human being has a long tradition carried out by Herodotus (484-425 BC), Hippocrates (460-377 BC) and Aristotle (384-322 BC). The word Anthropology was used by Aristotle and was used to designate knowledge for the study of spiritual human nature, that is, doctrine.

Anthropology is the scientific study of man and his culture, contemplating social behavior, beliefs, languages, modes of behavior. In addition, it considers the origin and historical evolution of the human being. In fact, anthropology has been consolidated as a social science with the colonization processes. For example, Menéndez (1996) asserts that the industrial revolution caused deep anthropological transformations in the context of organizations based on modes of industrial production and capitalist development processes because of colonial expansion that led to the international division of intellectual labor.

Importance of the Study

The conceptualizations of organizational anthropology to define the object of study are framed in the capitalist international division of intellectual labor. Anthropological metaphors such as character, tribe, clan, etc., among others, are attributed to Ohnismo, considered a folkloric trap by Berg and Faucheux (1982) and Alvesson and Berg (1992), leaving aside the capitalist concepts of performance and efficiency based on the Toyota organizational paradigm.

Smirnova (2016) states that anthropology has developed in physical and organizational settings to include administrative, cultural, and social anthropology. On the other hand, there are other types of anthropology such as industrial, organizational and business anthropology which, according to Roca i Girona (2001), make up a discipline whose unit of study is the industrial organizational business environment. For his part, Roca (1998) specifies that industrial anthropology is different from economic anthropology. Industrial anthropology refers to the economy of societies that is, to their activity as a social individual who produces, buys, sells and interacts with others in their economic environment. It is also known as business anthropology.

For Roca (1998) industrial anthropology limits specialization beyond the anthropology of work with an interest in social aspects based on productive labor practices, which lead to industrial anthropology being an anthropology of industrial society with an interest in the historical problems that are related to industrialism and its social anthropology. Therefore, the work of anthropology deals with industrial and non-industrial work, being the object of study the industrial organization, store, farm, artisan workshops, inserted either in the formal or informal economy.

The applied concepts of anthropology in industrial societies can be defined in relation to their practical use in a historical setting. Anthropology's interest in studying complex industrial societies includes interventions in different areas of organizational studies influenced by ideological and material power in industrial organizations (Maestre Alfonso, 1983). Thus, the process of formation and development of organizational anthropology under the approach of applied anthropology is linked to the phenomena of industrialization of societies.

Organizational anthropology studies human organizations, and through empirical work, it is possible to explain the opportunities and limitations associated with the use of anthropological methods in organizations and management. However, the texture of organizational anthropological research also includes actor-centered context, history, and process. That is, organizational anthropology separates between research and intervention.

On the other hand, García Canclini (1995) explains that sociology, psychology, anthropology, communication studies and other social sciences converge in multidisciplinary research on organizations. That is, the study of organizations must be framed in a multidisciplinary approach from a micro perspective to human groups subject to anthropology, paleontology, historiography, sociology pointing to the anthropology of organizations.

Method

This analysis begins in the first place by describing, analyzing and reflecting on issues and concerns related to the emerging topic of organizational anthropology in organizational studies, to continue with the topic of organizational ethnography, as the relevant methodology to use. Finally, some final comments are made from the reflective analysis.

Organizational Anthropology

Organizational anthropology is considered an emerging field, which has emerged as a discipline in convergence with sociology and psychology and the intersections between the local and the global to analyze the organizational components of complex societies, as well as their transformative effects on cultural dynamics in traditional models of capitalist organization. The connection between anthropology and organizational studies in a discipline of organizational anthropology accounts for the social diversity of the meanings of the human being. In addition, these types of studies are applicable to all types of organizations regardless of their nature and identity.

Authors such as Corsín Jiménez (2007), Caulkins, & Ann (2013) and Garsten, & Anette (2013), mention that administrative and organizational anthropology, also known as organizational anthropology, is a science that studies the interactions between objects and people of management. For Kottak (2011) organizational anthropology studies the diversity of human conditions that entails the adaptability in space and time of organizations, biology, society, culture and language, etc.

About the fundamental concepts of the theoretical framework of organizational anthropology, these are oriented to analyze the reality of organizations as an object of study of anthropology leading to processes of change in professional programs of various disciplines tending to apply anthropology in the organizational studies of industrial societies. Specifically, organizational anthropology provides support to human realities, such as social constructions, symbolic, cultural and ideological aspects of organizations. The theories and methodologies of organizational anthropology must be compatible with the reality of organizations developed through processes of transformation and formation of companies and companies.

Likewise, organizational anthropology contributes to analyze the perspectives of the actors, contributing to the human side of organizations made up of human beings. Organizational anthropology is a means of providing a background for the study of human beings in organizations that focuses on management and on profitability, efficiency, and effectiveness. For Richardson (1955) anthropology in organizations supports the focus on human relations in organizations, along with psychology and non-systematized knowledge.

About the field of organizational anthropology Roca (1998) considers that this focuses on the investigation of human relations, behaviors and cultures between the different processes of organizations, businesses, industries, companies, ventures, corporations, etc., as systems to provide knowledge, reveal its nature and contribute to criticize, change, improve, denounce, etc. It should be emphasized that the production of organizational anthropology knowledge focused on the diversity of applied organizations requires changes towards more collaborative efforts in professional tasks. The production of one's own knowledge in the anthropological organization as a discipline with its various approaches requires collaboration with change and professional work in parallel.

Regarding the above, Chanlat (1994) emphasizes that the anthropology of organizations is a symbolic ideological, cultural, meaning and identity aspect that creates and develops multiple realities. In other words, the anthropology of organizations is perceived through symbols that reveal internal relationships such as unified elements for work, social culture, organizational and corporate culture, and subcultures within the members of the organization. In such a way, that the theoretical knowledge of organizational anthropology is provided in objective tools to industrial psychology aimed at understanding the problems and human aspects in organizations.

The study of organizations from anthropology considers behavior, structure, group values, etc., which leads to analyzing the functioning of organizations (Jordan, 2013). Rather, organizational anthropology describes the sociopolitical relations in the structures of organizations aimed at modifying and transforming forms of commitment, times and new spaces, information and communication technologies. It should be emphasized that the dimensions of organizational anthropology have been modified by information technologies from the perspective of actors within related disciplines who are interested in working in organizations.

Organizational anthropology studies human organizations. That is to say, the anthropological dimension of the human being accounts for a more humanistic organization and the social sense and identity, giving rise to the diversity of human groups. Which leads to the creation and development of mostly human organizations.

Anthropology emphasizes the specificities of human groups in organizations, differentiating itself from sociology by participating with the people studied. The classical theory of anthropology in organizations described as political entities in which various groups pursue their interests and objectives, analyzes the existence of competition between multiple cultural groups, forming a social structure designed to translate demands into culture.

Classical anthropology claims an anthropology of the current world with critical positions and methodological crossovers in both materialist and idealist versions of interpretativism in common core on the familiarization of the exotic to build otherness as a form of practical construction of knowledge for participatory practices as proposed by the approach ethno methodological (Menéndez, 2006). The foregoing allows building processes of reflection and questioning of classical anthropological theories and their role in society framed in the scientific approach of Marxism.

For Baer (2014) the anthropological vision of organizations provides a perspective that big data fails to fully analyze and interpret the data related to the different organizational stakeholders as customers think, since the human sciences allow us to understand human subjectivity as for Decipher the functions of the technology used to create goods and services.

The concept of business anthropology supported by Jordan (2013) leaves anthropological practice not only for the benefit of organizations on issues related to group behavior, work processes, organizational change, diversity, globalization, etc. In this regard, Caulkins & Jordan (2013) and Morales Inga & Morales Tristán (2018) point out that organizational anthropology is a dynamic field in organizational studies that, more than a unified theory, is made up of multiple theoretical approaches with various methodologies developed and used in various contexts.

In line with the above, the organizational anthropology methodology aims to collect and use primary information to design an experiential and feedback workshop supported by classic tools such as the SWOT, the group interview, the problem tree, etc., that lead to diagnose problems and find solutions. In turn, the analytical tools of organizational anthropology are used to analyze hierarchies and relationships between and within groups and organisms (Lomnitz, 1975). In addition, the quantitative methodology of organizational anthropology is the conjunction of techniques such as participant observation and psychometrics to achieve the necessary qualifications to obtain objective numerical data on the participants and obtain comprehensive individual results.

From organizational anthropology, the imaginary is the individual perception and beliefs that build the process of social construction of reality generated by interactions between humans, enabling the organizational anthropological perspective created by humans in society of the symbolic world beyond the reality (Cely-López, & Gómez-Niño, 2016). In this regard, Jaumier (2020) warns that anthropology plays a role in understanding alternative organizations and the acts of imagining new ones that lean towards the local experiences and meanings of the members of the organization as a field of problematization rather than theory driven.

The role of organizational anthropology by focusing more on human relations than on production processes. It indicates that the organization is a community aimed at building and strengthening an identity, which, sustained through an organizational culture, values, norms, rites, myths, etc., develops a vision to generate value. Individuals and communities in organizational anthropology promote intervention practices to identify the necessary community perceptions about program design processes to foster the development of community organizations.

Regarding the anthropology of organizations and history, according to Llobera (2009) these contribute to appreciate epistemic cycles. Giving rise to flexible epistemic shelters focused on the construction of alterity supported by other disciplines tending to question relativistic ethnocentric rationalities that lead to the context of creative imagination.

For Czarniawska (2012), organizational anthropology is positioned in business and management research programs, by focusing on analyzing practices in co-evolution with market institutions. In turn, organizational anthropology has reached a stage of maturity focusing on the analysis of organizational theories, based on the emergence of the discipline that provides historical characteristics in the development of theories, traditional and innovative methodologies, and philosophical approaches to organizations and management research. Kunda (1986) and Weeks (2004) state that anthropological journeys establish explicit connections between anthropology and the study of organizations.

In this regard, Fotaki et al. (2020) claim that the analysis of spirituality, symbolism, and storytelling in organization studies are explicitly committed to anthropology. That is, organizational anthropology prioritizes symbolic meanings over more rational thought, makes the human side of the organization relevant and contributes to a holistic perspective of human behavior in organizations (Páramo, 2018; Roca i Girona, 2001). Ultimately, anthropology

Interpretive research in organizational anthropology has an emerging and symbolic role rooted in social processes and without a priori assumptions, with explanations and categories defined by organizational actors (Cely-López, & Gómez-Niño, 2016). The symbolic magical meanings on human rationality lead to show the human side of organizations. On the other hand, the lack of interest of symbolic anthropology in the organizational process is because technocracy is obsessed with efficiency and effectiveness has imposed organizational thinking (Chanlat, 1994).

Anthropology and sociology have the social aspect in common, but differentiating between them is that the anthropological approach makes the concerns of each human group more specific, leading to a better analysis of organizational phenomena such as organizational culture, which goes against the positive approach. Both anthropology and sociology study and analyze human and social issues and concerns in organizations leading to establishing general and universal social laws. However, anthropology is not concerned with the general laws that account for the diversity of human groups manifested in specific characteristics, analyzing social and cultural details, giving them identity and meaning.

The sociology and anthropology of organizations have the social aspect in common, although the latter gives meaning to the cultural and ideological identity specificities of the various groups that build multiple realities (Chanlat, 1994). Anthropological and sociological sensitivity analyzes human beings in contemporary organizations responsible for the future. Anthropology accounts for the social aspect of the diversity of individuals and human groups and studies, searching for the hidden differences that lead to their meaning and characteristics, with emphasis on specificities.

The specialties of organizational anthropology aim to study various aspects of the constitution of the human being. In other words, an organizational anthropology applied in organizational settings is concerned with organized individuals. Well, it focuses on the study horizon of organizations through intervention and research processes to generate new knowledge with the aim of solving social problems. For Thomas Barfield (2000) applied anthropology focuses on solving practical problems, creating guidelines, providing information and taking action, in categories of applied research and intervention.

Consequently, apply the knowledge of organizational anthropology to the different fields of organizational action, focusing on the analysis of the development of organizational life within the sociocultural context; if the researchers are participants, they contribute to the creation of theoretical knowledge. On the other hand, both anthropology and sociology deal with the social aspect of the organization, the universal and general laws of the social considering the positivist aspect. For example, anthropology studies the social organization of societies, language, beliefs, etc., in organizations. Thus, the analysis of organizational anthropology contributes to the study of issues related to the company and entrepreneurs, tools, methods, categories, etc.

The pioneering analysis in organizational and business anthropology was in the analysis of simple societies to complex societies. Business anthropology studies as a social science aim to explain the behavior of elites by addressing theoretical and methodological challenges using anthropological methods and tools to analyze practices and referents of positions of power whose study subjects are marginal subordinates (Cerutti, 2003; Hernández, 2013). In other words, the studies of entrepreneurship under an organizational anthropology had the objective of explaining the behaviors of the elites.

Socio-anthropological sensitivity removes the administration theory from linear causality of action-benefit (Muñoz, 2011) and provides the elements reproducing the logic of the organizational management leading to the agency of financialization of the economy as the protagonist of social creation instead of considering it as a fatality. Administration is supported by anthropology, sociology, psychology, etc. The administrative thought includes the socio-anthropological sensitivity leading to sharpen the vision for sustainable action contextualized and modulated of the dialectic public – private interests.

The organizational factors are analyzed in the analytical theoretical approaches of organizational and administrative anthropology and symbolic interactionism that deal with the categories of environments and organizational contexts that come from the information and confirmation emanating from semi-structured interviews, dimensions and sub dimensions (Cely-López, & Gómez-Niño, 2016).

In this regard, Cely-López & Gómez-Niño (2016) emphasize that organizational anthropology contributes to the administrative process of planning, organization, integration, direction and control; to social accounting that deals with issues related to employees, social community, social responsibility, environmental and ethical issues, etc. For Baba (2012), organizational management structures are supported by social and organizational anthropology to seek effectiveness in private companies and public organizations. In other words, public administration influenced by anthropology has the purpose of humanizing training in organizations.

Anthropological and sociological sensitivity identifies the phenomena and objects of the complexity of human beings who carry organizational collective life. Studies like that of Jamie Uys lead to the theoretical and methodological accumulation of anthropology and organizational sociology. Moreover, although the interaction time to study groups in organizational sociology is shorter and sporadic than in organizational anthropology that is dedicated to an intimate study of the group for a longer period. Institutional time management was able to fulfill the positional functions with advantage to plan from an anthropological perspective of organizations.

Traditional and organizational anthropology link technology to broaden the organizational focus and apply knowledge that contributes to the generation of initiatives for the construction of local and autochthonous meanings. It should be noted that technologies contribute to organizational systems in the creation and promotion of new companies, evaluation of technological intervention projects through the formulation of policies and strategies framed in organizational anthropology, contribute to the creation and capture of value in public-private partnerships, etc.

In this regard, Roberts & Grabowski (1996) state that organizational anthropology analyzes different technologies with emphasis on traditional technologies developed contextually with their own resources, and Western technologies classified as mechanical, human, and knowledge. And it is through the theoretical study through documentary and bibliographical analysis that it is intended to explore the relationships between organizational anthropology and traditional technology as part of the organizational space.

François Auguste Péron, a French naturalist and explorer (1775-1810), coined the term anthropology. In addition, it refers to the science born of the 19th century, which studies man. At present, research on the relationships between anthropology and organizational studies, introducing the theory and management of organizational anthropology, begins in the middle of the last century, anthropology displaced from its traditional core of the object of study based on knowledge. From pre-industrial times and non-industrial communities towards a disciplinary interest in more organizational concerns and problems (Marzal, 1996). It might be worth noting that the development of organizational, labor, and industrial anthropology are interrelated. Moreover, that, as a scientific discipline, anthropology becomes an applied science that is proposed as an applied industrial anthropology to study problems of the anthropology of work and its functional relationship with society, such as the phenomenon of rural migration to urban areas (Esteva, 1984, 1955; Capel, 2009).

The history of organizational anthropology and business organizations in the academic field are complementary developments to the theoretical knowledge in the development of organizational psychology applied to specific practices such as the diversification of products and services. In relation to the above, Harvey (2004) declares that historical reality prompted science and technology to establish the Fordist production system that strengthened the bureaucratic organizational system to control production from the perspective of rationality characterized as instrumental by the perspective criticism.

For authors such as Corsín Jiménez (2007), Caulkins, & Ann (2013) and North & Gita (2014), organizational studies require new concepts, approaches and technologies such as organizational and management anthropology, creative and knowledge management, etc..., conducive to personal and social development. A review of organization theory and organizational studies and their different approaches and relationships with anthropology highlights the anthropological perspective that leads to the humanistic aspect of organizations.

Organizational anthropology was established in 1927 with the Western Electric Company project, at industrial plants in Hawthorne, Chicago, as a scientific discipline led by sociologist and industrial psychologist Elton Mayo of the Harvard Business School. And it is related to the school of administration called neo-human relations or human resources created and developed by the same psychologist with his research in the Hawthorne plants between 1927 and 1932 (Chanlat, 2019; Roca i Girona, 2001).

Mayo's interest was to study workers' job satisfaction from the socio-psychological perspective. Authors such as Malinowski (1944), Radcliffe-Brown (1952) and Lloyd Warner (1952) participated in this project, laying the foundations of the theory of organizational anthropology. Considering the latter as the father of organizational anthropology for the work carried out as an ethnologist and sociologist (Bélanger and LeBlanc, 2011). The studies and analyses built from organizational anthropology contribute to clarify the differences between the referents to support arguments and solve problems that arise between management and workers. In addition, organizational anthropology includes questions and issues related to the welfare of workers assumed as political development organizations.

Based on experiments with the workforce and its productivity, Mayo develops industrial psychology to support the human dimension of organizations, a milestone that marks the beginning of organizational anthropology. Organizational anthropology demonstrated that job satisfaction and worker productivity are determined by their human relationships developed by the contribution of anthropological, ethnographic and participant observation techniques (Richardson 1955). Given the concept of organizational anthropology, organizations train internally for the productivity, motivation and training of members to create and develop an identity based on organizational capacity.

Organizational anthropology topics began to gain relevance from the famous Hawthorne research project and later with the Society Applied Anthropology research; giving rise to the Applied Anthropology Journal renamed Human Organization (Santibáñez, 1994). This emerged in the early 1950s as an expected priority in organizational research interrupted by the crisis in the human relations school that led to the adoption of the managerial perspective. Caudill (1958) carried out the first anthropological studies in a psychiatric hospital.

Munizaga (1988) carried out the first organizational anthropology. During the 1970s, organizational anthropology presented unfavorable academic and scientific production, struggled to become institutionalized and implementing programs to train organizational anthropologists, to study processes of organizational work dynamics, transculturation in organizational fields, social development, etc.

Organizational anthropology was established as a social science discipline based on ethnographic research methodologies during the 1980s (Bate, 1997) with the aim of studying and analyzing the nature and functioning of public and private organizations. Some classics in the business anthropology literature are Holzberg and Maureen (1981), Pérez-Lizaur (2010), Basaldúa (2005) and Urban and Koh (2013).

Year's later, organizational anthropology became a subdiscipline in management research, focusing on working conditions, the burden of work and schedules, the management of organizational processes, etc. Among the new knowledge interests attract the development of the disciplines of organizational and management anthropology, knowledge management and creativity aimed at promoting the formation of people development, creating skills and relationships between personality and the socio-ecological system including society and nature. Organizational anthropology carries out the organizational analysis of the development of organizational management.

The perspectives of organizational psychology in the analysis of organizational behavior are thought more as dysfunctional behaviors, fears and dilemmas, etc., to be addressed as problems and options to strategically position consistently to deal with anthropology for management. While anthropology contributes to satisfy the management needs and demands of organizations, giving rise to organizational anthropology from the management perspective, methods, tools and instruments for management. In other words, organizational anthropology should contribute to designing and developing managerial tools and instruments for the analysis of the organization.

The orientation of organizational anthropology towards the managerialist approach distances itself from the humanist approach that leads to practical application outside of the tensions between labor and capital, prioritizing the maximization of benefits and profitability. The relationships between both disciplines, anthropology and organizations, are a consequence of the interactions found in the management of behavioral limits to make potential contributions to learn and apply on issues of people's well-being aligned with capital and work.

Organizational anthropology broadens the interactions between individuals and the complicated social environment exerting the impact of human formation, care and respect for people. Therefore, the organizational anthropology approach is complementary to the organizational approach to assess job competencies by producing different types of information and data than if only one were used.

Concerning the instrumental conception of the human being, Chanlat (1994) describes it as manipulative, although other anthropologists maintain that organizational behavior has been strengthened with homo economicus as the dominant conception. It is precisely because of these differences that the categories of the economic model endorsed to understand the characterization of symbolic, mythical, magical, normative and religious phenomena, of organizational life and family affairs that can coexist simultaneously. Where the focus of the anthropological organization in the selection of personnel alleviates some of the problems.

In other words, an anthropological approach to organizations contributes to expanding and complementing knowledge in talent management. For this reason, practical organizational anthropology serves management in the management of knowledge of the specific problems of organizations from the theoretical and methodological frameworks of anthropology and anthropological techniques. What makes them necessary for organizational development.

Anthropological organizational facilitation is the professional external intervention aimed at improving the institutional management practices of the actors who pursue their own objectives based on the concepts and objects of study of organizational anthropology, such as the construction of alterity and reflexivity. Moreover, it is assigned as a function of organizational management urging higher education institutions to prepare knowledge.

From an organizational anthropology perspective with a specific contribution to organizational facilitation through a reconversion of ways of positioning in the face of problems. There is participatory action in social processes, collective actions with specific formal and informal purposes. Participatory and facilitation processes as transfer instruments are methodological challenges that present themselves as opportunities and difficulties to situate non-traditional actions as objects of organizational anthropology from different asymmetric rationalities. These challenges must be addressed in accordance with the anthropological contribution of methodological principles to facilitation and organizational participation aimed at creating and changing the organizational and management culture.

Reflections on management practices lead the framework of organizational anthropology to the point of becoming a discipline in organizational studies. This alternative must be included in the academic questions and concerns strategically position itself in the theoretical and practical deepening of an anthropology for management. The theoretical framework of organizational anthropology and the referents involved have a place in the anthropology of practice. Well, the practice of anthropology in organizational dynamics confronts processes between management and workers in order to change the methodological approach, affecting the entire human being inscribed in organizational behavior, demanding commitment and responsibility with oneself.

Social anthropology studies social relationships and structures. The analysis from the social anthropology of the family, the businessperson and the company are linked actors. Studies on simple societies in anthropology analyze the kinship systems of society, such as the case of Lebanese businesspersons in southeastern Mexico (Ramírez Carrillo, 1992), the determinants of the family pattern of businesspersons (Nader, 1972) in a comparative analysis. Practice for social agents applying anthropological imagination (Gravano, 1995) and the case method in organizational management in institutions, organizations and movements.

Organizational anthropology studies of organizations, entrepreneurship and the family refer to the family-organization. The family and the company from the perspective of anthropology is resolved around analyzing the articulation of the company and the labor participation of the family members and the relationships established between them and pointing to issues related to the members of the family. Family who are workers and owners at the same time in organizations. An analysis from the social anthropology of the family business is a business domestic unit that emphasizes the functions of the family as a primary network. Organizational anthropology firms equate the family as the domestic unit of members who contribute relationships, resources, practices, etc.

The field of social management through the anthropology of organizations contributes to build the options, including the relevant methodological and ideological ones. Organizational anthropology seeks to describe and analyze the structuring of social relationships at work, presentation and body appearance, duration, forms of commitment, experiences, new spaces and times, and other elements in the management of organizations.

Mexican anthropology, like the Manchester School of Anthropology, tries to overcome the prejudice of the managerial approach of organizational anthropology. Regarding the above, the organizational crisis coincided with the emergence of the Manchester School in organizational anthropology influenced by Gluckman (1940) on the research carried out on industrial organizations, including participant observation that led to the contradiction of harmony in the work proposed by the School of Human Resources, the social fit situations from a broader structure. Where the link between two organizations, the economic unit and the domestic unit, expands that family in the analysis of social networks characterized as a structure and represented by individuals or other networks since 1960 according to García and Oliveira.

Mexican anthropology has recent origins, but it has obtained a high impact and scope in economic, social, political and cultural achievements. Anthropological studies in Mexico originated with the colonization process in the 16th century followed by social and cultural contradictions in the need to describe and interpret indigenous cultures. In the independent Mexico of the 19th century, anthropology focused on issues and concerns related to the interpretation of the existing social reality in search of a common identity, creating a stable and strong state and the origin of the professionalization of anthropology.

At the beginning of the 19th century, physical anthropology and ethnology began in Mexico. Moreover, with this at the end of the same century, the development of empirically applied organizational anthropology begins, articulating work niches, although professional practice is more related to management actions of academic institutions. In 1910, the National School of American Archeology and Ethnology was founded, introducing the paradigm of indigenous anthropology with Manuel Gamio, becoming one of the lasting currents of anthropological thought (González, 2003; Villanueva, Serrano & Vera, 1999; Matos, 1987). . In this, themes such as the issues, problems and concerns of applied anthropology in Mexico aimed at recovering national identity and local history revolving around the analysis to understand one's own were developed.

In the 1920s and 1930s, the integrationist conception of anthropology was formed, called New Anthropology committed to nationalist interests with the teaching of anthropology in the academic programs of the National Polytechnic Institute and the National School of Anthropology and History (Olive, 1987). In which the traditional limits of anthropology as a discipline focused on the study of social groups such as peasants, migrants, workers, etc., during the 1970s, complementing the Mexican anthropology carried out by Esteban Krotz (1993) and García &Krotz. (1988) with an emphasis on the cultural heritage of the national state.

Marxist theory and critical perspective have a strong influence on the theoretical framework that supports the development of Mexican anthropology. While critical organizational studies are inspired by anthropology, it has not been credited that, the contributions remain implicit and elusive, revealing an incomplete story (Mir &Fayard, 2021). However, anthropological criticality contributes the focus on the dynamics of power and front, and its empirical focus on managerial practices in the contexts of indigenous organizations and informal settings. In turn, the contributions of the organizational anthropological approach complement feminist economies by making unpaid domestic work visible (Domínguez Forgueras, 2019).

In correspondence with the above, Roca i Girona (2001) indicates that the study of anthropology in organizations is considered more complex for anthropologists because they are implicitly under criticism for being involved in a contractual relationship for a salary in exchange for work. Nonetheless, despite organizational anthropology's imperfections in organizational studies that are characterized by the potential for opportunities for further cross-fertilization and scholarly scrutiny. This approach should focus on the organizational sciences that can benefit from organizational anthropology and ethnography as a method (Bate, 1997).

Latin American organizations and work situations are a laboratory of organizational anthropology aimed at researching, analyzing, formulating and applying policies in public and private formal structured organizations (Bermúdez, 2017). Well, the organizational anthropological production in Latin America is at the beginning of a dialogue and discussion based on the differences between history, regions, ethnic groups and other specificities of methodologies, research practices, convergences and detected differences.

In addition, organizational anthropology is an interdisciplinary professional whose specificity begins to develop by focusing on the design of an integral model considering the neighborhood as a symbol, and the semiotic mechanisms established in the construction of meaning. Hence, the anthropology consultancy of organizations needs a global and more objective tool capable of shortening the time to develop field research for comprehensive results with an emphasis on organizational analysis.

Gravano (1992) describes organizational anthropology as the intervention and facilitation of organizational processes using methodological tools that are not necessarily applied and practical anthropology for the implementation of listening, interpolation, objectification and transfer caused by the practices of the participants to make decisions about actions to achieve effectiveness. Likewise, Cely-López & Gómez-Niño (2016) affirm that organizational anthropology ventures into the analysis of behaviors, values, beliefs, customs in all organizational practices and activities related to work life, lifestyles, human development, education and training, etc. That is to say, trends in educational disciplines are aimed at sharing knowledge on organizational anthropology assigned as a separate subject on administrative, cultural and social anthropology.

To summarize, the agency of people and social movements in social structures is the new current in anthropological studies to reveal dynamic changes with the commitment to explain integration processes through research.

Organizational Ethnography

Organizational anthropology and organizational sociology are privileged in the referential framework of management by the methods of ethnography and ethnology to carry out research on their respective objects of study tending to acquire useful anthropological and sociological sensitivity to organizational administration and management. The ethnography of sociocultural anthropology in organizational contexts supports problem solving and provides theoretical-conceptual elements of organizational anthropology oriented to the analysis of behaviors and institutional relationships.

Organizational anthropology and ethnography offer a theoretical and conceptual framework and practical tools for studying and analyzing organizational functions, practices, activities, processes, and relationships. In the words of Bate (1997), organizational anthropology is a discipline that uses ethnographic research methodologies aimed at analyzing the nature and functioning of organizations as an object of study established since the 1980s. For its part, ethnography is the technique most representative anthropological and ethnographic research aimed at understanding and holistic observation of the system of phenomena and organizational behavior through the description of the elements that interact (Hammersley & Atkinson, 2007).

Therefore, organizational ethnography is the application of methodological techniques developed by anthropologists Malinowski and Radcliffe Brown. Thus, organizational anthropology and ethnography have become relevant in the use of methodological insights into organizational and management theory and research. Therefore, organizational ethnography and anthropological studies have created the field of organizational behavior by taking it into a separate field and losing touch with the essential qualities of anthropology. Anthropology remains the forgotten science in organizational studies (Bate, 1997).

There is a growing interest in the ethnographic methodology used in organizational anthropology to be applied in a formal and structural way in organizations, policies and public and private structures such as associations, companies and cooperatives. The anthropological reflexivity of organizations conceives ethnography to investigate and implement intervention processes capable of facilitating the understanding of behaviors and practices to record the voice of the voiceless.

The writing of anthropological ethnographies of organizations is distinguished from organizational science. Regarding the above, Van Maanen (1987) indicates that the influence of research is reflected in organizational anthropology and organizational ethnography. In addition, Turco (2016) and Anteby (2013) consider organizational ethnography as fertile in anthropological research in organizational and management studies in the use of ethnographic methods as indicated by Barley (1986) and Orlikowski (2002), in sharing meanings in organizational communities (Bechky (2003).

Hawthorne's study evidences the anthropological approach to the study of culture using the ethnological method applied by Warner under the direction of Mayo to the analysis of the human side of the organization in a group of workers as a small society. It should be noted that Mayo's ethnographic work is a practical approach to the study of human problems and behaviors in organizations, which supports important contributions to organizations such as objective observation, the participatory method, the social group, etc.

Organizational ethnographies contribute to theoretical development. It also improves organizations and businesses by resorting to the study of anthropology to collect the information that big data is not capable of obtaining to understand people's life patterns (Lebeau, 2017). In relation to the ethnographic approach to organizational improvement, it was nourished by a dialectical-institutional project towards a conflict theory model centered on contradiction and negativity (Lourau, 1979).

Organizational anthropology studies began with tools and methodologies developed by traditional ethnography, which have been criticized by Roca i Girona (2001), as poorly defined and as the result of heresy or contradiction.

On the other hand, the new tools of organizational ethnography and anthropology today represent the foundations for theoretical empirical research in the economic atmosphere to analyze patterns, perspectives, and rhythms of organizational life incorporated into mainstream organizational research.

Lastly, the ethnographic study of gender politics in the global movement like the published work on para-ethnography in business organizations making gender equality policies by Fisher, (2012a, b), remains an organizational research challenge.

Conclusion

The objective of the study was to analyze some of the theoretical, conceptual and methodological implications and contributions between organizational anthropology and ethnography, based on the assumption that the ethnographic analysis of organizations and interpretative research on organizational anthropology have an emerging and symbolic role. Rooted in social processes and without a priori assumptions, with explanations and categories defined by organizational actors. The analysis concludes that the ethnographic methodology is pertinent to be used in the analysis of its interactions with organizational anthropology as a new specialty in organizational studies.

The anthropological contribution to organizational studies highlights the human dimension, allowing for individual understanding and contextual meaning. In addition, organizational anthropology has contributed to the advancement of organizational studies, the company, business, management and business anthropology. The main contributions of organizational anthropology are academics and professionals who complement each other in organizational analysis to clarify the vision of organizations and apply them to specific products and services under new paradigms.

Organizational anthropology studies reality over time while contributing to the development of more humane organizations and improved social skills in management. (Greater coherence). Likewise, it analyzes the reality of social behavior to capture the integral and general character of organizational social life. In short, it rescues the dimensions of the human being, relying on anthropological tools to study and analyze the specific details of human groups as the dimensions of being in the organizational phenomenon.

Recommendations

The construction of a conceptual framework of organizational anthropology to study and analyze the phenomenon in theoretical depth supported by widespread methodological contributions to give meaning to organizational studies. This organizational anthropological conceptual framework must be put into practice and applied to organizational management issues.

In the anthropological organization, knowledge transmission processes and events using ethnographic methods require a lot of time to be considered as a laboratory for organizational anthropology. What makes it necessary to incorporate anthropological components such as artifacts and processes full of meanings to structure organizational transformations that facilitate the creation, transmission and reproduction of knowledge. Hence, its usefulness, since organizational, business, corporate or industrial anthropology is characterized by an ethnographic approach focused on shared meanings that include spiritual and material manifestations.

For their part, higher education institutions should promote the humanization of management by supporting new concepts, technologies and approaches to influence self-development and social development. In other words, the new fields of knowledge are organizational anthropology, knowledge, and creative management that contribute to human formation, the development of social relationships, and creative abilities.

Finally, the anthropology of organizations contributes to the study that allows deepening, detailing and revealing the basic individual dimensions of the human being. That is, the dimensions of the human being that account for the human side of organizations are anthropological contributions to the analysis of human behavior in the context of organizational studies. For example, a research object is the analysis of organizational anthropology related to traditional technology as a space for reflection to generate future research.

References

Alvesson, M. and Berg, P. O. (1992). *Corporate culture and organizational symbolism: An overview*. Berlin: Walter de Gruyter.

Anteby, M. (2013). *Manufacturing morals: The values of silence in business school education*. Chicago, IL: University of Chicago Press.

Baba, M. (2012). Anthropology and Business: Influence and Interests. *Journal of Business Anthropology*, 1(1), 20-71.

Baer, D. (27 de marzo de 2014). Business Insider. Recuperado de https://www.businessinsider.com/heres-why-companies-aredesperatetohireanthropologists-2014-3

Barfield, T. (Ed.). (2000). *Diccionario de Antropología*. México: Siglo XXI Editores.

Barley, S. R. (1986). Technology as an occasion for structuring: evidence from observations of CT scanners and the social order of radiology departments, *Administrative Science Quarterly*, Vol. 31 No. 1, pp. 78-108.

Bate, S. P. (1997). Whatever happened to organizational anthropology? A review of the field of organizational ethnography and anthropological studies. *Human Relations*, 50 (9), 1147–1175. https://doi.org/10.1177/001872679705000905.

Basaldúa, M. (2005) Los empresarios de la compañía industrial cerillera de san Juan del Rio: Antropología de la industria cerillera. Tesis de doctorado en antropología s/p Universidad Iberoamericana. México.

Bechky, B. A. (2003). Sharing meaning across occupational communities: The transformation of understanding on a production floor. *Organization Science*, 14(3), 312–330.

Bélanger, A. et LeBlanc, M-N. (2011). Socio-anthropologie de la culture populaire. *Séminaire de Doctorat en sociologie*. SOC 9004-40. Montréal: Université du Québec à Montréal (UQÀM). [inédito].

Berg, P. O. and Faucheux. C. (1982). *The Symbolic Management of Company Cultures*. Unpublished book manuscript, INSEAD, Fontainebleau,

Bermúdez, H. L. (2017). Sociology and Anthropology in administrator training. In Forum Doctoral (No. 7, pp. 27-27).

Caudill, W. (1958). Some Uses of Anthropology: Theoretical and Applied. *American Anthropologist New Series*, Vol. 60, No. 4 (Aug., 1958), pp. 762-764 (3 pages).

Caulkins, D. D., & Ann, J. (2013). *Companion to Organizational Anthropology*. England: Blackwell Publishing.

Caulkins, D., & Jordan, A. T. (eds.) (2013). *A Companion to Organizational Anthropology*. Chichester: Wiley-Blackwell.

Chanlat, J. F. (2019). *Antropología de las organizaciones*. Revista del Centro de Estudios de Sociología del Trabajo (11), pp. 17-39.

Chanlat, J. (1994). *Hacia una antropología de la organización. En Gestión y política pública*, Vol. III, núm. 2, segundo semestre, pp. 317-364, México.

Cely-López, C. L., & Gómez-Niño, O. (2016). An anthropological perspective of organizations from sociocultural characterization, management, and social accounting. The case of a tertiaryeducationinstitution. *Cuadernos de Contabilidad*, 17(43). 184 / vol. 17 / no. 43 / enero-junio 2.

Cerutti, M. (2003) Los estudios empresariales en América Latina ¿el debate interminable?.Boletín de Historia Económica, año 1, 2, junio. México. (Pp 3-9). Disponible en: http://www.audhe.org.uy/Boletin_Audhe/Boletin_2/Boletin_02_Cerutti.pdf.

Corsín Jiménez, A. (2007). The Anthropology of Organizations. England: Ashgate Publishing Limited.

Czarniawska, B. (2012). Organization theory meets anthropology: A story of an encounter. *Journal of Business Anthropology,* 1 (1), 118–140.

Domínguez Folgueras, M. (2019). ¿Cuánto vale el trabajo doméstico en España? Observatorio Social de La Caixa. Accedido 11 de enero de 2020. https://bit.ly/2Rmnhyg.

Esteva Frabegat, C. (1984) [1973]. *Antropología industrial.* Barcelona: Anthropos

Esteva Fabregat, C. (1955). Carácter social y familia obrera en México. Tesis de Maestría en etnología, presentada en la Escuela de Antropología e Historia de México.

Fisher, M. (2012a), Wall Street Women, Duke University Press, Durham, North Carolina. Fisher, M. (2012b), Toward a feminist para-ethnography on gender equality policy making in business, *Collaborative Anthropologies,* Vol. 5.

Fotaki, M., Altman, Y., & Koning, J. (2020). Spirituality, symbolism, and storytelling in twentyfirst-century organizations: Understanding and addressing the crisis of imagination. *Organization Studies*, 41 (1), 7–30.

García Canclini, N. 1982: *Las Culturas Populares en el capitalismo.* Nueva Imagen, México.

García Mora, C. &Krotz, E. (1988). *La antropología en México: panorama histórico.* Vol. 9. México: Instituto Nacional de Antropología e Historia.

Garsten, Ch., & Anette, N. (2013). *Organizational Anthropology: Doing Ethnography in and Among Complex Organizations.* London: Pluto Press.

Gluckman, M. (1940) Analysis of a Social Situation in Zululand, ManchesterManchester University.

Gonnet, J. (junio de 2012). Cultura, organizaciones y antropología. Una revisión crítica. Avá. Revista de Antropología (21), pp. 151-170. Recuperado de http://www.redalyc.org/articulo.oa?id=16903026800.

Gonzàlez Gamio, A. (2003). Manuel Gamio: una lucha sin final. México: Universidad Nacional Autónoma de México.

Gravano, A. (1995). La imaginación antropológica; interpelaciones a la otredad construida y al método antropológico. *Publicar en Antropología y Ciencias Sociales.* 5: 71-91.

Gravano, A. (1992). Antropología Práctica, muestra y posibilidades de la Antropología Organizacional. *Publicar en Antropología y Ciencias Sociales*, Buenos Aires, n. 1, p. 95-126, 1992.

Hammersley, M. & Atkinson, P. (2007). *Ethnography.* NY: Routledge.

Harvey, D. (2004). La condición de la posmodernidad. Amorrortu editores.

Hernández, V. (2013) Genealogía de una elite rural: elucidación antropológica de una práctica de poder. Mundo Agrario, vol. 13, nº 26, junio. Argentina. Disponible en: https://www.redalyc.org/pdf/845/84527468004.pdf.

Holzberg, C. y Maureen, G. (1981) Anthropology and Industry reappraisal and new directions. Ann. Review of Anthropology vol 10. Estados Unidos. (Pp. 317-360). https://doi.org/10.1146/annurev.an.10.100181.001533.

Jaumier S (2020) Why does the study of alternative organizations (so badly) need anthropology? In: Mir R and Fayard A. L. (eds) *The Routledge Companion to Anthropology and Business.* Pp. 414-432. New York: Routledge. doi:- 10.4324/9781003052456-22.

Jordan, A. (2013). *Bussines Anthropology.* Waveland Press, Inc.

Kottak, C. P. (2011). *Antropología cultural.* México: McGrawHill.

Krotz, E. (1993). Antropología y antropólogos en México: elementos de balance para construir perspectivas: (pp. 361-380). En: Balance de la Antropología en América Latina y el Caribe Universidad Nacional Autónoma de México. México.

Kunda, G. (1986). *Engineering culture: Control and commitment in a high-tech corporation.* Philadelphia, PA: Temple University Press.

Lomnitz, L. (1975). *Anthropology of scientific research at UNAM, in Science and Development 6.* Mexico: CONACYT

Lourau, R. (1979). *El análisis institucional.* Buenos Aires: Amorrortu.

Lebeau, S. (24 de julio de 2017). *Minnesota Business.* Recuperado de https://www.minnesotabusiness.com/anthropology-business.

Llobera, J. (Comp.): *La antropología como ciencia.* Madrid: Anagrama, 1975.

Maestre Alfonso, J. (1983). *Introducción a la Antropología social.* Madrid, Akla.

Malinowski, B. (1944). *A scientific theory of culture and other essays*. University of North Carolina Press.
Marzal, M. M. (1996). Historia de la anthropologìa. Volume I. Anthropologìaindìgena. Ediciones Abya-Yala.
Matos Moctezuma, E. (1987). Román Piña Chan y la Escuela Nacional de Antropología e Historia: (pp. 81-90). En: *Homenaje a Román Piña Chan Universidad Nacional Autónoma de México* – Instituto de Investigaciones Antropológicas. México.
Menéndez, E. (2006). Participación social en salud: las representaciones y las prácticas. In: Menéndez, E.; Spinelli, H.: *Participación social ¿para qué? Buenos Aires: Lugar Editorial*, 2006. p. 81-115.
Menéndez, E. (1996). *Fundamentals of economics*. Buenos Aires.
Mills, W. (1961). *La imaginación sociológica*. México: Fondo de Cultura Económica, 1961.
Mir, R., &Fayard, A.-L. (2021): Anthropology and organizational studies: A symbiotic connection. In: R. Mir & A. L. Fayard (eds.) *The Routledge Companion to Anthropology and Business*. New York: Routledge, 1–13.
Morales Inga, S., & Tristán, O. M. (2018). Capturando la cultura: tres aportes de la antropología a la selección de personal. *Palermo Business Review*, (18), 261-280.
Munizaga B., J. (1988). La violencia doméstica y la sociedad. *Revista De Sociología*, (3), 35–43. https://doi.org/10.5354/0719-529X.1988.27565.
Muñoz, R. (2011). Formar en administración. Por una nueva fundamentación filosófica. *Bogotá: Siglo del Hombre*. Fondo Editorial Universidad EAFIT.
Nader, L. (1972) Up me anthropologist: perspectives gained from studying up, mimeo, 28p. Disponible en: https://files.eric.ed.gov/fulltext/ED065375.pdf.
North, K., & Gita, K. (2014). *Knowledge Management. Value Creation through Organizational Learning*. New York: Springer International Publishing
Olive Negrete, J. C. (1981). Antropología Mexicana. México: Plaza y Valdés – *Instituto Nacional de Antropología e Historia* – Colegio Mexicano de Antropólogos.
Orlikowski, W. J. (2002). Knowing in practice: Enacting a collective capability in distributed organizing. *Organization Science, 13*(3), 249–273.
Páramo, D. (2018). Antropología organizacional. *Revista científica Pensamiento y Gestión*, 1(45).
Pérez-Lizaur, M. comp. (2010) *Empresa y Familia en México, una visión desde la antropología*. Universidad Iberoamericana, México.
Radcliffe-Brown, A. (1952). *Structure and Function in Primitive Societv*. London: Oxford Univ. Press.
Ramírez Carrillo, L. (1992) Estratificación, clase y parentesco: empresarios libaneses en el sureste de México. *Nueva Antropología,* vol XIII no 43. México. (Pp. 123). Disponible en: https://www.redalyc.org/pdf/159/15904311.pdf.
Richardson, F. (1955). Anthropology and Human Relations in Business and Industry. *Yearbook of Anthropology,* pp. 397-419. Recuperado de http://www.jstor.org/stable/3031158.
Roberts, K., & Grabowski, M. (1996). Organizations, Technology and Structuring. En S. Clegg, C. Hardy & W. Nord, *Handbook of Organization Studies* (pp. 409-423). Sage.
Roca i Girona J. (2001) Antropólogos en la empresa? A propósito de la mal llamada cultura de la empresa. Etnográfica, Vol. 1. Colombia. (Pp. 69-99). Disponible en: http://ceas.iscte.pt/etnografica/docs/vol_05/N1/Vol_v_N1_69-100.pdf.
Roca, J. (1998). *Antropologia Industrial y de la Empresa*. Barcelona: Ariel
Santibáñez, D. (1994) Una aproximación sistémico- cultural a la organización com unitaria Memoria para optar al título profesional de Antropólogo social, Universidad de Chile, Santiago.
Smirnova, V. (2016). *Organizational culture.* Moscow: Yurayt Publishing, p. 42-43.
Turco, C. J. (2016). *The conversational firm: Rethinking bureaucracy in the age of social media*. New York: Columbia University Press.
Urban, G. & Koh, K. (2013) Ethnographic research on modern business corporation. *Annual Review Anthropology*, vol 42. Estados Unidos. (Pp 139-158).: https://doi.org/10.11.
Van Maanen, J. (1987). *Tales of the field: On writing ethnography*. Chicago, IL: University of Chicago.
Villanueva, M.; Serrano, C. & Vera, J. L. (1999). Cien años de antropología física en México: inventario Bibliográfico. México: Universidad Nacional Autónoma de México – Instituto de Investigaciones Antropológicas.
Warner, W. L. (1952). *Structure of American Life*. Edinburgh University Press.

Weeks, J. (2004). *Unpopular culture: The ritual of complaint in a British bank*. Chicago, IL: University of Chicago Press.

Chapter 8

Psychoacoustics and Perception: Delivering Healthy and Sustainable Acoustic Environments

Laura de Azcárate[1,*]
and Ana Mombiedro[2]

[1]Architectural Association School of Architecture, Environmental and Technical Studies Department, Lecturer/Design tutor in Architecture and Acoustic Design, London, UK
[2]University of Alicante, Neuroarchitecture Masters coordinator, Alicante, Spain

Abstract

Human behavior is directly related to the appropriate use of the space, as space functionality and comfort are a "call" to the user in Architecture. Neuroscience and Architecture are connected through emotions, space, and body. Human behavior can change drastically when encountering acoustic problems once inhabiting the space. Acoustics can compensate for many factors that other disciplines cannot address at a particular milestone in the design process. (e.g., Speech intelligibility can be compromised when natural ventilation is required due to the external noise ingress. The designer should take advantage of decoration and interior design arrangements to improve sound insulation between rooms or most appropriate reverberation time values in a room. Hence, acoustic design is fundamental to the quality of buildings. The same way noise can be defined as "unwanted sound," pleasant sounds help create a sense of well-being (Music can be used to treat pathologies). Psychoacoustics explains how the human auditory system perceives sounds, as sound affects us both physiologically and psychologically. Stress and health problems are consequences of inappropriate design decisions and can be alarming for different project typologies. Noise can increase heart rate, blood pressure, respiration rate and even blood cholesterol levels. Once key health outcomes associated with environmental noise are identified, their relevance can be rated for assessing environmental noise issues. The use of biomaterials in architecture has a relevant impact on the environment throughout the life cycle of the buildings, but also Bioconstruction, as a new technique, influences people's health. Toxic chemicals released by materials can lead to inhalation, ingestion, dermal absorption producing cancer, asthma, or other diseases. New resources for designers are necessary to make healthier places for all people to live. Bio acoustics influences auditory perception and health. Good acoustic conditions delivered

* Corresponding Author's Email: lauradeazcarate@gmail.com

In: Psycho-Environmental Variables That Ensure People's Well-Being and Health …
Editors: Roberto Alonso González Lezcano and Guadalupe Cantarero García
ISBN: 979-8-89530-831-8

© 2025 Nova Science Publishers, Inc.

along with bio-construction techniques are key to healing and successful treatments, as well as resolving office or educational noise distraction or stress.

Keywords: comfort, neuroscience, human behavior, acoustic design, psychoacoustics, health, bio-construction, bio-materials, bio-acoustics, perception, well-being

Introduction

This chapter aims to gain insight into the relationship between Subjective perception, psychoacoustics and neuroarchitecture.

Analytical Framework

Subjective Acoustics from Auditory Perception

Subjective acoustics and auditory perception play an important role in comfort and well-being. Through cognition humans tend to perceive, recognize, and conceive. This mechanism allows us to interact with the surrounding space that creates emotions and hence, affects human behavior inside buildings. Perception is the ability to interpret information received by our different senses from the environment. This is an active process that depends on our cognitive process and prior knowledge. Auditory perception could be defined as the ability to receive and interpret information that reached the ears through audible frequency waves (Lebowitz, Dams-O'Connor and Cantor 2012).

Auditory perception is a multi-step process:

1. Detection: if the sound has enough intensity and is within an audible range, it will reach the ears and brain will be able to extract some information (position of the sound source, movement…)
2. Discrimination: differentiation between background noise and a particular sound
3. Recognition; sound localization, and differentiation (voice…)
4. Comprehension: understanding of the sound we hear means decoding a message

The world of acoustics allows us to have two different visions from reality, which can be either objective or subjective. Noise is perceived as "unwanted sound" (Namba. 1987). The same scene can be perceived as positive or negative just by the nature of its content and situation (e.g., a rock concert can be pleasant despite its high sound pressure levels). Sounds are complex with rapidly changing complex vibration, and human hearing exhibits non-linear characteristics that simplify the information and conclude on a human response to stimuli, which makes them the final arbiters of an acoustic environment.

The human hearing system has an average frequency range of 20-20.000Hz. (Figure 1) however this can vary between individuals. This frequency range changes because of a normal aging process (the upper limit tends to reduce), as well as a decline in hearing sensitivity at all frequencies (Howard y Angus 2013).

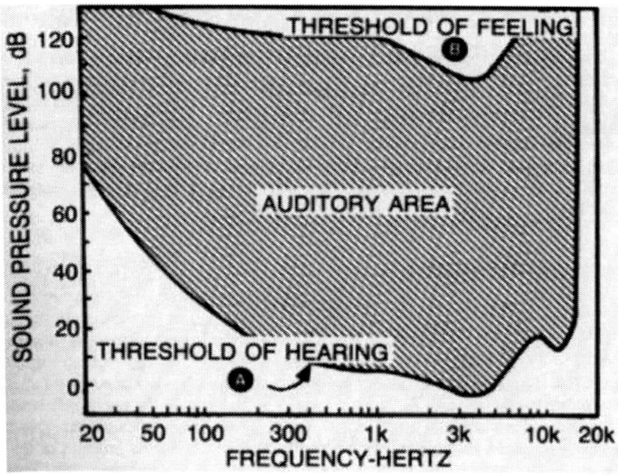

Figure 1. Human hearing system average auditory area.

In order to predict noise effects on people, it is necessary to know the relationship between subjective attributes and physical characteristics of noise. While analyzing acoustic perception we can describe the four central quantities or dimensions of psychoacoustics, which according to (Pulkki y Karjalainen 16/01/2015) are the "basic quantities of sound measured by the hearing system "pitch, loudness, timbre, and subjective duration (Table 1). Identifying these basic quantities is the first step in recognizing different types of sounds, such as speech, natural sounds, and musical instrument sounds.

Table 1. The four central quantities or dimensions of psychoacoustics (Pulkki y Karjalainen 16/01/2015)

PSYCHOACOUSTIC PARAMETER	PHYSICAL PARAMETER
Pitch	Frequency
Loudness	Level (intensity)
Timbre	Magnitude spectrum
Duration	Time

The theory describing loudness perception is one of the central theories of psychoacoustics. Although the perceived loudness of an acoustic sound is related to its amplitude, there is not a simple one -to-one functional relationship. As a psychoacoustic effect it is affected by both the context and nature of the sound, and it is difficult to measure because its dependent on the interpretation by listeners of what they hear (Howard y Angus 2013) (Table 2).

Psychoacoustic Parameters

From a subjective point of view, we could describe some parameters that define how a human perceive sound:

Loudness

Loudness is the subjective intensity of sound, independent of any meaning of the sound (Kryte 1970). When sound is very loud, it easily becomes unwanted, noisy, and annoying, disturbs conversation, and causes temporary threshold shift (TTS). If the sound is not loud, it usually has no serious effect on most people. (Namba. 1987) Findings in Psychophysical experiments may be influenced by the judgment methods used (categorical judgment, magnitude estimation, etc.) and the types of stimuli (pure tones, complex sounds, artificial sounds, actual sounds, etc.)

Table 2. Typical sound levels in the environment (Howard y Angus 2013)

EXAMPLE SOUND/SITUATION	DB (SPL)	DESCRIPTION
Long range gunfire at gunner's ear	140	Ouch
Threshold of pain	130	
Jet take-off at approximately 100m	120	
Peak levels on a night club dance floor	110	Very noisy
Loud shout at 1m	100	
Heavy truck at about 10m	90	
Heavy car traffic at about 10m	80	Noisy
Car interior	70	
Normal conversation at 1m	60	
Office noise level	50	Quiet
Living room in a quiet area	40	
Bedroom at nighttime	30	
Empty concert hall	20	Just audible
Gentle breeze through leaves	10	
Threshold of hearing for a child	0	

Four psychological/physical relations contribute to loudness (Meunier, Van Eeckhoutte y Moore 2021)

1. The intensity level required to make each tone or frequency appear equally loud subjectively.
2. The time required to achieve a stable perception of loudness (critical summation time)
3. The growth of loudness as the bandwidth widens.
4. The growth of loudness as the intensity increases

Attribute	Concept	Major factors	
Loudness	Subjective intensity	Steady physical factors	· Sound energy · Frequency
Noisiness	Unwantedness by auditory factors	Non-steady physical factors	· Duration · Spectal complexity Tone components · Temporal complexity Intermittency Impulsiveness
Annoyance	Unwantedness by non-auditory factors	Non-physical factors	· Meaning of sound · Personality & liking · Adaptation · Situation · Relation to source

Figure 2. Factors affecting Loudness, noisiness, and annoyance (Namba. 1987).

Primary acoustic factors	Sound level Frequency Duration
Secondary acoustic factors	Spectral complexity Fluctuations in sound level Fluctuations in frequency Rise-time of the noise Localization of noise source
Nonacoustic factors	Physiology Adaptation and past experience How the listener's activity affects annoyance Predictability of when a noise will occur Is the noise necessary? Individual differences and personality

Figure 3. Factors that affect individual annoyance to noise (Namba. 1987).

Time is a crucial variable when differentiating noisiness and loudness. (noise annoyance is mainly influenced by loudness). According to (Kryte 1970), the duration of noise usually has much to do with its acceptability, unwantedness, or noisiness (Figure 2). The critical duration of the temporal summation of loudness is less than 1 s, while the critical duration of noisiness seems to be longer. Noise annoyance is mainly influenced by loudness, because, in most situations, the louder the sound, the more annoying it is (Figure 3).

The pressure amplitude of a sound wave does not directly relate to its perceived loudness (Howard y Angus 2013), being possible for a sound wave with a larger pressure amplitude to sound quitter than a sound wave with a lower pressure amplitude (i.e., human hearing varies as the frequency varies).

Equal loudness contours (Figure 4) show the sound pressure levels across the frequency range at which the sound is judged to be equally loud. The curves describe how loud a sound must be in terms of the measured sound pressure level to be perceived as being of the same loudness as 1kHz tone of a given level. These identify the non-linearities of the human auditory system using simple sinusoidal input signals. The graphical illustration of auditory performance trends provides a visual representation of these non-linearities with respect to both frequency and amplitude across the range of auditory perception (Charbonneau, et al. 2012). The ear is not flat and is also dependent on sound level (e.g., a sound level which is audible at 20Kz would sound much louder if it was a 4kHz).

The "phon" scale is a subjective scale of loudness based on judgements of listeners to match the loudness of tones to reference tones at 1kHz (Howard y Angus 2013). The table below (Figure 5) shows two frequency weightings which are commonly used to perform a compensation for the variation of sensitivity of the ear as a function of frequency. The "A" weighting is most appropriate for low frequency sound as it compensates for the low-level sensitivity versus frequency curve of the ear, its measured in dBA. On the other hand, the "C" weighting is more suited to sound at higher absolute sound pressure levels and its more sensitive to low-frequency components.

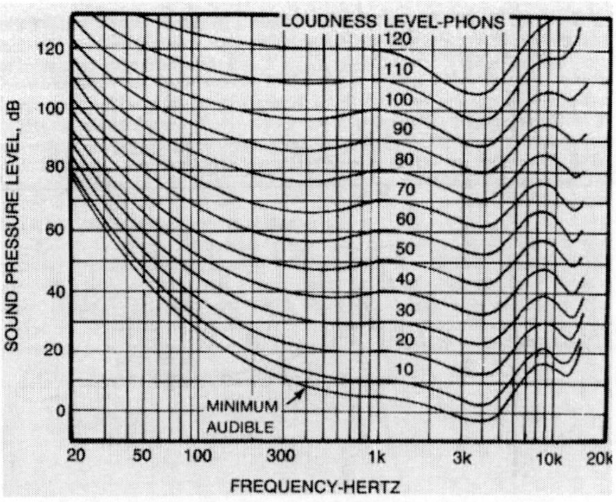

Figure 4. Equal Loudness Contours (Phons) for the human ear.

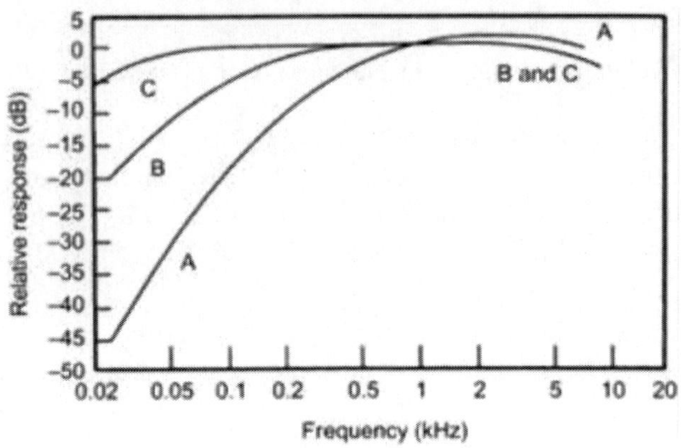

Figure 5. The frequency response "A" and "C" weightings.

Pitch

Pitch is defined by the American National Standards Institute as 'that auditory attribute of sound according to which sounds can be ordered on a scale from low to high' (American National Standards Institute (ANSI) 2013) Pitch is perceived from many types of sounds, such as sinusoids, vocals, instrument sounds, and noisy sounds. However, the definition is problematic in the sense that not all sounds have clear pitch, and some of them have more than one pitch. In Musical acoustics pitch relates to issues such as notes on a score, key, melody, harmony, tunning systems and intonation in performance (Howard y Angus 2013)

Timbre

"Timbre is that attribute of auditory sensation in terms of which a listener can judge two sounds similarly presented and having the same loudness and pitch as being dissimilar" (American National Standards Institute (ANSI) 2013) Timbre emerges more rapidly than loudness, pitch and perceived location from the process of auditory-unit formation (It only takes a few milliseconds to identify vowel sounds or the sounds of musical instruments, whereas loudness and pitch have integration times of more than 10 ms).

To reduce the complexity of the problem, the study of timbre is often limited to a relatively well-defined category of sounds (Hermes 2023). Timbral descriptors are used to indicate the perceived quality or tonal nature of a sound which can have a particular pitch and loudness also (Howard y Angus 2013). There is no subjective rating scale for timbre judgements, unlike pitch and loudness which can, on average, be reliably rated by listeners on scales from "high" to "low."

Duration

"Subjective duration "(Pulkki y Karjalainen 16/01/2015) is the subjective attribute that quantifies a set of sounds from "short" to "long", can be done in a similar manner to quantifying the loudness and pitch of sound. The unit of subjective duration is the dura, which corresponds to the perceived duration of 1 s of a 1-kHz tone (Fastl y Zwicker 2007)

When two sounds have the same pitch, loudness, and duration, timbre is what makes one particular musical sound different from another.

Physical Parameters

Acoustics can be also measured and analyzed through several physical parameters from an objective point of view

Frequency

The ear can hear frequencies between 20Hz and 20.000 Hz. The ear canal has a natural frequency of 3000 Hz due to its shape, which causes an increase of SPL in the eardrum relative to the entrance of the canal. These frequencies are important for speech.

(Level) Intensity

The limits of audible intensities of sound are called "threshold of hearing." This varies for each individual with frequency and with its duration.

Time

There is a minimum duration for a sound to be perceived. If two signals arrive within 10 msec they cannot be distinguished. However, if one of them is delayed by more than 30 msec it can be heard as an individual sound.

Direction

People's ears are 12 cm apart. Differences in the sound received by each ear define "sound localization." Above 1500 Hz the ear is not sensitive to phase.

Indoor auditory perception is in direct relationship with space geometries, and hence the acoustics of it. In crowded spaces such as public transports (underground, bus, aeroplanes…) human comfort is the result of a particular environmental factors (quality of air, temperature, relative humidity) but also it is a result of the acoustics that these environmental factors cause. Together with vision and visuals when human contact and concentration happens during an event, is the noise associated with it. Subjectively, concentration of people can be seen as positive or negative, if that is something pursued by the designer for the final user. Architectural typologies and materials proposed in early designs are crucial to respond to human comfort for different activities that require concentrated public (events, transport, seminars…). According to (Hasman 2023) Acoustic comfort is greatly influenced by geometry, volume, and layout of a space, as well as the sound absorption, transmission and reflection characteristics/properties of building features, materials, and interior finishes

Neuroscience and Architecture: Human Behavior Compromised

Architecture plays a fundamental role in shaping the built environment in which we live and work. It not only impacts our physical surroundings but also influences our behavior, emotions, and well-being. As neuroscience has advanced, researchers have delved into understanding how certain attributes of architectural designs affect the human brain and behavior. Exploring the intricate relationship between neuroscience and architecture is shedding light on how architectural choices can either support or compromise human behavior. By examining existing research from high-impact journals, we can gain insights into how architectural design principles can enhance or hinder various cognitive and emotional processes.

The links between architecture and neuroscience are not well understood jet (Eberhard, 2008) more likely, Neuroarchitecture is turning into a whole new discipline in which researchers are studying on one end the specific needs of people, according to their neuropsychological development, and on the other the potential space has to facilitated comfort to the user. Focusing on the space potential, some of the key attributes are the artificial lighting (lx), the temperature (°C), the humidity (RH%), and noise (dB) (Bower, 2019) Among the mentioned features, the noise, studied from the discipline of acoustics, assumes a pivotal role in addressing multifaceted considerations within the design process that may elude other design disciplines. For instance, the compromise of speech intelligibility due to the provision of natural ventilation, necessitating mitigation against external noise ingress, highlights the intricate challenges faced by designers. To address this, designers strategically leverage decorative elements and interior design configurations. This includes optimizing sound insulation between rooms and attaining optimal reverberation time values within a given space. The incorporation of such acoustic design principles emerges as a foundational aspect influencing the overall quality of architectural structures (Spence, 2020).

Psycho-Environmental Frameworks of Neuroarchitecture of Sound

The neurobiological foundations of auditory perception encompass a series of intricate processes within the nervous system, particularly the auditory system. Commencing with the capture of sound waves by the outer ear, the auditory pathway orchestrates a symphony of events. Vibrations in the eardrum lead to the movement of the middle ear ossicles, transducing mechanical vibrations into fluid movement in the cochlea—a spiral-shaped structure in the inner ear. Specialized hair cells within the cochlea convert these fluid movements into electrical signals, subsequently transmitted to the auditory nerve. As auditory signals traverse through the brainstem, thalamus, and auditory cortex, complex analysis and interpretation of auditory stimuli unfold. This neural processing not only enables the perception of basic auditory qualities but also extends to emotional and cognitive integration, cross-modal interactions, and the adaptive plasticity of neural circuits, allowing for learning and preference development. This comprehensive understanding contributes to our appreciation of how the brain processes auditory information, thereby shaping our sensory experience and emotional response to the surrounding soundscape.

However, humans make sense of the world not only via single sets of sensory information, but rather merging together all sensory cues that define the dwelled space. Therefore, human experience in the built space, cannot be explained and understood by studying single sets of sensory stimuli –visual, auditory, haptic, light, heat, sound, touch…– instead, human behavior needs to be investigated as a whole, in which emotions and rational thinking play a major role. Which could be seen as a handicap for providing specific design parameters which could lead to accurate –but unreal– relationships between environment and human behavior, in the following chapter a set of daily space-behavior situations are explained. The neurobiological bases of sound perception in architectural space may be a useful framework for interior designers and architects to take advantage of design in acoustics, improving sound insulation between spaces and providing most appropriate reverberation time values.

Spatial Layout and Navigation

Wayfinding is the discipline that studies how people make sense of where they are. Using this knowledge architects and designers plan how people navigate in buildings such as hospitals, airports, malls or even cities. The way architectural spaces are organized can significantly impact an individual's ability to navigate within a built environment. In a study published in the Journal of Cognitive Neuroscience (Marchette, A. S., Vass, L. K., Ryan, J., & Epstein, R. A., 2015), functional MRI scans were used to examine the neural mechanisms underlying human navigation. The findings revealed that the brain's hippocampus, which is crucial for spatial memory and navigation, is highly sensitive to spatial layout and configuration. Although humans perceive the environment as a whole, in which the whole is more than the sum of its parts (Sternberg, 2021), researchers need to study independent variables and its impact (Bower, 2019) . Sound is one of the variables that sheds light on navigation since humans can rapidly tell where they are by the sounds they hear or by the reverberation time of the space, like when humans enter a Cathedral (Eberhard, 2006) and they know immediately where they are. Therefore, an architectural design that lacks clear soundscape design may compromise navigation abilities and lead to cognitive stress.

Biophilic Design and Stress Reduction

Biophilic design, which incorporates natural elements into the built environment, has gained attention in recent years due to its potential to reduce stress and enhance overall well-being. A study in the Journal of Environmental Psychology (Ryan, C. O., Browning, W. D., Clancy, J. O., Andrews, S. L., & Kallianpurkar, N. B., 2014) investigated the impact of biophilic elements in office spaces. The research found that exposure to nature-inspired design elements, such as greenery and natural materials, led to reduced stress, increased creativity, and improved cognitive performance. Sound plays a crucial role in biophilic design too, as irregular surfaces, as the ones provided by greenery, absorb sound waves and make a major contribution to physiological comfort by reducing the number of vibrating particles entering the inner ear.

Spatial Layout and Social Interaction

The layout and design of spaces can either promote or hinder social interaction. Social interaction, except for situations in which only deaf humans are involved –such as the case of

Gallaudet University–, needs adequate acoustic arenas to facilitate communication between individuals. A study in the Journal of Environmental Psychology (Appleyard, D., Lintell, M., & Lynes, J., 1977) examined the influence of urban design on social interaction. The findings showed that architectural designs with clear spatial organization and defined public spaces fostered greater social interaction among residents. In contrast, spaces with poor layout and limited public areas compromised social engagement and community well-being. In urban environments, sound design is key to mitigate uncomfortable noises such as traffic or construction works.

Color and Emotional Responses

Color is a critical aspect of architectural design that can evoke various emotional responses. A study in the journal Color Research & Application (Ou, L. C., Luo, M. R., Woodcock, A., & Wright, A., 2004) explored the psychological and physiological effects of color on individuals. The research revealed that different colors can elicit distinct emotional responses, with warm colors like red and yellow being associated with increased arousal and excitement, while cool colors like blue and green are linked to calmness and relaxation. A similar study, in which the oxygen saturation (SpO_2), pulse rate, and quantitative electroencephalogram were measured to evaluate the impact of color perception, published after the Annual International Conference of the IEEE Engineering in Medicine and Biology Society (Sroykham, W., Wongsathikun, J., & Wongsawat, Y., 2014) showed that there was a greater brain activity when individuals were exposed to red or yellow rooms. Nevertheless, monochromatic atmospheres are uncommon in everyday situations, plus the measures taken in laboratories do not take into account the impact that other sensory cues that define the experience of the space, like sounds, may have in human's behavior.

Architects shall use this knowledge with regards to color to create environments that promote specific emotional states, but, once more, design must be faced in a multisensory approach, having sound a crucial role in the way or body maps the space.

Geometry, Beauty and Approach-Avoidance Decisions in Architecture

The shape of the space humans dwell matters when it comes to making decisions. Curvilinear spaces were judged more beautiful –activating the anterior cingulate cortex of the brain– than flat or angular spaces but they don't impact approach-avoidance decisions (Vartanian et. al 2013). Results extend the known impact of contour on aesthetic preferences to architecture, emphasizing the role of emotion in favoring curvilinear designs. Having curved surfaces can as well, lead to better acoustic properties of the space, reverberation time values in the room with curved surfaces will improve sensory experience. These decisions are especially relevant in situations where crowds of people share space, like in the cities' subway, corridors of concert halls, restaurants or hospitals waiting rooms.

Psychoacoustics: Health Outcomes Associated with Noise

People's mental health and social wellbeing are determined by a lifestyle (behaviors, feelings, emotions, genetics…) along with environmental factors. Determinants of these factors can have short or long-term impacts, which can lead to a Lifestyle Diseases (LD) (Hasman 2023). Stress and health problems are consequences of inappropriate design decisions and can be alarming for project typologies. Noise can increase heart rate, blood pressure, respiration rate and even blood cholesterol levels. Once key health outcomes associated with environmental noise are identified, their relevance can be rated for assessing environmental noise issues.

The same way noise can be defined as "unwanted sound," pleasant sounds help create a sense of well-being (Music can be used to treat pathologies). Psychoacoustics explains how the human auditory system perceives sounds, as sound affects us both physiologically and psychologically. Knowledge in psychoacoustics is based on listening tests in order to find out how humans perceive sounds and hence to be able to evaluate health consequences. There is a cognitive dimension (higher level processing) that is unique to each listener in terms of pitch, loudness, and timbre (Howard y Angus 2013).

Our knowledge on psychoacoustics is therefore based on listening tests that are tested through carefully designed experiments with controlled variables. This process is called "controlled experimentation." This allows us to explore which aspects of a sound affect listening experiences and how. Psychologists call a behavioral response such as a listening experience, the dependent variable, and those aspects that might affect it are called the independent variables.

Subjective testing is a complex subject. For many psychoacoustic experiments the "Psychoacoustic rating scales" are used, where the listener is invited to choose the point on the scale that best describes what they hear (Table. 3). Several rating scales exist for the evaluation of the quality of the speech signal and the following are examples:

- Absolute category-rating (ACR) test
- Degradation category-rating (DCR) test
- Comparison category-rating (CCR) test

Table 3. Rating scale and descriptions for the Comparison category-rating (CCR) test (Howard y Angus 2013)

RATING	DESCRIPTION
3	Much better
2	Better
1	Slightly better
0	About the same
-1	Slightly worse
-2	Worse
-3	Much worse

Hearing Damage

The ear is a sensitive and accurate organ of sound analysis. Hence it can be damaged by exposure to excessive levels of sound or noise (Howard y Angus 2013).

This damage can be described in two forms:

- *A loss of hearing sensitivity*

  The effect of noise exposure causes the efficiency of the transduction of sound into nerve impulses to reduce. This shift in the threshold can be temporary, but ultimately becomes permanent as their hair cells are damaged due to long-term exposure, which does not allow them to recover

- *A loss of hearing acuity*
  This is more subtle and severe than the first effect. The damage is not only to reduce the threshold between critical bands, but also to increase the bandwidth of our acoustic filters. This produces impairment on our ability to separate the different components of a sound, and as a consequence, to reduce our speech understanding.

The amount of hearing loss suffered by an individual depends on a number of factors, including the following (Table. 4):

Table 4. Factors affecting the degree of hearing loss (Dance y Zepidou 2019)

Intensity of the noise	Time interval between exposures
Frequency spectrum of the noise	Individual susceptibility
Duration of the noise	Leisure pursuits
Character of the noise	

Noise Exposure

The Control of Noise at Work Regulations 2005 (Health and Safety Executive 2005) ensures that workers' hearing is protected from excessive noise at their place of work. The level at which employers must provide hearing protection and hearing protection zones is 85 dB(A) (daily or weekly average exposure) and the level at which employers must assess the risk to workers' health and provide them with information and training is 80 dB(A). There is also an exposure limit value of 87 dB(A), taking account of any reduction in exposure provided by hearing protection, above which workers must not be exposed.

Noise Criteria

The objective of an acoustical criteria is to guide the design of an occupied space, so that it meets a specified acoustical standard (Health and Safety Executive 2005) There are two components to be considered in complying with acoustical criteria:

- limiting the noise emission into the space
- designing the acoustics of the space

The dimensions, materials and furnishings determine the acoustics of a space. In HVAC design the compliance is to acoustical criteria with the absence of activity noise: no office machines, telephones, printers etc. The widespread use of A weighted decibels for environmental noise assessment is influencing room noise criteria (Table 5).

NR curves Kosten & van Os developed the criteria for assessing the effects of external industrial and other noises on people in their homes. So, the work was aimed at domestic premises, especially night time disturbance. NR is a tangent assessment, where the rating is given to the highest NR curve which is tangential to an octave band analysis of the noise. In their validation of NR curves, the acceptable spectra. Kosten and van Os's data did not test the NR curves at the lower frequencies for which they are used. Consequently, circumstances arise in HVAC applications in which an objectionable low frequency noise satisfies the NR design criterion.

Whilst it would be possible to modify NR in order to increase its stringency at low frequencies, there are other criteria, described below, which already do this, and which should be used as an alternative to NR (Table 6).

Table 5. Noise criteria according to space functionality

RECOMENDED	NR/NC index
Workshops	60-70
Mechanised offices	50-55
Gymnasia, swimming baths	40-50
Restaurants, bars, café	35-45
Office, library, courtroom	30-40
Cinema, small conference room	25-35
Classroom, studio, large conference room	20-30
Concert hall, theatre	20-25
Diagnostic clinic, audiometric room	10-20

Table 6. Noise Rating and Noise Criterion curves

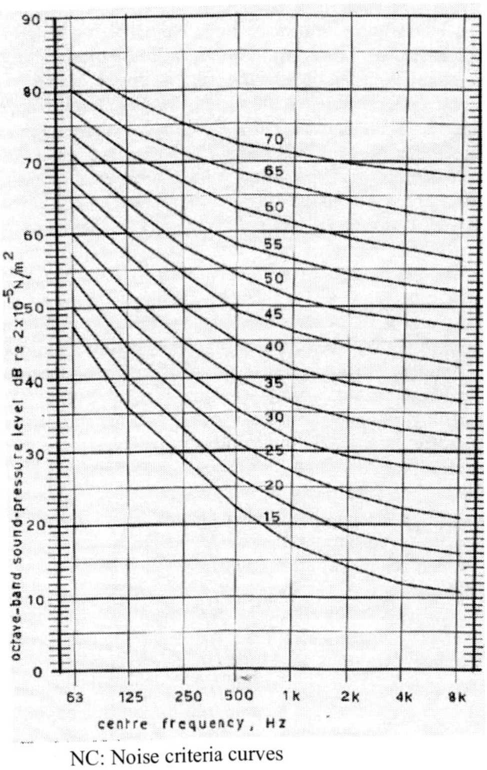

NC: Noise criteria curves

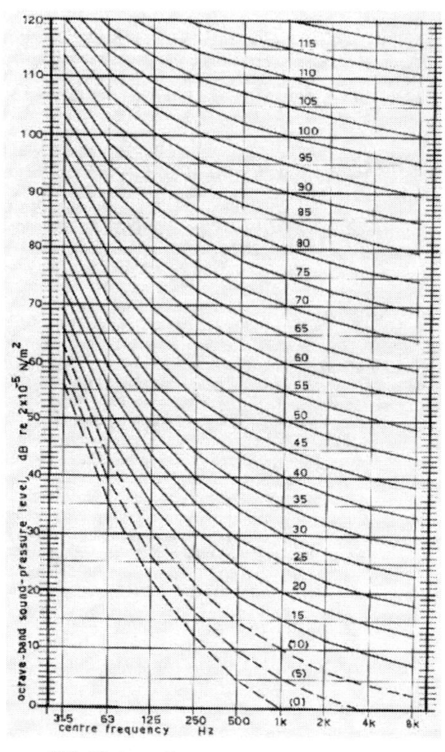

NR: Noise rating curves

NC curves: Beranek developed these criteria to ensure good speech intelligibility, typically measured speech communication between colleagues in offices where background noise interfered. for non-sensitive spaces. Baranek determined "acceptable" conditions. This led to NC curves. NC is a 'tangent' approach similar to NR. It was found that a noise spectrum closely following an NC curve, and therefore satisfying the basis for the curves, does not itself give a pleasant sound, but rather has both throb (rumble) and hiss.

The NR criterion (noise rating) is not safe to use under all circumstances since it permits unacceptable levels of low frequency noise. It is recommended that use of the NR be phased out. The NC criterion is an improvement on the NR, although it is no longer recommended by ASHRAE except for non-sensitive locations.

According to (Hasman, 2023) people's health and wellbeing are influenced more by their physical and social environments than by their genetics and medical conditions. Research on wellbeing, and multisensory design evidence the fact of the relationship between humans and nature is more than needed in nowadays projects. There is a connection between a physical space and human's psychological and physiological response to it. The introduction of natural inputs in architectural projects such as water, natural daylight, changes of temperature, shadows, natural forms and textures, natural materials, are positive aspects to create a better and healthier environment, which affect Psychoacoustics and hence how sound affects us both physiologically and psychologically.

Bioacoustics: Delivering Healthy and Sustainable Acoustic Environments

Delivering "healthy experiences" in architecture is a broad topic. Aligned with the mission of the United Nation's third Sustainable development Goal (SGD) for 2030: "Good Health and Wellbeing, architects and designers are called for bringing a social value for the long-term wellbeing of communities. With the aim of promoting health and wellbeing, it is very important to integrate nature within the architectural process.

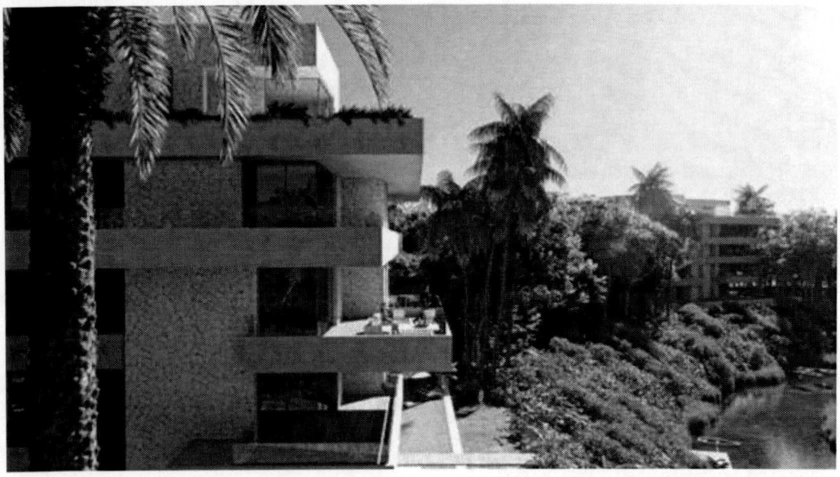

Figure 6. Soundscape as part of the big open terraces at the residence" The Reserve at Mayakobá", Mexico. L35 Architects.

Acoustics, as a branch of architectural design, can be integrated into that design process from the concept design stage, raising auditory perception as a value that the user experience can have, or even can suffer if it is not understood as a part of the project. Depending on the site selection, and the architectural typology chosen, acoustics can have a positive or negative impact on the delivered space as an "experience". Acoustics can be a determining factor for the space arrangements allowing a particular soundscape to break in the building or can be even immersed into a thermal or interior design strategy using biomaterials (Figure 6).

The Benefits of "Silence": Soundscapes

What "silence" means, depends on the "room" or physical space we are in. Silence is not the "complete absence of sound", because this would alter our proprioception (this is what happens in anechoic chambers) (Mombiedro 2022). The Japanese practice of Shinrin-yoku, or forest bathing, is the simple and therapeutic act of spending time in a forest, immersing ourselves in a particular soundscape. "Spending more time around trees" by just contemplating (and not exercising) is a technique that has been proven to improve health. Japan launched a national health program of "Shinrin-yoku" in 1982 (Park, y otros 2009) where the physical and psychological effects of "forest bathing" have been studied: trees emit oils (phytoncydes) as protection from germs and insects which help our immune systems (Li Q, y otros 2009) forests also lower our heart and blood pressure and reduce stress hormones, depression is reduced while boosting energy walking in a forest. Walking in nature provides a balm for urban children and for those who want to escape technology according to the World Economic Forum (Livini s.f.).

Physiological effects of Shirin-yoku were analyzed against environmental factors. The Profile of Mood States (POMS) was used to gauge the psychological response pf the patients according to six effective dimensions (Table 7).

Table 7. Six effective dimensions to gauge psychological response of the patients according to the Profile of Mood States (POMS) (Park, y otros 2009)

T-A (tension and anxiety)	C (confusion)
D (depression and dejection)	F (fatigue)
A-H (anger and hostility)	V(Vigor)

Significant differences were seen between the changes resulting from viewing or walking in a forest landscape and those from a city landscape (Figure 7). The POMS measurements show that forest environments can relieve human psychological tension, depression, anger, fatigue, and confusion, and moreover, that they can enhance human psychological vigor. (Park, and others 2009) reported that a relationship exists between the POMS score and the physical environmental factors (Figure 8).

From this research we could conclude that environmental factors can have a significant psychological effect. In terms of acoustics, positive or negative Soundscapes that activate the auditory perception, have a significant health consequence as a result, hence this should be considered in the design process when aiming to deliver healthy and sustainable acoustic environments. What a soundscape is could be described as a combination of sounds that can be heard in a particular environment, and is unique for a specific location, changing by the minute. The soundscape (as defined in the WSP's Handbook for Acoustic Ecology as 'An environment of sound (or sonic environment) with emphasis on the way it is perceived and understood by the individual, or by a society') needs to be treated as a whole, not merely its component elements; this is a recognition that sound creates relationships and meaning, not just effects.

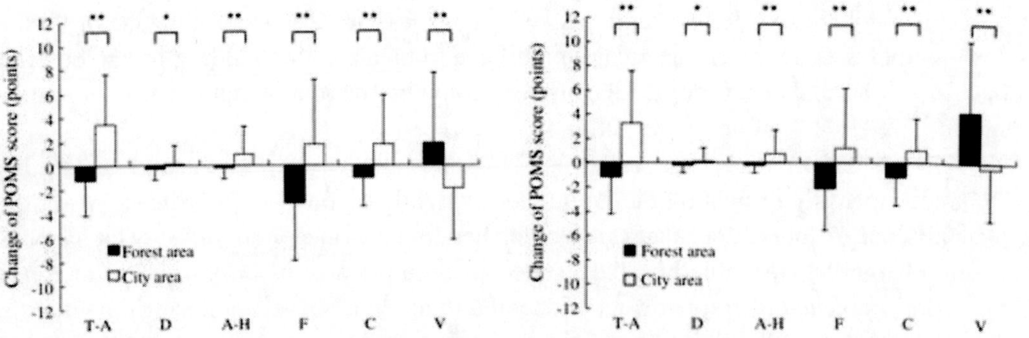

Figure 7. The changes in the average POMS subscale scores after the viewing (left) or walking (right) are presented (city vs forest) (Park , and others 2009).

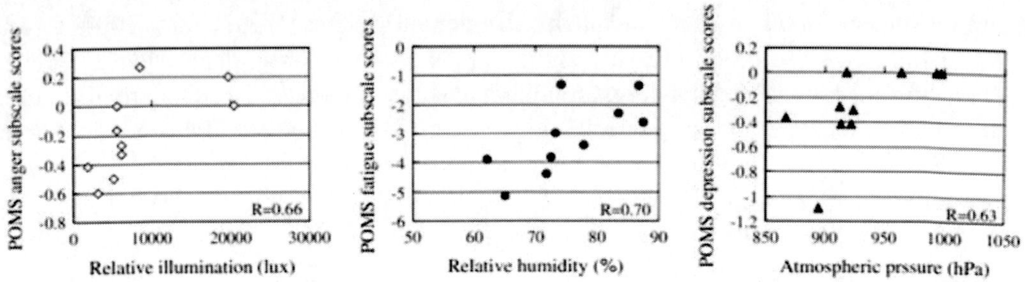

Figure 8. Relationship between POMS and physical environmental factors in forest areas - (Park , and others 2009).

Murray Shaffer wrote about the Natural Soundscape, and the subjective perception that exists between different geographical locations due to the nature of the sound sources it contains (Schafer 1994). He describes how the same physical location can create different emotions just due to the sound behavior of its natural elements (snow that absorbs the sound, the absence of life or sound…). He supports the idea the modern Western culture has neglected the psychology of aural perception. Binaural hearing, sound localization and auditory fatigue (the effect of prolonged exposure to the same sound) has been studied. His study and research group aim to determine in what significant ways individuals and societies of various historical areas listen differently (Table 8).

Table 8. The relationship between three terms that involves soundscapes (Schafer 1994)

TERM	CORRESPONDENCE	EXAMPLE/SITUATION
The figure	The signal or the sound mark	A bull roaring
The ground	The ambient sounds around it	The riverbank
The field	The place where all the sounds occur (the soundscape)	A mellow in Australia

The World Soundscape Project (WSP) was established as an educational research group by R. Murray Schafer during the late 1960 and early 1970 at Simon Fraser University. The group studied the Soundscapes of Canada, as well as in different European cities in Sweden, Germany, Italy, France and Scotland (School of Communication Simon Fraser University s.f.) The World Forum for Acoustic Ecology, founded in 1993, is an international association of affiliated organizations and individuals who share a common concern for the state of the world's soundscapes.

From this research, Barry Truax suggests some guiding principles for the qualitative aspects of urban acoustic design and sustainability that address quality of life issues (Table 9).

Together with climate change and the increasing growth of cities, soundscapes are being modified having a direct consequence on people's health and behavior (psychological responses could differ from other historical moments). Progress in technology, such as electric car motors or the fact of moving factories to metropolitan areas have a significant positive impact on the new soundscapes from XXI century, however the increasing population and densification can balance negatively technological changes (further research and studies will indicate significant quantities and conclusions). As an objective fact, connecting with nature independently from the historical moment we are, humans perceive in a different manner, acknowledging positive multisensory experiences which play a key role on the use of the space. According to (Hasman, 2023) exposure to nature reduces cognitive fatigue and improves biological health by accelerating psychological and physiological restoration up to 37% after a psychological and /or an "environmental stressor."

Acoustics and Biophilia

Soundscapes are in direct relationship with biophilic and sensory design. For the purpose of understanding the context of Biophilic Design, we describe the use of biomaterials in architecture as something that has a relevant impact on the environment throughout the life cycle of the buildings. "Bioconstruction" as a new technique has an effect on people's health. Toxic chemicals released by materials can lead to inhalation, ingestion, dermal absorption producing cancer, asthma, or other diseases. New resources for designers are necessary to make healthier places for all people to live. Bio-acoustic materials are being investigated (p.e PET fibers from recycled plastic bottles) and used to improve acoustic comfort and wellbeing in buildings.

According to (Hasman 2023), Biophilic and Sensory Design has a restorative influence on people's mental wellbeing. Human-nature relationships can be cultivated with the support of multisensory design, which daylights the dynamic relationship between a physical space and human's psychological and physiological responses in that space and further defines how human experience can be amplified with the integration of natural elements, natural light, water, and sound into the built environment.

Biophilia appears in design since the earliest human structures (Browning, Ryan y Clancy 2014). Inspiration from nature is seen adorning Greek temples, porcelain fish bowls in China, or gardens in Arabic Spanish architecture. Evolution of art styles such as the Art Nouveau designs of the 19th century progress show the importance natural elements have in intermittent trends, always present in human everyday concerns.

Biophilic design can be organized into three categories providing a framework for understanding and enabling thoughtful incorporation of a rich diversity of strategies into the built environment (Table 10).

Table 9. Guiding principles for the qualitative aspects of urban acoustic design and sustainability that address quality of life issues between three terms that involves soundscapes (Truax s.f.)

Principle	Description
1	The soundscape needs to be treated as a whole, not merely its component elements; this is a recognition that sound creates relationships and meaning, not just effects
2	Listening as the embodied interface between the individual and the acoustic environment needs to be a central concern. What still needs to be developed are methodologies for documenting how information and meaning are created for residents, not merely the affective qualities of the soundscape
3	Soundscape design can respond to and create 'quality of life' improvements and 'acoustic sustainability' issues that go beyond traditional risk assessment and legislation; these benefits affect everyone, not just those with particular sensitivities to sound, as valuable as such people's experiences are in order to focus attention on particular issues. Given the vulnerability of soundscapes to changes that threaten the balance of elements that comprise them, careful consideration needs to be given to maintaining soundscapes on a human scale, as argued above, in order to preserve their role in encouraging a sense of belonging, identity and social relatedness, as well as to minimize the risks to physiological and psychological health
4	Soundscape design inherently deals with interdisciplinary issues, and can benefit from a wide range of expertise across the sciences, healthcare, the social sciences, the arts, and many related professions.
5	Acoustic ecology needs to be integrated within other environmental concerns that have a high public profile today, both because of the importance of the soundscape as an 'acoustic habitat' and for the positive, listener- centered approaches and examples it has created; its practices can deepen our understanding and experience of both acoustic and technologically mediated environments, as well as providing alternative sonic worlds we may find inspiring and possibly therapeutic

Table 10. Nature-design relationships: three categories within Biophilic design (Browning, Ryan y Clancy 2014)

Nature in the Space	1	Visual Connection with Nature	A view to elements of nature, living systems and natural processes.
	2	Non-Visual Connection with Nature.	Auditory, haptic, olfactory, or gustatory stimuli that engender a deliberate and positive reference to nature, living systems or natural processes
	3	Non-Rhythmic Sensory Stimuli.	Stochastic and ephemeral connections with nature that may be analyzed statistically but may not be predicted precisely
	4	Thermal & Airflow Variability.	Subtle changes in air temperature, relative humidity, airflow across the skin, and surface temperatures that mimic natural environments
	5	Presence of Water	A condition that enhances the experience of a place through seeing, hearing or touching water.
	6	Dynamic & Diffuse Light	Leverages varying intensities of light and shadow that change over time to create conditions that occur in nature.
	7	Connection with Natural Systems	Awareness of natural processes, especially seasonal and temporal changes characteristic of a healthy ecosystem
Natural Analogues	8	Biomorphic Forms & Patterns	Symbolic references to contoured, patterned, textured or numerical arrangements that persist in nature.
	9	Material Connection with Nature	Materials and elements from nature that, through minimal processing, reflect the local ecology or geology and create a distinct sense of place
	10	Complexity & Order.	Rich sensory information that adheres to a spatial hierarchy similar to those encountered in nature.
Nature of the Space	11	Prospect	An unimpeded view over a distance, for surveillance and planning.
	12	Refuge.	A place for withdrawal from environmental conditions or the main flow of activity, in which the individual is protected from behind and overhead.
	13	Mystery.	The promise of more information, achieved through partially obscured views or other sensory devices that entice the individual to travel deeper into the environment.
	14	Risk/Peril	An identifiable threat coupled with a reliable safeguard.

- Nature in Space addresses the direct, physical, and ephemeral presence of nature in a space or place. This includes plant life, water and animals, as well as breezes, sounds, scents and other natural elements (e.g., a butterfly garden). Experiences are achieved through the creation of meaningful, direct connections with these natural elements, particularly through diversity, movement and multi-sensory interactions.
- Natural Analogues address organic, non-living and indirect evocations of nature. Objects, materials, colors, shapes, sequences, and patterns found in nature, manifest as artwork, ornamentation, furniture, décor, and textiles in the built environment. The strongest Natural Analogue experiences are achieved by providing information richness in an organized and sometimes evolving manner.
- Nature of the Space addresses spatial configurations in nature. This includes our innate and learned desire to be able to see beyond our immediate surroundings, our fascination with the slightly dangerous or unknown; obscured views and revelatory moments; and sometimes even phobia inducing properties when they include a trusted element of safety. The strongest Nature of the Space experiences are achieved through the creation of deliberate and engaging spatial configurations commingled with patterns of Nature in the Space and Natural Analogues.

These goals aim to integrate nature perceptually in design delivering a holistic experience, demonstrating immediate benefits to health. As a case study, Fallingwater house designed by Frank Lloyd Wright (Pennsylvania, USA) recreates a harmonic equilibrium between people, the physical and natural environments. The architect used locally source materials with a limited color palette for a better integration and used low ceiling heights intentionally to enhance people's visuals into the horizontal landscape through long windows. Light, textures, colors, sounds… all aspects influence the multisensory experience of the user. Architectural elements such as a stairway connected to the exterior allow to create a physical connection to natural elements. Furniture and finishes inside imitate colors of surrounding nature and continue in the outside terraces.

This experience at 360 degrees delivered by an American architect in 1939 is very representative as a case study of A biophilic design, but the designer's goal nowadays is very different from what an Architect from the XXI century must encounter. Passive strategies, globalization (non-local material resources) and restrictive international environmental criteria position Biophilic strategies within a different point. Specifically acoustic and thermal insulation from interior to exterior (specially in extreme climates where mechanical ventilation is required in order to satisfy energy demands) produce an" invisible barrier" for the user, having a physical and psychological connection with nature (e.g., if natural ventilation is not allowed, or acoustic levels outside impede opening windows and free movements in and out), the architectural experience changes. Multisensory design should be achieved maybe by recreating outdoor soundscapes into the inside, enhancing interior design arrangements connected/unconnected between them, as well as reproducing natural elements in interior design (as it was done with Art Nouveau).

There is a risk that "Biophilic style" could be limited to cost and hence to a selected public ("shaping" in XXI century is more expensive and has a different approach than in other historical moments) New techniques such as digital fabrication or Artificial Intelligence introduce a high level of efficiency and productivity in manufacturing processes. Potential errors in fabrication (filling a mold, printing, machining etc.) are eliminated. The Forbes Magazine (Forbes Magazine s.f.) explains how digital manufacturing methods are supported by artificial Intelligence (AI) as a revolutionary method which helps operational teams simplifying decisions, improving effectiveness and does not affect final costumer cost. AI uses computers programmed to assess huge streams of data and make decisions that maximize speed and quality, which equate to reliability.

A potentially resulting "biophilic space" has in addition a direct impact with room acoustics, as shapes, textures and forms of the construction elements influence how the acoustic waves spread and behaves in an enclosed space. Many of the "natural analogues "such as Biomorphic Forms & Patterns mentioned before, affect how the sound behaves in the room. The interior "style" significantly affects the acoustics depending on the function. Rational architecture that raised in 1920 with pure geometries such as cubes, double heights, and flatness in general, solved structural and material problems, but has consequences for the normal use of the space due to the unsuitable acoustics it provided.

Biophilia also has an acoustics impact at a urban scale. As a case study "Caixa Forum Madrid" designed by Herzog and De Meuron. the project's goal is to step back off the main street to create a public square. The designers imagined the urban space as a meeting point and considered a 460m2 green wall of 15000 plants and species, which masks negative soundscapes such as traffic road noise with positive soundscapes such as birds, animals and leave movements. Natural shapes also dump traffic acoustic waves reducing reverberation time in a critical point where people could suffer direct reflections from an extremely large façade.

Conclusion

Subjective acoustics and auditory perception play an important role in comfort and well-being. Through neuroscience and architecture, we understand how humans tend to perceive, recognize, and conceive, when inhabiting spaces. Subjective and objective attributes of sound affect people on their routines. Evaluation and perception of nature vary from user to user according to individual preferences, including thermal, lighting, and acoustic comfort. New research is being conducted in relation to Bio design and acoustics. Biophilic design and stimuli prediction are key when defining interior space arrangements at early stages. It is very important to separate noisy from quiet areas, introducing acoustic lobbies when sound insulation is a concern, consider main forms, shapes, and volumes, as well as the nature of the sound sources to be controlled (frequency content) that will scatter the sound, or concentrate it according to a multidisciplinary design strategy. Finishes and furniture, even the introduction of natural features (leaves, trees, plants…) will affect the acoustic conditions. The introduction of "positive soundscapes" as an alternative to negative sounds or "negative silence" needs to be further studied. Appropriate acoustic and new bio-designs bring benefits in terms of comfort, as well as improved efficiency and better health conditions. Guidance on the design, installation and operation of specialized building and engineering technology - along with AI and robotic manufacturing for new bio-construction products - is needed to ensure people's well-being and health in sustainable indoor spaces.

References

American National Standards Institute (ANSI). 2013. *"ANSI webstore."* Accessed 2023. https://webstore.ansi.org/standards/asa/ansiasas12013r2020.

Bower, Isabella, Richard Tucker, and Peter G. Enticott. "Impact of Built Environment Design on Emotion Measured via Neurophysiological Correlates and Subjective Indicators: A Systematic Review." *Journal of Environmental Psychology*, Volume 66, 2019.

Browning, W, Catherine Ryan, and Joseph Clancy. 2014. "14 Patterns of Biophilic Design: Improving Health and Well-Being in the Built Environment". *Terrapin Bright Green.*

BSI British Standards Institution. 1967. "BS 4198:1967 Method for calculating Loudness." *BSI Group*. 09 14. Accessed 2023. doi:https://doi.org/10.3403/00050046.

Charbonneau, Jeremy, Colin Novak, Robert Gaspar, and Helen Ule. 2012. "A-weighting the equal loudness contours." *The Journal of the Acoustical Society of America (Publi med)* Volume131(4):3502. doi:10.1121/1.4709236.

Dance, S., and G Zepidou. 2019. "Sound Exposure of Choristers". *National Library of Medicine NIH.* doi:https://doi.org/10.4103/nah.nah_40_19.

Eberhard, John Paul. Brain Landscape: *The Coexistence of Neuroscience and Architecture*. Chicago: Oxford University Press, 2008.

Fastl, Hugo, and Eberhard Zwicker. 2007. *Psychoacoustics: Facts and Models*. Vol. Volume 22 of. Springer Science & Business Media. ISBN 3540688889.

Forbes Magazine. n.d. *"The Forbes Magazine"*. Accessed 11/11/2023. https://www.forbes.com/sites/forbestechcouncil/2020/06/12/artificial-intelligence-powers-flexibility-in-digital-manufacturing/?sh=7ddbdace32aa.

Hasman, Mina. 2023. *RIBA Climate Guide*. RIBA publishing.

Health and Safety Executive. 2005. "Control of Noise at Work Regulations." https://books.hse.gov.uk/.

Hermes, D J. 2023. "Timbre Perception". *The Perceptual Structure of Sound. Current Research in Systematic Musicology*". Vol. vol 11. Springer, Cham. doi:https://doi.org/10.1007/978-3-031-25566-3_6.

Howard, David M, and Jamie A. S. Angus. 2013. *Acoustics and Psychoacoustics*. Focal press Taylor & Francis Group. ISBN 978-0-240-52175-6.

Kasetani, T., N. Takayama, B. J. Park, K. Furuya, and Kagawa. 2008. "Relation between light/thermal environment in the forest walking road and subjective estimations for taking in the atmosphere of the forest (in Japanese)". *Journal of The Japanese Institute of Landscape Architecture.* Volume 71,Issue 5. Pages 713-716

Kryte, Karl D. 1970. *The effects of noise on Man*.r. Vol. 1 p. 112. Standford Research Institute, Menlo Park California: Elsevier Inc. doi:https://doi.org/10.1016/C2013-0-11015-X.

Lebowitz, M., K. Dams-O'Connor, and J. Cantor. 2012. "Feasibility of computerized brain plasticity-based cognitive training after traumatic brain injury." *Journal of rehabilitation research and development.*

Li Q., M. Kobayashi, Y. Wakayama, H Inagaki, and M. H. Katsumata. 2009. "Effect of phytoncide from trees on human natural killer cell function. *International Journal of Immunopathology and Pharmacology."* doi:10.1177/039463200902200410.

Livini, Ephrat. n.d. *"The World Economic Forum"*. Accessed 22/10/2023. .https://www.weforum.org/agenda/2017/03/the-japanese-practice-of-forest-bathing-is-scientificially-proven-to-be-good-for-you.

Marchette, S. A., Vass, L. K., Ryan, J., & Epstein, R. A. "Outside looking in: Landmark generalization in the human navigational system" *The Journal of Neuroscience*, 35(44), 14896–1490 (2015)

Meunier, S., M. Van Eeckhoutte, and BCJ Moore. 2021. "Loudness: From Neuroscience to Perception." *Frontiers in Psychology* 12. doi:10.3389/fpsyg.2021.785093.

Mombiedro, Ana. 2022. *Neuroarquitectura: Aprendiendo a través del espacio*. Edited by Ediciones Khaf. Grupo editorial Luis Vives. ISBN 978-84-15995-54-8.

Namba., Seiichiro. 1987. "On the psychological measurement of loudness, noisiness and annoyance: A review." *Journal of the Acoustical Society of Japan* (E) 8,6.

Ou, Li-Chen & Luo, Ming & Woodcock, Andrée & Wright, Angela. (2004). "A study of colour emotion and colour preference. Part I: Colour emotions for single colours". *Color Research & Application.* 29. 232 - 240. 10.1002/col.20010.

Park, Bum Jin, Yuko Tsunetsugu, Tamami Kasetani, Takahide Kagawa, and Yoshifumi Miyazaki. 2009. "The physiological effects of Shinrin-yoku (taking in the forest atmosphere or forest bathing): evidence from field experiments in 24 forests across Japan". *Environ Health Prev Med*, 15(1):18-26. doi:10.1007/s12199-009-0086-9.

Pulkki, Ville, and Matti Karjalainen. 16/01/2015. *Communication Acoustics: An Introduction to Speech, Audio and Psychoacoustics.* Vol. Chapter 10: Basic Psychoacoustic Quantities. John Wiley & Sons. doi:10.1002/9781119825449.ch10.

Ryan C. O., Browning W. D., Clancy J. O., Andrews S. L., Kallianpurkar N. B. "Biophilic design patterns. Emerging Nature-Based Parameters for Health and Well-Being in the Built Environment" *International Journal of Architectural Research*, Volume 8 - Issue 2 – July 2014 (62-76).

Schafer, R Murray. 1994. *The Soundscape: our sonic environment and the tuning of the world.* Rochester, Vt.: Destiny Books.

School of Communication Simon Fraser University. n.d. "*The World Soundscape Project"* (WSP). The Sonic Research Studio & WSP. https://www.sfu.ca/sonic-studio-webdav/WSP/index.html.

Spence, C. "Senses of place: architectural design for the multisensory mind" *Cognitive Research: Principles and Implications*. Volume 5, Article number: 46 (2020).

Sroykham, W., Wongsathikun, J., & Wongsawat, Y. (2014). "The effects of perceiving color in living environment on QEEG, oxygen saturation, pulse rate, and emotion regulation in humans" in *Annual International Conference of the IEEE Engineering in Medicine and Biology Society*, 2014, 6226–6229.

Sternberg, Robert J., Sternberg, Karin (2012). *Cognitive Psychology* (6th ed.). Belmont, CA: Cengage Learning.

Truax, Barry. n.d. "Acoustic sustainability in urban design: lessons from the World SoundScape Project, *Cities and Health." 5:1-2,122-126.* doi.org/10.1080/23748834.2019.1585133.

Biographical Sketches

Laura de Azcárate

Affiliation:

Architectural Association School of Architecture, Environmental and Technical Studies Department. Lecturer, Design tutor in Architecture and Acoustic Design. London, UK

Education:

- 1995-2008 Bachelor of Music (Piano). Conservatorio Profesional de Música de Majadahonda, Madrid.
- 2005 2013 Graduated with honors from the Architecture Faculty of Universidad San Pablo CEU, Madrid
- 2009 -2010– Erasmus in Liège, Belgique. Institut Supérieur d'Architecture Saint Luc de Wallonie
- 2015-2017– Masters in Environmental and Architectural Acoustics, London South Bank University
- 2024-2025 Masters in Teaching, Universidad Politécnica de Madrid

Business Address:

Calle Candamo, 118. Hoyo de Manzanares. 28248. Madrid, Spain

Research and Professional Experience:
Professor at Architectural Association School of Architecture since 2016.

Professional Appointments:
Lecturer in Environmental Acoustics at Master en Eficiencia Energética de la Edificación, Universidad CEU San Pablo, Madrid since 2023

Publications from the Last 3 Years:

1. De Azcárate, L. (2023) *Sustainable Acoustics for a better livability and wellbeing.* IGI Global.
2. De Azcárate, L and others. (2024) *Confort y bienestar:la arquitectura de los sentidos.* Aretha

Ana Mombiedro

Affiliation:
University of Alicante, Neuroarchitecture Masters coordinator. Alicante, Spain

Education:

- 2006 – 2014 Graduated with honors from the Architecture Faculty of Universidad San Pablo CEU
- 2015 – Certificated course, The Brain and Space, Neuroscience, Duke University
- 2017 – Certificated course, Visual Perception and The Brain, Neuroscience, Duke University
- 2018-2019 Masters in Teaching, Universidad Internacional de Valencia
- 2023 – Certificated course, The Science of Well-Being for Teens, Yale University, Psychology
- 2023 – 2024 Masters in Neuropsychology of Learning

Business Address:
Parque del Huécar, 2, 16001, Cuenca, Spain

Research and Professional Experience:
Professor at Universidad de Alicante since 2023.

Professional Appointments:
Coordinator of the Masters of Neuroarchitecture, Universidad de Alicante, since 2023
Director of Postgrado Neuroarquitectura Escola Sert, 2022-2025

Honors:
Applied research project, *Jugar el Espacio*, displayed at the Venice Bienalle, 2021.

Publications from the Last 3 Years:

1. Mombiedro, A, (2022). *Neuroarquitectura. Aprendiendo a través del Espacio.* Edelvives.
2. Mombiedro, A, (2024). *Espacio cuerpo y mente.* Fundación ARQUIA

Chapter 9

Telemedicine: The New Era of the Internet of Things. Portable Medical Devices as a Solution for Health Monitoring of Patients at Risk of Social Exclusion

Guillermo Sáez Cruz[1]
Natalia García-Tenorio Fernández[1]
and Daniel Arranz-Paraíso[2,*]
[1]Universidad San Pablo CEU, Alcorcón, Madrid, Spain
[2]R&D Development Manager at Pinisan SL. C/Gran Canaria, Madrid, Spain

Abstract

The evolution of technology is enabling an instant connection between patients and healthcare professionals. This enables closer and real-time monitoring with continuous collection of biometric data. Patients now take on the role of self-monitoring using user-friendly, painless, portable, and cost-effective devices. Access to this data is crucial for patients living in sparsely populated areas or with limited access to healthcare services due to distance, lack of transportation to medical centres, and issues with communication and travel systems. Cardiac monitoring is one of the best examples, as biometric electronic wristbands can track the condition of patients with heart diseases. Device readings, such as detecting sinus arrhythmia, can activate alarm systems to mobilize medical services, reducing the risks associated with delayed interventions during critical time periods. The ability to continuously collect data enables the creation of comprehensive patient profiles, allowing precise identification of high-risk episodes, such as nocturnal apnea. The prospects are promising, as the implementation of these technologies will enable interventions that extend the quality of life in the next human generations.

Keywords: telemedicine, telehealth, medical devices, wearable devices, IoT, health monitoring

---

* Corresponding Author's Email: daniel.paraiso@pinisan.com

In: Psycho-Environmental Variables That Ensure People's Well-Being and Health …
Editors: Roberto Alonso González Lezcano and Guadalupe Cantarero García
ISBN: 979-8-89530-831-8
© 2025 Nova Science Publishers, Inc.

Introduction

What Is Telemedicine?

The term "telemedicine," as we know it today, was first coined by Bird and his colleagues between 1967 and 1969. They defined telemedicine as the delivery of healthcare services without the physical doctor-patient contact typical of this discipline [1]. Despite this, there is no globally accepted, exclusive definition of telemedicine and its derivatives [2, 3].

Telemedicine arose thanks to the development of ICT (Information and Communication Technology), which was introduced in the healthcare field, seeking to end its physical limitations. Technological advances have allowed the simultaneous evolution of telemedicine, together with the emergence of new concepts that are based on the initial idea of telemedicine and that develop it, always adapting to modern technologies. These new concepts include telehealth, e-health, and m-health [3].

Telehealth: extension of the concept of telemedicine to include new activities, including the education of both patient and healthcare professional, as well as patient care. In addition, its objectives are aligned with those of Public Health, which has made it possible to change the previous paradigm, carrying out epidemiological studies, health education, health services management and policy, environmental health, industrial health, and biostatistics, digitally [4].

Thanks to the development of the internet and mobile devices, the technology industry coined the novel terms e-health and m-health, which were created to highlight technological innovations and their increasing integration in the healthcare sector (especially in medical care), expanding the initial concept of telemedicine.

E-health is considered a novel area of research that aims to increase patient's accessibility to the healthcare system and to reduce its cost, by means of the combination of public health, medical informatics, and health services management. It can be defined as "any health service, platform, tool, or intervention delivered electronically," internet-driven and that do not overlap with other domains (m-health) [5, 6]. Este concepto incluye, tanto los sistemas de apoyo a decisiones clínicas y sistemas de entrada de orden médicas, como los registros médicos electrónicos.

M-health is the most modern concept, as it arose as an adaptation of telemedicine to the entry into the market of smartphones. This has greatly improved the global population's access to medical care, especially in areas at risk of social exclusion. It represents a revolution in the concept of telemedicine as it allows individualized and personalized medical care for each patient.

Telemedicine has evolved into different subclasses, which are indeed a projection of the four fundamental pillars that compose it: consultation, diagnosis, monitoring, and mentoring [3].

Within the taxonomy of telemedicine, consultation involves remote interactions between healthcare professionals or providers and patients. This enables the exchange of medical information and expert guidance, improving collaboration and accessibility in medical care.

Diagnosis in telemedicine involves the remote assessment of a patient's medical condition by healthcare specialists. Typically, this is based on the transmission of medical images, records, and laboratory results, enabling accurate diagnoses when geographic distances separate the patient from the specialist.

Monitoring plays a significant role in telemedicine and encompasses the continuous follow-up of patients' health, especially those with chronic diseases or requiring ongoing care. This includes remote monitoring of vital signs, chronic disease management and telemetry, which reduces the need for frequent in-person visits and allows for early intervention.

Mentoring involves experienced healthcare professionals providing remote guidance to less experienced colleagues, often during complex medical procedures. Despite being less developed than other components, it has the potential to improve medical training, knowledge transfer and skills development, especially in surgical and specialized fields.

COVID-19 as the Onset of the Telemedical Revolution in Health

Since the late 20th century, telemedicine has gradually developed and, especially in the last decade, has been increasingly integrated into medical practice. However, it never gained real relevance for two main reasons: a) reluctance from both healthcare providers and patients to integrate it into their daily healthcare routine; and b) economic barriers, including outdated healthcare IT infrastructure and lack of reimbursement, particularly in private healthcare systems [7, 8].

It was not until the COVID-19 pandemic that telemedicine gained relevance, significantly impacting the healthcare system and global society [8]. The World Health Organisation (WHO) Emergency Committee declared on March 11, 2020, the COVID-19 pandemic, infection caused by SARS CoV-2 virus [9]. This situation triggered a forceful implantation of a new, ever before reached, digitalisation of the healthcare system, which took place in both inpatient and outpatient care. Regarding the latter, teleconsultations (i.e., virtual consultations) were implemented as part of the patient ambulatory control, limiting patient inflow into the emergency room. On the other hand, a series of telemedicine applications were implemented for inpatient management, such as: tele-triage, which allowed to assess the patient condition, so that only those patients that required emergency care and whose condition was rapidly progressing, would be referred to the hospital, whereas the rest of the patients would remain in in-home health monitoring. This telemedicine service experienced a strong acceptance with a rapid exponential growth; teleconsultations with hospitalised patients, avoiding personal contact with healthcare providers and interhospital virtual communications, which allowed an enrichment of medical expertise and served as a method of counselling for certain administrative and medical decisions [10, 11].

Triage has always been necessary under disastrous events, to ensure a correct patient care. The repercussion of an insufficient triage leads to Emergency Department (ED) overcrowding, which has been associated to increased waiting times or even to patients leaving the ED without receiving their proper assessment or treatment. Patient under-care due to this ED overload is linked to chronification of diseases and even to patient death. Emergency triage depends on several factors, such as the number of patients and their health state, the presence of critical patients and the availability of medical staff [12]. During COVID pandemic, the ER was extremely overloaded with thousands of new daily cases, and triage played a pivotal role in diminishing risks regarding both patient and physicians' safety. Some fundamental measures were implemented in the ED and hospitals, such as infrared thermal cameras and COVID-19 rapid antigen testing in those suspected cases, as well as enhancement of social distancing by the reconfiguration of the waiting room areas. Moreover, telehealth services (such as teleconsultation, tele-triage, and tele-emergency) suffered an exponential growth and application in the medical setting and were essential as they allowed the reduction in patient inflow in the ER, risk of infection and physicians' workload, as well as the conservation of personal protective equipment (PPE). During the pandemic, the main goal of tele-triage shifted from the management of overcrowded ED to ensure patient care, to the protection of physicians (by decreasing patient overload in the ED) due to the staff shortages that medical centres suffered at the time. It allowed a prior screening by means of telehealth applications, so patients could be or not forwarded to another triage setting in the hospital or ED, for example, outdoor tents [13].

In terms of tele-triage, a 2023 systematic review examined 14 cohort studies on tele-triage interventions during the COVID-19 pandemic. Key findings obtained from this study include the positive impact of tele-triage on correctly discerning the need of the patient to be hospitalized or not, as well as improving waiting times and visit durations using telephone consultation and medical apps as the main tele-triage methods. It was noted that, the use of virtual triage services helped healthcare institutions to reduce its workload by minimizing the inappropriate use of emergency services while improving patient safety and satisfaction [14].

Regarding interhospital virtual communications, they were crucial to ensure a correct everyday patient care. It allowed an interdepartmental collaboration, so physicians were able to carry out medical interventions remotely. This was crucial at that time when the entire world was under lockdown. There are some examples in the literature, which include the remote monitoring during neurointerventional procedures, specially focusing on three cases of endovascular aneurysm treatment. In response to the challenges posed by the COVID-19 pandemic and logistical limitations, a novel high-resolution, low-latency streaming technology facilitated the guidance of interventional teams by a remote neurointerventional specialist. The cases, conducted in distant cities, demonstrated a successful application of the Woven Endobridge (WEB) embolization system, with the streaming technology enabling effective communication and supervision [15].

The Woven Endobridge (WEB) is a medical device used for treating intracranial aneurysms. It diverts blood flow within the aneurysm by deploying a self-expanding double-layer nitinol mesh, suitable for various aneurysm types [16]. The live-streaming platform displayed features such as a remotely controlled high-definition camera and secured, encrypted data transfer. This technology not only overcame the challenges imposed by the pandemic but also highlighted its potential to enhance the learning experience for neurointerventionalists by providing real-time support and fostering effective communication between remote proctors and on-site treating physicians. As the field continues to advance, the adoption of such remote support systems emerges as a decisive strategy for overcoming logistical barriers to on-site proctoring, contributing to improved patient safety in neurointerventional procedures [15].

During the pandemic, these services were accepted by the population, as it allowed to overcome essential barriers, the distance one. However, this period also served to determine some important weaknesses of the first telemedicine implementations. For instance, phone consults do not allow non-verbal communication analysis, which is fundamental in some disciplines, such as psychiatry. In this sense, in Ireland, a survey analysed the confidence with which psychiatrists diagnosed their patients during the pandemic by means of phone consults, and it showed that 92% of these professionals were not confident in their diagnosis as they were not able to assess the body language of their patients. This demonstrated how necessary the transition from a telephone consultation to a video consultation was [17].

A New Astonishing Era for Telemedical Devices

The pandemic caused by the COVID-19 virus marked a turning point, enabling the unprecedented expansion of telemedicine horizons. This paved the way to the evolution of the pre-existing concept of IoT (Internet of Things), which plays a pivotal role in the overall advancement of telehealth and the creation of a smart environment. The concept of "Internet of Things," coined by Kevin Ashton in 1999, involves connecting data on the Internet to a developing global service architecture. Since this moment, IoT technologies such as Wi-Fi or Bluetooth have allowed to connect and coordinate diverse systems, which in turn contributes significantly to the creation of intelligent and efficient solutions, promoting innovation on a great scale. This new era of computational processing and telemedical device sensing is contributing to the creation of a global smart environment, vastly improving urban residents' quality of life. With a rapidly increasing global population and a rise in chronic diseases, there is a heightened need for cost-effective healthcare systems that can efficiently manage and deliver diverse medical services while minimizing overall expenses [18, 19].

Examples of IoT include networked devices to control airflow and temperature in operating room. Incorporation of IoT in the healthcare system has transformed it, offering several advantages. It enables the automatization of previously laborious processes (administrative tasks and paper-data recording), consequently minimising human errors. Other improvements include cost reduction in healthcare, overcoming geographical limitations, early detection of chronic diseases, improved medication management, quick access to healthcare, and ultimately, enhanced treatment outcomes. The transformative impact of IoT promises to optimize healthcare delivery across various facets of the industry [20].

IoT application to human health is an extension of the telemedicine concept, especially e-health. Many different technologies have emerged since then to fill different gaps that were unaffordable years ago in terms of continuous monitoring of vitals and disease progression without being hospitalized. In this sense, medical devices have evolved into telemedical devices, which enable the in-home monitoring and, sometimes, diagnosis. This is a great tool, especially for those populations in risk of social exclusion. This type of telemedical devices include wearable devices (in contact with the outer body) and ingestible biosensors.

Wearable Devices

Definitions

Wearable devices can be defined as exogenous sensors that are placed in different structures, from smartwatches, clothes, patches… that continuously collect data (functional or physiological) that is then processed and analysed. This data can be used with a monitoring, preventive, diagnostic and even treatment aim [21].

Wearable devices are in contact with the body surface to carry out their functions. However, novel approaches have developed interfacing wearable devices, known as bio-integrated wearable devices, and both will be covered in this chapter.

Design of Medical Devices

Wearable devices are characterised by five main qualities: a) wireless mobility; b) portability; c) simplicity of use d) interactivity and intelligence; e) durability. Implementation of wearable devices in the medical setting fulfils the "4P medical model" [22], that is, preventive, predictive, personalised, and participatory medicine [23].

These devices are meant to be used in any body part and have been consequently classified in three main areas: 1) head, which include smart glasses (e.g., virtual reality glasses may be useful for medical training and intraoperative guidance) and contact lenses; 2) limb wearable devices, which are mainly placed in the upper limbs (e.g., smartwatch, smart-bracelet, which allow a constant monitoring of vitals such as heart rate), although they can also be worn in legs and feet; and 3) torso wearable devices, which may include belts and clothes (e.g., underwear). This is possible due to the integration of electronic products within the fabric [22].

The integration of sensors with the soft and curvilinear surfaces of the human body requires careful materials design to ensure seamless and non-invasive interfaces. Conventional inorganic materials used in planar electronic devices are ill-suited for bio integration due to their high modulus and brittle mechanical properties. To address this, there is ongoing research to develop alternative materials and device designs that are flexible, allowing for reversible bending, which can be achieved through thickness reduction. Flexible devices encompass materials like nanomembranes/nanowires/nanoribbons of silicon and thin films of conjugated small-molecule organics. While flexibility enables integration across small body regions, accommodating the complex textures and natural motions of the skin requires stretchability [24].

Applications of Medical Devices

One of the most recent telemedicine branches is m-health, which uses mobile devices to collect data (e.g., vital). In this sense, m-health is tightly linked to innovative medical devices. One of the most evolving areas regarding the use of electronic medical devices is cardiovascular health, where wearables play a key role in the correct patient telemonitoring and prevention of cardiovascular events, such as heart failure [21].

A typical form of monitoring heart health is by means of a heart rate monitoring device, which can record heart rate by either one of two approaches: a) electrical, which relies on electrocardiography (ECG) sensors that record electrical signals, generating bio-potentials; and b) optical, which involves photoplethysmography (PPG) sensors that record the blood volume being pumped by means of light-base technology (light is emitted through the skin by a light-emitting diode and its dispersion off blood vessels is gauged). Electrical devices comprise two components: a monitor or transmitter, and a receiver. Upon heartbeat detection, the monitor transmits a radio signal, enabling the receiver to assess and display the current heart rate. EGC sensors are mainly used in chest-worn straps equipped with integrated electrodes, whereas PPG are mainly included in smart watches and smartphones [25]. There are several studies assessing the suitability of electronic medical devices in cardiovascular health.

The 2019 Apple Heart Study engaged almost 240,000 participants over a period of eight months, in which heart rate was monitored by means of a commercial smartwatch. They observed that, if an individual experienced an irregular pulse and received a subsequent notification about it, there was a positive predictive value of 84% for the detection of atrial fibrillation when verified via an electrocardiogram patch (worn for 13 days post-notification). From all the participants, merely 0.52% received the irregular-rate notification. Despite the study's low representation of patients with heart failure (less than 4%), this technology shows potential in assessing heart failure patients who do not require electrocardiographic monitoring or cardiac implantable electronic devices (CIED) [26].

Smartwatches can be also employed for monitoring Parkinson's disease (PD) patients by analysing tremor and balance dysfunction through a gyroscope or accelerometer. Roberto's group assessed smart watches for quantifying tremors in PD patients, evaluating clinical correlation, and assessing acceptance and reliability as a monitoring instrument. The findings suggest that smartwatches have the potential to serve as a clinical tool and are well-received by patients [27].

Researchers have conceived a novel strategy to improve dielectric sensors, resulting in the creation of a trilayer radiofrequency tooth-mounted sensor designed specifically for monitoring food consumption. This sophisticated device becomes functional upon the incorporation of analyte-sensitive layers. Composed of biocompatible materials, the dielectric sensor is well-suited for placement in the mouth and stands out for its capability to detect a diverse range of analytes, including alcohol, pH, salinity, sugar, and temperature. Demonstrator devices showcase the versatility of the interlayer material, including a porous silk film and a modified PNIPAM hydrogel that responds to changes in pH or temperature. In a noteworthy real-world application, the device is attached to tooth enamel for real-time detection of ingested foods [28].

Many other studies have analysed the viability and usefulness of different wearable devices. For example, in terms of the application and advantages of connected hearing technologies which can be classified into smartphone-connected hearing aids, direct-to consumer devices, and smartphone-based hearing aid applications. By incorporating Bluetooth features, such as Listen Live and StreamLine Mic on smartphones, it broadens options for users with hearing loss, providing cost-effective alternatives to traditional remote microphone systems. Smartphone-connected hearing aids, with their Bluetooth capabilities, present a promising avenue for user-centric adjustments and potential innovations in adult aural rehabilitation [29].

One increasing concern nowadays is mental health. There is an increased prevalence of acute stress, particularly connected to diseases like cardiovascular issues, and the growing incidence of mental health problems such as anxiety and depression, especially in low- and middle-income countries. Researchers are actively developing compact, portable, and precise technologies to monitor stress and mental health by analyzing vital signs and neural activity. Understanding these issues, is primal since the recent surge in commercially available smart devices and wearables. Despite advancements, monitoring stress and mental health remains challenging, leading to a focus on non-intrusive wearables with regulatory approval and user tolerance. People prefer practical devices like smartphones and wearables over large monitoring tools [30, 31].

Altered heart rate variability (HRV) measurements are linked to autonomic nervous system (ANS) dysregulation, impacting cardiovascular diseases and mental health conditions. In 2018, Hernando et al. utilized the Apple Watch, revealing that HRV measurements, especially the R–R interval series, outperform heart rate (HR) alone in detecting stress. Most commercially available devices rely on average HR, heavily influenced by the autonomic nervous system, which can be significantly altered in various physiological and pathological circumstances. HRV metrics are considered superior, particularly in situations of altered autonomic function such as depression, as they provide a more accurate reflection of physiological changes [32, 33].

However, using only one device to measure such a complex state was not sufficient. Many studies explored the use of multiple devices to achieve this goal. The research by van Kraajj et al. (2020) supports this idea, using two different wearables: an unspecified chest patch to monitor heart rate and a wristband (Chillband) to track activity. The study emphasizes a significant connection between heart rate and the intricate interplay of chronic stress, gender, and circadian rhythm [34].

Anxiety is characterized by an unpleasant emotional reaction that is disproportionate to a specific stressor, or even in its absence. This reaction may or may not be prolonged, leading to tension and physical manifestations [35]. To explore the feasibility of using wearables for assessing anxiety, Balconi et al. (2019) employed wearable EEG (electroencephalogram) and ECG devices, such as the MuseTM headband (InteraXon Inc., Toronto, ON, Canada) or the Lowdown Focus glasses (SmithOptics Inc., Clearfield, UT, USA). The study aimed to examine the effects of mindfulness exercises on both the objective and subjective levels of stress and anxiety in individuals. Although the study provided limited details on the specific EEG signatures utilized on subjects, the authors suggested that the wearable brain-sensing device holds the potential to improve objective stress response by increasing awareness of EEG signatures associated with dysfunctional hyperactivation [36].

Even if cardiac activity has been objectively associated to anxiety as a measurable physiological parameter, different approaches must be studied. A good example is the study conducted by Sano et al. (2018), in which two sensors were employed to assess the accuracy of skin conductance, skin temperature, and three-axis acceleration using the Q-sensor (Affectiva, Boston, MA, USA) and the Motion Logger (AMI, Ardsley, NY, USA), which records activity levels. The study found that skin temperature and skin conductance were more effective in detecting stress and mental health conditions [37].

Depression, or major depressive disorder, is a prevalent and significant medical condition that has adverse effects on your emotions, thoughts, and behaviours. Depression leads to feelings of sadness and a diminished interest in activities that were once pleasurable. Its incidence is increasing year by year and is especially notorious in teenagers, in which literature shows that 34% of adolescent at a global scale are in risk or suffering depression episodes, with a higher prevalence in Africa, Asia and The Middle East [38].

Despite being a complex pathology that is more challenging to assess and diagnose using wearables compared to stress or anxiety, it is crucial to explore novel approaches. This is particularly important because wearables are more likely to be adopted by teenagers and are generally easier for the general population to use. To achieve this, Narziev et al. (2020) [39] identified five factors related to depression symptoms, derived from the DSM-5 questionnaire: mood, physical activity, sleep, social activity, and food intake (for appetite information). These factors were monitored to detect depression using the "Short-Term Depression Detector" (STDD) framework, which utilized sensors from a smartwatch (Galaxy S3) and an Android smartphone. Participants received in their smartphones the surveys necessary to analyse their subjective state, whereas the smartwatch utilized a heart rate monitor and accelerometer to gauge subjects' physical activity levels. All this information was analysed and interconnected by employing Machine Learning. This enabled to determine the participants' mood based on a combination of these factors. Notably, the smartwatch showed that physical activity levels tend to be lower in individuals experiencing depression [39].

The STDD demonstrated an impressive accuracy of 96% in classifying individuals in the depressive group [39]. This research underscores the challenges of objectively recognizing depressive symptoms through wearable technologies and suggests the potential utility of smartphone apps for gathering metrics and qualitative data to aid in depression detection.

Bio-Integrated Wearable Devices

Seamless integration of wearable devices with the body demands careful consideration of material composition, structure, and interface requirements. Ensuring biocompatibility is crucial, especially for materials in direct contact with the body, to prevent irritation, allergic reactions, or toxicity. Commonly used materials include noble metals like gold and medical-grade silicones. Advances in material compositions often prioritize performance, though there is growing academic interest in understanding the biological reactions to materials, particularly at the nanoscale [40, 41].

Bio-integrated wearable devices must establish interfaces with the body for both short-term and long-term durations under various environmental conditions. One good example is Gelderm, a versatile wound care solution which integrates 3D-printed alginate fibres with color-changing pH sensors and drug-eluting scaffolds. It undergoes UV sterilization, ensuring effective bacterial eradication without compromising drug efficacy. The colour-changing sensors are characterized using ImageJ and a smartphone application for real-time monitoring of wound conditions [42].

Adhesive coupling is a common method, requiring attention to adhesion strength, strategies for minimizing physical damage during application or removal, and designs to prevent interfacial contaminants or trapped moisture [43]. This aspect is a focal point of intense research interest, as detailed in a comprehensive topical review. The goal is to create wearable devices that not only perform well but also ensure comfort and safety during extended periods of use.

Detection of biomarkers associated with body conditions provides in-depth healthcare information and benefits to disease management, where the key challenge is to develop a minimally invasive platform with the ability to directly detect multiple biomarkers in body fluid. Dermal tattoo biosensor holds the potential to simultaneously detect multiple health-related biomarkers in skin interstitial fluid because of the features of minimal invasion, easy operation, and equipment-free result reading. Herein, a colorimetric dermal tattoo biosensor fabricated by a four-area segmented microneedle patch is developed for multiplexed detection of health-related biomarkers. The biosensor exhibits colour changes in response to the change of biomarker concentration (i.e., pH, glucose, uric acid, and temperature), which can be directly read by naked eyes or captured by a camera for semi-quantitative measurement. It is demonstrated that the colorimetric dermal tattoo biosensor can simultaneously detect multiple biomarkers in vitro, ex vivo, and in vivo, and monitor the changes of the biomarker concentration for at least 4 days, showing its enormous potential for long-term health monitoring. This innovative biosensor offers a promising solution for real-time and continuous monitoring of various biomarkers, contributing to personalized healthcare and disease management [44].

In the realm of tissue engineering and regenerative medicine, the synergy of biomaterials and living cells has paved the way for innovative solutions, with extrusion bioprinting emerging as a transformative technique. Bioinks, formulations of biomaterials and living cells, play a pivotal role in this process, along with growth factors and other biomolecules. Bioinks are applied to the human body by extrusion bioprinting, a method that deposits bioinks layer by layer, which has gained prominence in the fabrication of three-dimensional constructs mimicking native human tissue. The mechanical forces employed in this technique, namely pneumatic, piston, and screw-driven mechanisms, offer varying levels of control and precision in the deposition of bioinks [45, 46].

Bioprinted constructs find diverse applications in tissue engineering and combatting infectious diseases. In tissue engineering, these constructs, also referred to as scaffolds, are cultured in bioreactors and grown into functional 'artificial' tissue or organ substitutes. These substitutes are then implanted into patients to aid in the repair or treatment of tissue and organ injuries. On the other hand, in the realm of combating infectious diseases, bioprinted constructs serve as in vitro models, mimicking human tissue and organs to test and validate newly developed therapeutics and vaccines prior to human use [47, 48].

The novel approaches in extrusion bioprinting aim to mimic the complex structures of native tissues, incorporating multiple cell types, extracellular matrix components, and bioactive molecules. One key focus is on multiple-biomaterial printing, utilizing various techniques such as multiple print heads, co-axial printing, and chaotic bioprinting to enhance construct complexity. Another approach involves mimicking heterogeneous structures through coaxial printing, creating tubular channels for bioinks. Chaotic bioprinting blends varied materials to create strands with aligned microstructures, promising increased biological similarities. Embedded bioprinting, including methods like Freeform Reversible Embedding (FRE), enables printing directly into a supportive medium, overcoming challenges in viscosity and allowing for complex designs. Hybrid bioprinting combines extrusion-based bioprinting with other techniques like electrospinning to produce scaffolds with varying structures and environments, enhancing biological function. These advancements highlight the potential for further developments in extrusion bioprinting for tissue regeneration and complex scaffold fabrication [49].

Another novel approach is for the treatment of diabetes mellitus by the development of islet organoids which holds significant promise for advancing diabetes treatment and pancreatic tissue engineering. Digital Light Processing (DLP) bioprinting, known for its precision and speed, has been crucial in constructing these organoids. In addressing the need for tailored bioinks, a specialized formulation was created, incorporating Gelatin Methacryloyl (GelMA), pancreatic extracellular matrix (ECM), and platelet-rich plasma (PRP). This bioink demonstrated notable potential in promoting angiogenesis and favorable macrophage polarization. In both in vitro and in vivo assessments, the 3D printed organoids maintained the activity of islet β-cells with enhanced glucose sensitivity. The orchestrated immune-regulation response, marked by abundant M2-polarized macrophages, reduced inflammation, and improved angiogenesis, establishes this specific bioink as a promising foundation for 3D printed islet organoids in diabetes treatment [50].

Ingestible Biosensors

Wearable sensors were originally designed to monitor a physiological indicator continuously, providing information about human physiology outside of the hospital setting. However, these show a main limitation: they cannot reach innermost regions of the body. Alternately, ingestible biosensing capsules (IBCs) have been designed. While they travel through the GI tract, these IBCs can monitor a wide range of parameters and even offer targeted approaches for surgical and pharmaceutical therapy.

IBCs can be classified in two main types: passive and active devices. Passive IBCs travel along with the natural peristaltic motion of the gastrointestinal tract, which presents a challenge as their locomotion cannot be controlled. Most commercially available ingestible biosensors follow this design and are intended mainly for monitoring physiological parameters (e.g., temperature, pH, gas) and capsule endoscopy (which can integrate several types of cameras) [51].

Active devices aim to control their locomotion. There are different approaches for this, such as magnetically controlled devices, whose movement depend on magnetic fields stablished by permanent, surgically implantable, magnets. Nevertheless, these devices come with inherent risks and limitations that should be considered, such as the exertion of substantial forces on surrounding tissues or the possibility of IBCs becoming trapped in collapsed segments of the gastrointestinal tract, such as the intestines. Other approaches involve the direct integration of locomotion systems (e.g., anchoring or propeller systems). Active IBCs are still being developed and have been tested on animal models, but they are not yet commercialised [52].

Proteus Digital Health™ Inc. (Proteus) developed an ingestible event marker that is approved in the USA and EU. The wearable sensor securely transmits recorded data via Bluetooth to compatible computing devices, which can be even linked to a cloud database for comprehensive analysis and accessibility. The system comprises ingestible sensors, a skin-worn receiver patch, and a mobile user interface. The ingestible sensor allows a safe and accurate monitoring of medication intake, as it tracks drug intake times, measuring medication adherence and allowing assessment of other physiological and behavioural parameters in relation to medication. The sensor, powered by gastric fluid (which also allows communication), opens possibilities for measuring various physiological factors within the body. These include detecting chemical species, gastric transit times, gastrointestinal activity, and even properties like hydration and fat content [53].

Capsule endoscopy allows a wireless approach based on the use of a pill integrating a camera that captures different images throughout the gastrointestinal tract. The first authorised capsule endoscopy by the FDA (Food and Drug Administration) was in 2001. The initial pill camera, known as the M2A capsule (mouth to anus), was later rebranded as PillCamTM SB (small bowel). PilcamTM (Medtronic, USA) has developed several approaches, like PillCamTM ESO and PillCamTM COLON, which can diagnose small intestine lesions by transmitting 2 to 6 images per second. PillCamTM ESO, with a 20-minute battery life, transmits 18 images per second, while PillCamTM COLON activates after 2 hours for a complete colon evaluation. Despite a 16.5% failure rate due to limited battery life, capsule endoscopy is invaluable for localizing lesions, especially in cases of recurrent and obscure gastrointestinal bleeding. It aids in lesion localization before angiography, surgery, or additional endoscopic procedures, providing a superior diagnostic yield compared to other imaging studies [52, 54].

In a more novel approach, PillcamTM Crohn's Capsule has been recently introduced [55] to visualise small intestine and colon. It aims to record the entire gastrointestinal tract, from the mouth to the rectum. This capsule provides a comprehensive panoramic view of the mucosa, allowing the assessment of inflammatory response, stenosis, ulcer formation, extent of the disease, and effectiveness of treatment [56].

Novel Approaches

Artificial Intelligence

Artificial intelligence (AI) replicates human intelligence in learning and problem-solving to handle complicated tasks. Two fundamental areas of AI are machine learning (ML) and neural network (NN). ML uses mathematical models to enable a computer to learn from data on its own, without direct instructions. It leverages algorithms and vast amounts of data to make decisions and generate models that provide accurate results or predictions. However, NN is based on computer training. It aims to mimic the brain with this training, so that it can attain AI through deep learning (DL). There are several DL algorithms that have been applied in the healthcare field recently: deep neural networks (DNNs), convolutional neural networks (CNNs), spike neural networks, recurrent neural networks (RNNs) and its popular extension, long short-term memory (LSTMs). Of especial relevance is their use for ECG interpretation [57].

Several studies have assessed the implication of DL-based models in cardiovascular health monitoring, including the early detection of arrythmias, atrial fibrillation and myocardial infarction. In this sense, CNN is widely used for image analysis. It processes gridded data such as images, utilizing convolutional layers to identify features in diverse image regions. Their capability in extracting local features and correlating spatial-temporal signals makes them a suitable choice in a wide range of tasks, as they reduce spectral variance and demonstrate high discriminatory power.

CNNs models can be used to analyse and detect heart abnormalities. For example, this model can be used to detect several types of arrythmias (bradycardia, tachycardia, atrial fibrillation, and bundle branch block), by directly analyzing spectrogram-based images and therefore eliminating the need for visual analysis by a doctor [58]. Another example is the study carried out by Zhao and colleagues, through which they designed an AI-based STEMI autodiagnosis algorithm with an accuracy in STEMI detection of 99.01%. Moreover, this algorithm showed to have a greater performance than that of doctors [59]. Another CNN-based model was developed to analyse ECG rhythm (sinus, atrial, junctional, ventricular, and artificial pacemaker rithms) and conduction (bundle branch block, atrioventricular block and Wolff-Parkinson-White) abnormalities. This model also showed higher accuracy and F1 scores to that of the physicians [60]. Overall, CNN-based models constitute a promising tool in artificial intelligence-based ECG diagnosis.

Ingestible Biosensors

Recently, Italian researchers have designed Pillsid® (PILl-refiLled implanted System for Intraperitoneal Delivery), a device based to main components: an ingestible capsule, and an implantable device for intraperitoneal drug delivery. The intraperitoneal implantable robotic device acts as an insulin dispenser that aims to manage glucose levels in the patient suffering from type 1 diabetes and it is surgically implanted in the abdomen. It presents a wireless powering system, reducing the necessary doctor interventions for device maintenance. When it runs out of insulin to dispense, it is refilled with the correct medication by means of a magnetic ingestible pill. When ingested, the pill traves through the gastrointestinal tract until it reaches the region nearby the implantable device. The magnets allow it to rotate and uses a retractable needle to pierce and to deliver a supply of insulin into the reservoir and, once empty, it is excreted through the gastrointestinal tract. This device has been tested in pigs and has turned out to be functional, and, in a future, it could provide a better, less invasive form of treatment [61]. It would allow a more autonomous glucose level management [62].

TytoCare®

TytoCare® is an all-encompassing examination kit comprising a device that features as an exam camera and as a non-contact basal thermometer. Additionally, it includes a stethoscope adaptor for auscultating the heart, lungs, and abdominal sounds, as well as a tongue depressor adaptor for throat examination, and an otoscope adaptor for inspecting the ears. In a paediatric cardiology clinic, a study compared Tyto, an FDA-cleared telehealth examination tool, with standard digital devices. Tyto demonstrated superior image and sound quality, particularly for heart, lungs, and ears, enhancing its capacity for remote diagnosis. Clinicians accurately assessed abnormal clinical findings with Tyto, supporting its use in paediatric care and telemedicine. The study acknowledged limitations but emphasized its focus on comparing devices rather than making clinical diagnoses. Notably, Tyto's effectiveness in assessing heart sounds and tympanic membranes was highlighted, concluding that it provides high-quality data for telehealth examinations and supports screening for paediatric medical conditions [63].

Today's society has evolved into an always connected one via smartphones and the internet. This transformation has significantly benefited poorly communicated rural areas, particularly through improved telehealth services. Devices like TytoCare® enable individuals to conduct autochecks, including physician video calls, and assess various pathologies from the comfort of their homes. The device is already in use by many families, contributing to the advancement of telehealth and providing accessible healthcare options.

PEN3®

Electronic noses (e-nose) show promise in detecting cancer at initial stages due to their real-time analysis, low cost, portability, and user-friendly features, providing advantages over technologies like Gas Chromatography-Mass Spectrometry (GC-MS). An electronic nose is a device crafted to detect odors collectively, rather than individually. It commonly distinguishes between odors by utilizing an array of diverse chemical sensors. In a study focused on colorectal cancer (CRC), a portable electronic nose (PEN3®) and GC-TOF-MS were used to analyze gases and volatile organic compounds (VOCs) in the urinary metabolome. The investigation compared different cancer stages with non-cancerous conditions. Results from PEN3® and GC-TOF-MS exhibited high accuracy, with PEN3® separating CRC from non-cancer cases. The combined data from GC-TOF-MS identified 23 potential biomarker VOCs for CRC. Overall, both PEN3 and GC-TOF-MS demonstrated successful discrimination between the cancer and non-cancer groups [64].

Objectives

The objective of this chapter is to gather the most important home-used equipment utilized for diagnosing or monitoring diseases at a domestic level. This includes activity bracelets, GPS assistance or monitoring systems for geriatric patients, as well as the upcoming health landscape, where companion robots could be the solution to the unintended loneliness pandemics.

Material and Methods

A standardized literature search was conducted in the PubMed, ScienceDirect, and Scopus databases to conduct a systematic review of the scientific literature. The keywords "tattoo history," "diabetes," "bioink," "glycaemia," "Pen3®," "TytoCare®," "PillCamTM" and "Pillsid" were selected and combined with terms such as "medical device," "IA healthcare," "telemedicin," "COVID19" and "weareable devices."

Only original research articles published in the last 10 years, with DOI and in English were considered. Literature reviews, letters to the editor, and low-quality papers were excluded. The final selection of articles was carried out manually, applying the predefined inclusion and exclusion criteria. This process allowed the identification of a set of relevant articles for the systematic review, which were then analyzed in depth to obtain a comprehensive understanding of the impact of new medial devices and the telemedicine in the future human health and the next step in the future social relationships with the environment.

Discussion

Wearable medical devices and telemedicine converge in a common path, shaping the future of healthcare by the use and application of innovative technologies. The evolution of telemedicine adds a historical backdrop to the dynamic synergy between advancements in wearable devices and the ever-expanding realm of remote healthcare.

Telemedicine, which was born in the late 1960s, has undergone a great metamorphosis, giving rise to telehealth, e-health, and m-health, each a testament to its adaptability in a rapidly changing technological landscape. Telehealth extends beyond direct patient care, encompassing education for both patients and healthcare professionals, aligning its goals with bigger public health initiatives. The arrival of the internet and mobile devices had further encouraged the creation of e-health, focusing on electronically delivered health services to enhance accessibility and reduce costs. The latest addition, m-health, takes advantage of the ubiquity of smartphones, providing personalized medical care, particularly in areas with limited access to traditional healthcare resources.

The taxonomy of telemedicine, as previously explained, indicates its applications in terms of consultation, diagnosis, monitoring, and mentoring. Each pillar serves a unique purpose, promoting collaboration, accessibility, and knowledge-transfer across different departments of healthcare delivery. The COVID-19 pandemic acted as a catalytic force, that provided telemedicine an unprecedented relevance. Teleconsultations and tele-triage became indispensable tools, addressing historical barriers of reluctance and economic constraints. However, its increased use has also revealed some weaknesses, such as the limitations of telephone consultations, especially in disciplines such as psychiatry, underscoring the imperative need for continuous improvement due to lack of nonverbal communication analysis availability by the physicians.

Another term that was developed in the health care system during COVID-19 pandemic is the Internet of Things (IoT). This integration holds promises for automation, cost reduction, early disease detection, and improved treatment outcomes. Wearable devices, including smartwatches and ingestible biosensors, emerge as integral components of telemedical devices, enabling in-home monitoring and, in some cases, diagnosis.

Moving on to the focal point of wearable medical devices, this area unfolds with innovations ranging from smartwatches to bio-integrated sensors, propelling healthcare into an era of preventive, predictive, personalized, and participatory medicine. The classification of wearables into head, limb and torso categories reflects their diverse applications, from smart glasses that aid medical training to smartwatches that continuously monitor vital signs.

Ensuring seamless integration with the human body, researchers struggle with many challenges through the development of flexible and stretchable materials. Nanomembranes, nanowires, and thin films of organics contribute to the flexibility of wearable devices, accommodating the natural motions of the skin and anatomy of the user.

The applications of wearable medical devices span various healthcare domains, with a focus on cardiovascular health, Parkinson's disease monitoring, and innovative approaches such as tooth-mounted sensors and mental health monitoring. Stress, anxiety, and depression, measurable through altered heart rate variability and other physiological manifestations, become areas of exploration for wearables. Due to the huge prevalence of mental health pathologies these proposals seem interesting to help those patients, especially those in risk of social exclusion such as teenagers.

With the continuous expansion of these technologies, bio-integrated wearable devices, including dermal tattoo biosensors and ingestible biosensors, have been developed. These devices display the potential for long-term health monitoring and personalized healthcare. Although tattoo biosensors seem to be highly invasive, in the practice they help to monitor many parameters from home without the need of been in the clinic. Same happens with ingestible biosensors (ingestible pills), which provide valuable information reducing invasiveness compared to other traditional techniques.

Some projects implement the combination of wearable technology with artificial intelligence (AI), introducing sophisticated capabilities in healthcare. Deep learning algorithms, such as convolutional neural networks (CNNs), enhance the interpretation of medical data, enabling early detection of conditions like arrhythmias and atrial fibrillation.

Novel approaches, such as PILLSID for intraperitoneal drug delivery in diabetes treatment show the significant importance these devices will have in the near future. Also, the integration of TytoCare® in telehealth services, exemplify the acceptance of patients and comfort that can be provide to them, with especial consideration to those populations that have no access to the health care system due to geographical limitations. In conclusion, the integration of wearable devices, artificial intelligence, and innovative biosensing technologies marks the beginning of a new era in healthcare.

These technologies provide personalized, real-time monitoring and diagnostic capabilities, revolutionizing the way we manage health and lead the way into a future where healthcare is not only accessible but also tailored to individual needs. Wearable devices, with their diverse applications and potential for seamless integration into daily life, take protagonism in this healthcare revolution. As these wearable technologies continue to evolve, they have the potential to redefine healthcare delivery, making it more proactive, preventive, and patient-centered. The journey of telemedicine, from its emerging stages to its current convergence with wearable devices, announce a paradigm shift in how we approach healthcare, bringing us closer to a future where health is not merely managed but comprehensively understood and optimized through the marriage of technology and medicine.

These new advances bring healthcare personnel closer to patients, but it's important to consider that in the architecture of the new networks and systems, all of this must be supported correctly. New healthcare centers should consider having rooms with appropriate technology to enable telemedicine consultations in a comfortable space for healthcare staff. Moreover, these spaces should be where the consultation feels as realistic as if it were done in person. Implementing augmented reality systems and artificial vision glasses can be starting points for establishing this new medical system. The rooms should be conditioned to allow for proper assessment with sufficient space and without elements that could be harmful to the staff.

On the other hand, it's essential to consider a very important point, which is the need for the participation of computer engineers to maintain an adequate level of security to prevent the leakage of sensitive patient data. As well as to prevent identity theft. Artificial intelligence is advancing by leaps and bounds and is already capable of mimicking people's voices, generating videos practically identical to reality by basing them on one person and substituting their physical features for another, and even generating audios identical to the person with their characteristic voice traits. All of this makes it essentially necessary for an integral and joint collaboration of engineers, architects, healthcare professionals, and social agents to correctly integrate these new systems into the society of the near future.

Conclusion

- Telemedicine's dynamic evolution from the late 1960s adapts to changing technologies, giving rise to telehealth, e-health, and m-health.
- Telehealth extends beyond direct patient care to include education, aligning with broader public health goals.
- The COVID-19 pandemic transforms telemedicine, overcoming historical barriers and making teleconsultations indispensable.
- The integration of the Internet of Things (IoT) into telemedicine promises automation, cost reduction, and improved outcomes.
- Wearable devices, with their diverse applications and potential for seamless integration into daily life, play a leading role in this healthcare revolution.
- The intersection of wearable tech and AI introduces advanced capabilities, including deep learning algorithms and Brain-Computer Interfaces (BCIs).
- Ongoing innovation, exemplified by PILLSID and TytoCare®, shapes the future of wearable technology in healthcare.
- The convergence of telemedicine and wearable devices signifies a change in basic assumptions, promising a comprehensive understanding and optimization of health through technology and medicine.

References

[1] Freis, D. (2022). When Teleconferencing was the Future: The 1970 'Medizin Interkontinental' Transmission and West German Medicine in the Space Age. *European Journal for the History of Medicine and Health*, 79(1), 32–66. https://doi.org/10.1163/26667711-bja10018.

[2] Waller, M., & Stotler, C. (2018). *Telemedicine: a Primer. Current Allergy and Asthma Reports*, 18(10), 54. https://doi.org/10.1007/s11882-018-0808-4.

[3] Bashshur, R., Shannon, G., Krupinski, E., & Grigsby, J. (2011). The Taxonomy of Telemedicine. *Telemedicine and E-Health,* 17(6), 484–494. https://doi.org/10.1089/tmj.2011.0103.

[4] Becevic, M., Sheets, L. R., Wallach, E., McEowen, A., Bass, A., Mutrux, E. R., & Edison, K. E. (2020). Telehealth and Telemedicine in Missouri. *Missouri Medicine*, 117(3), 228–234.

[5] Delir Haghighi, P., & Burstein, F. (2022). Advances in E-Health and Mobile Health Monitoring. *Sensors,* 22(22), 8621. https://doi.org/10.3390/s22228621.

[6] Wilson, J., Heinsch, M., Betts, D., Booth, D., & Kay-Lambkin, F. (2021). Barriers and facilitators to the use of e-health by older adults: a scoping review. *BMC Public Health,* 21(1), 1556. https://doi.org/10.1186/s12889-021-11623-w.

[7] Greiwe, J. (2022). Telemedicine Lessons Learned During the COVID-19 Pandemic. *Current Allergy and Asthma Reports,* 22(1), 1–5. https://doi.org/10.1007/s11882-022-01026-1.

[8] Hincapié, M. A., Gallego, J. C., Gempeler, A., Piñeros, J. A., Nasner, D., & Escobar, M. F. (2020). Implementation and Usefulness of Telemedicine During the COVID-19 Pandemic: A Scoping Review. *Journal of Primary Care & Community Health*, 11, 215013272098061. https://doi.org/10.1177/2150132720980612.

[9] Acter, T., Uddin, N., Das, J., Akhter, A., Choudhury, T. R., & Kim, S. (2020). Evolution of severe acute respiratory syndrome coronavirus 2 (SARS-CoV-2) as coronavirus disease 2019 (COVID-19) pandemic: A global health emergency. *Science of The Total Environment*, 730, 138996. https://doi.org/10.1016/j.scitotenv.2020.138996.

[10] Frid, A. S., Ratti, M. F. G., Pedretti, A., Valinoti, M., Martínez, B., Sommer, J., Luna, D., & Plazzotta, F. (2020). Teletriage Pilot Study (Strategy for Unscheduled Teleconsultations): Results, Patient Acceptance and Satisfaction. *Studies in Health Technology and Informatics*, 270, 776–780. https://doi.org/10.3233/SHTI200266.

[11] Carrillo de Albornoz, S., Sia, K. L., & Harris, A. (2022). The effectiveness of teleconsultations in primary care: systematic review. *Family Practice*, 39(1), 168–182. https://doi.org/10.1093/fampra/cmab077.

[12] Alhaidari, F., Almuhaideb, A., Alsunaidi, S., Ibrahim, N., Aslam, N., Khan, I. U., Shaikh, F., Alshahrani, M., Alharthi, H., Alsenbel, Y., & Alalharith, D. (2021). E-Triage Systems for COVID-19 Outbreak: Review and Recommendations. *Sensors,* 21(8), 2845. https://doi.org/10.3390/s21082845.

[13] Uscher-Pines, L., Sousa, J., Mehrotra, A., Schwamm, L. H., & Zachrison, K. S. (2021). Rising to the challenges of the pandemic: Telehealth innovations in U.S. emergency departments. *Journal of the American Medical Informatics Association*, 28(9), 1910–1918. https://doi.org/10.1093/jamia /ocab092.

[14] Farzandipour, M., Nabovati, E., & Sharif, R. (2023). The effectiveness of tele-triage during the COVID-19 pandemic: A systematic review and narrative synthesis. *Journal of Telemedicine and Telecare,* 1357633X2211502. https://doi.org/10.1177/1357633X221150278.

[15] Bechstein, M., Elsheikh, S., Wodarg, F., Taschner, C. A., Hanning, U., Buhk, J.-H., McDonough, R., Goebell, E., Fiehler, J., & Bester, M. (2020). Interhospital teleproctoring of endovascular intracranial aneurysm treatment using dedicated live-streaming technology: first experiences during the COVID-19 pandemic. B*MJ Case Reports,* 13(10), e016722. https://doi.org/10.1136/bcr-2020-016722.

[16] M. Carter, A., Romero, B., Dai, H., Phuyal, S., Li, D., & Lucke-Wold, B. (2023). Woven Endobridge embolization: Indications and innovation. *Advanced Neurology*, 2(3), 293. https://doi.org/10.36922/an.293.

[17] Olwill, C., Mc Nally, D., & Douglas, L. (2021). Psychiatrist experience of remote consultations by telephone in an outpatient psychiatric department during the COVID-19 pandemic. *Irish Journal of Psychological Medicine,* 38(2), 132–139. https://doi.org/10.1017/ipm.2020.51.

[18] Vollherbst, D. F., Hantz, M., Schmitt, N., Do, T. D., Neuberger, U., Kauczor, H. U., Bendszus, M., Sommer, C. M., & Möhlenbruch, M. A. (2023). Experimental investigation of transvenous embolization of arteriovenous malformations using different in vivo models. *Journal of NeuroInterventional Surgery,* 15(7), 712–716. https://doi.org/10.1136/neurintsurg-2022-018894.

[19] Mori, H., Kundaliya, J., Naik, K., & Shah, M. (2022). IoT technologies in smart environment: security issues and future enhancements. *Environmental Science and Pollution Research*, 29(32), 47969–47987. https://doi.org/10.1007/s11356-022-20132-1.

[20] Abdulmalek, S., Nasir, A., Jabbar, W. A., Almuhaya, M. A. M., Bairagi, A. K., Khan, Md. A.-M., & Kee, S.-H. (2022). IoT-Based Healthcare-Monitoring System towards Improving Quality of Life: A Review. *Healthcare*, 10(10), 1993. https://doi.org/10.3390/healthcare10101993.

[21] Alvarez, P., Sianis, A., Brown, J., Ali, A., & Briasoulis, A. (2021). Chronic disease management in heart failure: focus on telemedicine and remote monitoring. *Reviews in Cardiovascular Medicine*, 22(2), 403. https://doi.org/10.31083/j.rcm2202046.

[22] Lu, L., Zhang, J., Xie, Y., Gao, F., Xu, S., Wu, X., & Ye, Z. (2020). Wearable Health Devices in Health Care: Narrative Systematic Review. *JMIR MHealth and UHealth*, 8(11), e18907. https://doi.org/10.2196/18907.

[23] Boffetta, P., & Collatuzzo, G. (2022). Application of P4 (Predictive, Preventive, Personalized, Participatory) Approach to Occupational Medicine. *La Medicina Del Lavoro*, 113(1), e2022009. https://doi.org/10.23749/mdl. v113i1.12622.

[24] Ray, T. R., Choi, J., Bandodkar, A. J., Krishnan, S., Gutruf, P., Tian, L., Ghaffari, R., & Rogers, J. A. (2019). Bio-Integrated Wearable Systems: A Comprehensive Review. *Chemical Reviews*, 119(8), 5461–5533. https://doi.org/10.1021/acs.chemrev.8b00573.

[25] Gajda, R., Gajda, J., Czuba, M., Knechtle, B., & Drygas, W. (2024). Sports Heart Monitors as Reliable Diagnostic Tools for Training Control and Detecting Arrhythmias in Professional and Leisure-Time Endurance Athletes: An Expert Consensus Statement. *Sports Medicine*, 54(1), 1–21. https://doi.org/10.1007/s40279-023-01948-4.

[26] Perez, M. V., Mahaffey, K. W., Hedlin, H., Rumsfeld, J. S., Garcia, A., Ferris, T., Balasubramanian, V., Russo, A. M., Rajmane, A., Cheung, L., Hung, G., Lee, J., Kowey, P., Talati, N., Nag, D., Gummidipundi, S. E., Beatty, A., Hills, M. T., Desai, S., Turakhia, M. P. (2019). Large-Scale Assessment of a Smartwatch to Identify Atrial Fibrillation. *New England Journal of Medicine*, 381(20), 1909–1917. https://doi.org/10.1056/NEJMoa1901183.

[27] López-Blanco, R., Velasco, M. A., Méndez-Guerrero, A., Romero, J. P., del Castillo, M. D., Serrano, J. I., Rocon, E., & Benito-León, J. (2019). Smartwatch for the analysis of rest tremor in patients with Parkinson's disease. *Journal of the Neurological Sciences*, 401, 37–42. https://doi.org/10.1016/j.jns.2019.04.011.

[28] Tseng, P., Napier, B., Garbarini, L., Kaplan, D. L., & Omenetto, F. G. (2018). Functional, RF-Trilayer Sensors for Tooth-Mounted, Wireless Monitoring of the Oral Cavity and Food Consumption. *Advanced Materials*, 30(18). https://doi.org/10.1002/adma.201703257.

[29] Maidment, D. W., & Amlani, A. M. (2020). Argumentum ad Ignorantiam: Smartphone-Connected Listening Devices. *Seminars in Hearing,* 41(04), 254–265. https://doi.org/10.1055/s-0040-1718711.

[30] Elgendi, M., & Menon, C. (2019). Assessing Anxiety Disorders Using Wearable Devices: Challenges and Future Directions. *Brain Sciences*, 9(3), 50. https://doi.org/10.3390/brainsci9030050.

[31] Can, Y. S., Chalabianloo, N., Ekiz, D., & Ersoy, C. (2019). Continuous Stress Detection Using Wearable Sensors in Real Life: Algorithmic Programming Contest Case Study. *Sensors,* 19(8), 1849. https://doi.org/10.3390/s19081849.

[32] Hernando, D., Roca, S., Sancho, J., Alesanco, Á., & Bailón, R. (2018). Validation of the Apple Watch for Heart Rate Variability Measurements during Relax and Mental Stress in Healthy Subjects. *Sensors*, 18(8), 2619. https://doi.org/10.3390/s18082619.

[33] Valenza, G., Garcia, R. G., Citi, L., Scilingo, E. P., Tomaz, C. A., & Barbieri, R. (2015). Nonlinear digital signal processing in mental health: characterization of major depression using instantaneous entropy measures of heartbeat dynamics. *Frontiers in Physiology*, 6. https://doi.org/10.3389/fphys.2015.00074.

[34] van Kraaij, A. W. J., Schiavone, G., Lutin, E., Claes, S., & Van Hoof, C. (2020). Relationship Between Chronic Stress and Heart Rate Over Time Modulated by Gender in a Cohort of Office Workers: Cross-Sectional Study Using Wearable Technologies. *Journal of Medical Internet Research*, 22(9), e18253. https://doi.org/10.2196/18253.

[35] Kalin, N. H. (2020). Novel Insights Into Pathological Anxiety and Anxiety-Related Disorders. *American Journal of Psychiatry*, 177(3), 187–189. https://doi.org/10.1176/appi.ajp.2020.20010057.

[36] Balconi, M., Fronda, G., & Crivelli, D. (2019). Effects of technology-mediated mindfulness practice on stress: psychophysiological and self-report measures. *Stress,* 22(2), 200–209. https://doi.org/10.1080/10253890.2018. 1531845.

[37] Sano, A., Taylor, S., McHill, A. W., Phillips, A. J., Barger, L. K., Klerman, E., & Picard, R. (2018). Identifying Objective Physiological Markers and Modifiable Behaviors for Self-Reported Stress and Mental Health Status Using Wearable Sensors and Mobile Phones: Observational Study. *Journal of Medical Internet Research*, 20(6), e210. https://doi.org/10.2196/jmir.9410.

[38] Shorey, S., Ng, E. D., & Wong, C. H. J. (2022). Global prevalence of depression and elevated depressive symptoms among adolescents: A systematic review and meta-analysis. *British Journal of Clinical Psychology*, 61(2), 287–305. https://doi.org/10.1111/bjc.12333.

[39] Narziev, N., Goh, H., Toshnazarov, K., Lee, S. A., Chung, K.-M., & Noh, Y. (2020). STDD: Short-Term Depression Detection with Passive Sensing. *Sensors,* 20(5), 1396. https://doi.org/10.3390/s20051396.

[40] Stauffer, F., Thielen, M., Sauter, C., Chardonnens, S., Bachmann, S., Tybrandt, K., Peters, C., Hierold, C., & Vörös, J. (2018). Skin Conformal Polymer Electrodes for Clinical ECG and EEG Recordings. *Advanced Healthcare Materials*, 7(7). https://doi.org/10.1002/adhm.201700994.

[41] Kwak, M. K., Jeong, H., & Suh, K. Y. (2011). Rational Design and Enhanced Biocompatibility of a Dry Adhesive Medical Skin Patch. *Advanced Materials,* 23(34), 3949–3953. https://doi.org/10.1002/adma.201101694.

[42] Mirani, B., Pagan, E., Currie, B., Siddiqui, M. A., Hosseinzadeh, R., Mostafalu, P., Zhang, Y. S., Ghahary, A., & Akbari, M. (2017). An Advanced Multifunctional Hydrogel-Based Dressing for Wound Monitoring and Drug Delivery. *Advanced Healthcare Materials*, 6(19). https://doi.org/10.1002/adhm.201700718.

[43] Bai, W., Kuang, T., Chitrakar, C., Yang, R., Li, S., Zhu, D., & Chang, L. (2018). Patchable micro/nanodevices interacting with skin. *Biosensors and Bioelectronics*, 122, 189–204. https://doi.org/10.1016/j.bios.2018.09.035.

[44] He, R., Liu, H., Fang, T., Niu, Y., Zhang, H., Han, F., Gao, B., Li, F., & Xu, F. (2021). A Colorimetric Dermal Tattoo Biosensor Fabricated by Microneedle Patch for Multiplexed Detection of Health-Related Biomarkers. *Advanced Science*, 8(24). https://doi.org/10.1002/advs.202103030.

[45] Zhang, Y. S., Haghiashtiani, G., Hübscher, T., Kelly, D. J., Lee, J. M., Lutolf, M., McAlpine, M. C., Yeong, W. Y., Zenobi-Wong, M., & Malda, J. (2021). 3D extrusion bioprinting. *Nature Reviews Methods Primers*, 1(1), 75. https://doi.org/10.1038/s43586-021-00073-8.

[46] Ning, L., Yang, B., Mohabatpour, F., Betancourt, N., Sarker, M., Papagerakis, P., & Chen, X. (2020). Process-induced cell damage: pneumatic versus screw-driven bioprinting. *Biofabrication,* 12(2), 025011. https://doi.org/10.1088/1758-5090/ab5f53.

[47] Zimmerling, A., & Chen, X. (2020). Bioprinting for combating infectious diseases. *Bioprinting*, 20, e00104. https://doi.org/10.1016/j.bprint. 2020.e00104.

[48] Murphy, S. V, & Atala, A. (2014). 3D bioprinting of tissues and organs. *Nature Biotechnology,* 32(8), 773–785. https://doi.org/10.1038/ nbt.2958.

[49] Chen, X. B., Fazel Anvari-Yazdi, A., Duan, X., Zimmerling, A., Gharraei, R., Sharma, N. K., Sweilem, S., & Ning, L. (2023). Biomaterials / bioinks and extrusion bioprinting. *Bioactive Materials*, 28, 511–536. https://doi.org/10.1016/j.bioactmat.2023.06.006.

[50] Zhu, B., Wang, D., Pan, H., Gong, T., Ren, Q., Wang, Z., & Guo, Y. (2023). Three-in-one customized bioink for islet organoid: GelMA/ECM/PRP orchestrate pro-angiogenic and immunoregulatory function. *Colloids and Surfaces B: Biointerfaces*, 221, 113017. https://doi.org/10.1016/j.colsurfb.2022.113017.

[51] Min, J., Yang, Y., Wu, Z., & Gao, W. (2020). Robotics in the Gut. *Advanced Therapeutics,* 3(4). https://doi.org/10.1002/adtp.201900125.

[52] Lu, T., Ji, S., Jin, W., Yang, Q., Luo, Q., & Ren, T.-L. (2023). Biocompatible and Long-Term Monitoring Strategies of Wearable, Ingestible and Implantable Biosensors: Reform the Next Generation Healthcare. *Sensors,* 23(6), 2991. https://doi.org/10.3390/s23062991.

[53] Hafezi, H., Robertson, T. L., Moon, G. D., Au-Yeung, K.-Y., Zdeblick, M. J., & Savage, G. M. (2015). An Ingestible Sensor for Measuring Medication Adherence. IEEE Transactions on Biomedical *Engineering*, 62(1), 99–109. https://doi.org/10.1109/TBME.2014.2341272.

[54] Robertson K. D, Singh R. Capsule Endoscopy. [Updated 2023 Aug 8]. In: StatPearls [Internet]. Treasure Island (FL): StatPearls Publishing; 2025 Jan-. Available from: https://www.ncbi.nlm.nih.gov/sites/books/ NBK482306/.

[55] Ferreira, J. P. S., de Mascarenhas Saraiva, M. J. da Q. e C., Afonso, J. P. L., Ribeiro, T. F. C., Cardoso, H. M. C., Ribeiro Andrade, A. P., de Mascarenhas Saraiva, M. N. G., Parente, M. P. L., Natal Jorge, R., Lopes, S. I. O., & de Macedo, G. M. G. (2022). Identification of Ulcers and Erosions by the Novel PillcamTM Crohn's Capsule Using a Convolutional Neural Network: A Multicentre Pilot Study. *Journal of Crohn's and Colitis*, 16(1), 169–172. https://doi.org/10.1093/ecco-jcc/jjab117.

[56] Toskas, A., Laskaratos, F.-M., Coda, S., Banerjee, S., & Epstein, O. (2023). Is Panenteric PillcamTM Crohn's Capsule Endoscopy Ready for Widespread Use? A Narrative Review. *Diagnostics,* 13(12), 2032. https://doi.org/10.3390/diagnostics13122032.

[57] Ferguson, T., Olds, T., Curtis, R., Blake, H., Crozier, A. J., Dankiw, K., Dumuid, D., Kasai, D., O'Connor, E., Virgara, R., & Maher, C. (2022). Effectiveness of wearable activity trackers to increase physical activity and improve health: a systematic review of systematic reviews and meta-analyses. *The Lancet Digital Health,* 4(8), e615–e626. https://doi.org/10.1016/S2589-7500(22)00111-X.

[58] Panganiban, E. B., Paglinawan, A. C., Chung, W. Y., & Paa, G. L. S. (2021). ECG diagnostic support system (EDSS): A deep learning neural network based classification system for detecting ECG abnormal rhythms from a low-powered wearable biosensors. *Sensing and Bio-Sensing Research*, 31, 100398. https://doi.org/10.1016/j.sbsr.2021.100398.

[59] Zhao, Y., Xiong, J., Hou, Y., Zhu, M., Lu, Y., Xu, Y., Teliewubai, J., Liu, W., Xu, X., Li, X., Liu, Z., Peng, W., Zhao, X., Zhang, Y., & Xu, Y. (2020). Early detection of ST-segment elevated myocardial infarction by artificial intelligence with 12-lead electrocardiogram. *International Journal of Cardiology*, 317, 223–230. https://doi.org/10.1016/j.ijcard.2020.04.089.

[60] Zhu, H., Cheng, C., Yin, H., Li, X., Zuo, P., Ding, J., Lin, F., Wang, J., Zhou, B., Li, Y., Hu, S., Xiong, Y., Wang, B., Wan, G., Yang, X., & Yuan, Y. (2020). Automatic multilabel electrocardiogram diagnosis of heart rhythm or conduction abnormalities with deep learning: a cohort study. *The Lancet Digital Health*, 2(7), e348–e357. https://doi.org/10.1016/S2589-7500(20)30107-2.

[61] Iacovacci, V., Tamadon, I., Kauffmann, E. F., Pane, S., Simoni, V., Marziale, L., Aragona, M., Cobuccio, L., Chiarugi, M., Dario, P., Del Prato, S., Ricotti, L., Vistoli, F., & Menciassi, A. (2021). A fully implantable device for intraperitoneal drug delivery refilled by ingestible capsules. *Science Robotics,* 6(57). https://doi.org/10.1126/scirobotics.abh3328.

[62] Tian, X., Zeng, Q., Kurt, S. A., Li, R. R., Nguyen, D. T., Xiong, Z., Li, Z., Yang, X., Xiao, X., Wu, C., Tee, B. C. K., Nikolayev, D., Charles, C. J., & Ho, J. S. (2023). Implant-to-implant wireless networking with metamaterial textiles. *Nature Communications*, 14(1), 4335. https://doi.org/10.1038/s41467-023-39850-2.

[63] McDaniel, N. L., Novicoff, W., Gunnell, B., & Cattell Gordon, D. (2019). Comparison of a Novel Handheld Telehealth Device with Stand-Alone Examination Tools in a Clinic Setting. *Telemedicine and E-Health*, 25(12), 1225–1230. https://doi.org/10.1089/tmj.2018.0214.

[64] Tyagi, H., Daulton, E., Bannaga, A. S., Arasaradnam, R. P., & Covington, J. A. (2021). Non-Invasive Detection and Staging of Colorectal Cancer Using a Portable Electronic Nose. *Sensors,* 21(16), 5440. https://doi.org/10.3390/s21165440.

Biographical Sketches

Guillermo Sáez Cruz

Student of double degree of Pharmacy and Biotechnology at CEU San Pablo University with 2 and half years of experience working with PGPR in Plant Biotechnology department and as a community pharmacist after been working for 7 months giving pharmaceutical advice to patients. Great interest in the study of novel approaches in the field of telehealth, medical devices and biosensors.

Student pursuing a double degree in Pharmacy and Biotechnology at CEU San Pablo University, with 2 years nad 6 months of hands-on experience in the Plant Biotechnology department specializing in PGPR. Additionally, I have served as a community pharmacist, providing pharmaceutical advice to patients for 7 months.

My academic and professional journey reflects a commitment to bridging biotechnology and pharmaceutical practice. Intrigued by innovative approaches, my focus extends to the dynamic realms of telehealth, medical devices, and biosensors. Eager to contribute my diverse skills and passion for emerging healthcare technologies to advance the intersection of pharmacy and biotechnology.

Natalia García-Tenorio Fernández

Student of Pharmacy and Biotechnology double degree at CEU San Pablo University, with 6-months experience in community pharmacy and over 3 years of experience in the Molecular Biology laboratory as intern. I carried out an Erasmus mobility at King's College London, where I earned some experience in both hospital and community pharmacies. My experience facing the public has grown great interest in the latest advances to improve patient's quality of life by means of new medical devices and biosensors.

Chapter 10

Telepharmacy and the Mediterranean Pharmacy Model: Challenges and Benefits of a Patient-Centered Care System

J. Huerto-Querejazu[1]
and Daniel Arranz-Paraiso[2,*]
[1]Universidad San Pablo CEU, Alcorcón, Madrid, Spain
[2]R&D Development Manager at Pinisan SL. C/Gran Canaria, Madrid, Spain

Abstract

Pharmaceutical management, custody, and medication dispensing or sales models vary by country, with governments and institutions adopting either liberal or interventionist approaches. The lack of government control over the prices of subsidized medications allows the free market to dictate the economic values of these products. Patients must cover these costs fully or partially if they lack insurance covering medical expenses for such conditions. However, in systems like the Spanish one, the concept is social, and these treatments are funded collectively by all citizens through tax revenue, under the common idea of a society where cooperation is holistic and comprehensive. Moreover, treatments regulated by government economic control incur lower expenses than in the free-market American system, allowing for more advanced and suitable treatments for patients. The establishment of these models stems from the intersection of economic and psychosocial factors. A Mediterranean-style system offers close and nearly daily or weekly follow-ups by pharmaceutical professionals for citizens. This is particularly important for the most vulnerable individuals who have entered social exclusion or are at risk of entering it. The loneliness pandemic resulting from the individualism pervasive in modern society often leads patients to view their pharmacist as more than just a dispensing or sales service. This is especially true for elderly patients living alone in a world where human affection and closeness are being dismantled in favour of economic considerations. The strong emphasis on psychosocial support and companionship gives the Mediterranean model a significant advantage over the liberal system.

Keywords: pharmaceutical care, pharmacy model, education, mental healthcare

* Corresponding Author's Email: daniel.paraiso@pinisan.com

In: Psycho-Environmental Variables That Ensure People's Well-Being and Health …
Editors: Roberto Alonso González Lezcano and Guadalupe Cantarero García
ISBN: 979-8-89530-831-8
© 2025 Nova Science Publishers, Inc.

Introduction

The pharmacy model present in Mediterranean countries, such as Spain, is known as the Mediterranean model. It is characterized by its focus on building proximity with patients and providing personalized pharmaceutical care. This active engagement between the patient and the pharmacist during medication dispensing, along with subsequent pharmacological follow-up, has become increasingly relevant in Spain in recent years. Consequently, this pharmacy model fosters trust-based relationships and allows for an understanding of everyone's unique needs to provide better pharmaceutical services [1, 2].

A key aspect of the Mediterranean model is its emphasis on patient proximity [1]. This means that the role of the pharmacist extends beyond merely selling medications over the counter; it involves developing empathy, fostering close communication, and understanding each patient's personal health concerns. Over the years, Spanish pharmacists have been encouraged to adopt this model to offer higher-quality services, promote health, prevent diseases, and educate the population [2-4].

Another noteworthy aspect of the Mediterranean model is the establishment of a trust-based relationship between the patient and their pharmacist. Individuals visiting a pharmacy should feel as if it's a "safe zone" where they can openly discuss their health concerns, seek information about medications, including interactions and potential side effects, without hesitation. This creates a favorable environment for providing personalized pharmaceutical care, as the pharmacist gains a better understanding of the patient's needs [5].

Pharmaceutical care in the Mediterranean model extends beyond community pharmacies to include hospitals and other healthcare settings. Physicians, nurses, and pharmacists collaborate to achieve better patient outcomes [6].

A critical component of this system is review and therapeutic monitoring following medication dispensing, aimed at identifying potential interactions, adverse effects, or issues that may arise while treatment. Therefore, in cases where errors or opportunities for improvement in the treatment plan exist, the pharmacist has a responsibility to communicate with other healthcare professionals to make the necessary adjustments to ensure proper dispensation [7].

In terms of patient education, pharmacists provide information on dosage, proper use, dosing schedules, administration, precautions, and other relevant details about medications. This approach ensures that patients understand the medications they are using and raises awareness about the importance of adherence to their treatment. Pharmacists' role extends beyond dispensing medications; it involves empathy, close communication, and understanding patients' personal health concerns [8].

Furthermore, in this pharmacy model, pharmacists are equipped to provide guidance on milder health conditions and offer recommendations to patients who are uncertain about their solutions. This approach to managing common health problems that can be resolved with over-the-counter medications helps alleviate the burden on the healthcare system and provides a quick and accessible solution to patients' concerns. As mentioned earlier, health education is essential not only for patients but also for professionals. According to the Mediterranean model, pharmacists require ongoing training to stay updated on pharmacological advancements.

The establishment of a national healthcare system that offers free and accessible coverage to all citizens has been a significant goal for the State. The primary objective is to ensure that individuals have unrestricted access to healthcare services, regardless of their social, economic, racial, or other backgrounds [9, 10].

The current national healthcare system was inspired by models in Europe, resulting in a wide array of hospitals, medical centers, and clinics. According to Article 44.2 of the General Health Law of 1986 in Spain, it is defined as the set of Health Services of the State Administration and the Health Services of the Autonomous Communities, as established in this Law. Furthermore, according to Article 46, which outlines the characteristics of the National Healthcare System, its services are extended to the entire population. Therefore, the National Healthcare System aims to provide universality, financing through public resources, decentralization by the State, and quality healthcare [9].

Each autonomous community assumes responsibilities for healthcare for the residents of its geographical area. However, healthcare coverage is provided throughout the Spanish territory. The National Health System identifies individuals through a unique personal code linked to a healthcare card, granting them access to healthcare institutions and services across Spain. As a result, healthcare establishments have a standardized system that facilitates the flow of information and patient medical records, regardless of the autonomous community in which they are located. According to the Ministry of Health, the National Health System comprises 3,055 primary care health centers, 10,067 primary care clinics, and 468 hospitals, with over 650,000 professionals working in healthcare facilities nationwide [11].

The National Healthcare System faces a series of challenges due to the aging population, which leads to increased healthcare demand. While an increase in life expectancy is a positive aspect for the country, as it signifies improved quality of life and health compared to previous years, it also means greater healthcare resource allocation. One of the fundamental principles of the National Healthcare System is to guarantee universal access for the entire population. In this way, healthcare is considered a right, not a privilege for those with higher economic means who can afford to pay for healthcare. This system also ensures comprehensive coverage, from primary care to specialized treatments, including medications, primarily funded through public taxes [9-11].

The Mediterranean model of pharmacy plays a crucial role in the detection and support of mental health disorders. Pharmacists are well-positioned to aid individuals with mental illnesses due to their expertise in medication management and their accessibility in the community [12]. The relationship between people with mental disorders and health professionals is shifting towards patient autonomy and active participation. This recognizes the importance of involving individuals with mental disorders in their own care and decision-making processes [13].

Pharmacists can offer a range of services in mental health care, including treatment management, drug information, counselling, and support for treatment adherence strategies. They can also contribute to the early detection of mental illness and support multidisciplinary teams in the delivery of mental health care [12]. Community pharmacies, in particular, have the potential to increase community awareness of mental health services and resources [14]. Training programs for pharmacy staff members have been shown to improve their understanding of mental illness and their confidence in engaging in conversations about mental health [15].

In this model, pharmacists have expanded roles and responsibilities beyond medication-related concerns. They can provide psychotherapy and other therapeutic techniques to help individuals develop effective coping strategies for emotional and psychological difficulties.

The training of pharmacists needs to align with the broadening scope of practice in mental health care [16]. Additionally, pharmacists can play a role in the management of cardiometabolic risk, metabolic syndrome, and related diseases in individuals with severe mental illness [17].

The integration of mental health into pharmacy curricula is essential for preparing future pharmacists to handle cases of mental illness. Students can benefit from courses that cover interviewing patients with mental health disorders, reviewing mental health-related medicines, and addressing social interactions [18]. The inclusion of mental health from the beginning of the curriculum and the enhancement of students' communication skills are also important considerations [19].

The Mediterranean pharmacy model plays a significant role in supporting families and managing neurodegenerative diseases. Pharmacists are well-positioned to provide guidance and support to families dealing with neurodegenerative diseases [20]. They can offer counselling and education on the importance of a balanced diet and a healthy lifestyle in the prevention and management of these diseases [21]. The Mediterranean diet, rich in antioxidants, fiber, and omega-3 fatty acids, has been associated with a lower risk of such degenerative diseases [22]. Pharmacists can provide information about the Mediterranean diet and its potential benefits to families [23].

In the context of neurodegenerative diseases, pharmacist nutritionists in the Mediterranean model can provide comprehensive care. This can lead to dietary consultations at community pharmacies, where pharmacists work alongside patients to address dietary concerns and provide personalized recommendations. Pharmacists can also educate families about the importance of regular health check-ups and medical examinations [24, 25].

The Mediterranean model of pharmacy plays a crucial role in medication management for patients with cognitive impairment, particularly in the context of personalized dosage systems. Geriatric patients often face challenges with traditional drug dosage forms, such as tablets and capsules, due to difficulties in swallowing. However, advancements in pharmaceutical technology, including the development of buccal drug administration systems, have provided alternative options for medication delivery [26]. These advancements are especially important for patients with cognitive impairment, as they may have difficulty adhering to medication regimens.

Patients with cognitive impairment, including those with dementia, often rely on strategies and support from caregivers to manage their medications. Community pharmacies play a vital role in assisting patients and their caregivers with medication acquisition and delivery. Patients and caregivers trust primary healthcare professionals, including pharmacists, to provide guidance and support in medication management. Community pharmacies also offer valuable resources and environmental support for patients with cognitive impairment [27].

Assessing the ability of patients, including geriatric patients, to self-administer medication is crucial for personalized medication management. Clinicians use validated lists and comprehensive geriatric assessments to evaluate the quality of medication regimens and assess patients' cognitive abilities, mobility, and functional status. The ability to self-administer medication is assessed through various tasks related to medication self-administration, which are recorded and rated by experts [28].

Person-centred care and patient safety are essential in geriatric hospitals. However, there may be differences in the focus of healthcare services between geriatric hospitals and care facilities. Geriatric hospitals tend to prioritize healthcare over well-being compared to geriatric care facilities. This distinction is important in the context of personalized patient care and highlights the need for policy efforts and practices that prioritize holistic care in geriatric hospitals. Impaired cognition significantly affects a person's ability to manage their medications. Studies have explored various aspects of medicines management by individuals with dementia or cognitive impairment living in the community. These studies have examined methods for assessing capacity, strategies for supporting independent medication management, and the role of healthcare professionals, including pharmacists, in assisting with medication acquisition and delivery [29-31].

Online pharmacy navigation skills are relevant to medication management, particularly in the context of chronic medical conditions. Neurocognitive functions, such as prospective memory, play a role in health-related internet navigation skills. Studies have shown that prospective memory is impaired in individuals with HIV disease and is related to medication management capacity. The increased use of online pharmacy services, especially during the COVID-19 pandemic, highlights the importance of understanding the role of neurocognitive functions in health-related internet navigation skills [32].

Convenience in medication management is a crucial factor in treatment adherence. Strategies such as synchronization using pill organizers or Smart medication management systems for all the medications patients use without having a pharmacy at home can enhance adherence and simplify medication management. [33, 34]. And all of this is also thanks to pharmacy technicians who play an increasingly important role in supporting pharmacists in medication management. They assist in medication dispensing, perform clinical functions, and provide administrative support in pharmacy operations. The role of pharmacy technicians has evolved to support the expanding responsibilities of pharmacists and enhance medication outcomes. [33, 34]. The role of pharmacy technicians in medication history programs has been successful in gathering accurate medication information. Standardized training, regular feedback, and education, as well as interdisciplinary collaboration, are key elements for the implementation and maintenance of medication history programs. Pharmacy technicians play a crucial role in supporting medication management and improving patient outcomes. [33, 34].

The American Geriatrics Society (AGS) Beers Criteria® provides guidelines for potentially inappropriate medication use in older adults. These criteria are widely used by healthcare professionals in the United States to ensure safe and appropriate medication management in older adults. Adhering to these criteria can help prevent medication-related issues and improve patient outcomes [35].

It should always be understood that polypharmacy is a common issue among older adults, and medication management plays a crucial role in ensuring the safe and appropriate use of medications. Cognitive impairment can affect external medication management, understanding of pharmacotherapy, and the use of over-the-counter medications. Further studies are needed to explore prescription approaches and optimize medication management for older adults. [36-38].

Currently, the co-payment system for prescription medications prescribed by physicians is common in many countries in our continent. Specifically in Spain, co-payment was introduced into public healthcare in 1967 and initially applied without differentiation in the amount contributed between the active workforce and pensioners. In 1978, the first change was implemented in the system, differentiating the contribution for treatments of a chronic nature. For all other medications, a 20% co-payment was established, except for pensioners, who were exempt from making this contribution.

In 1975, the General Mutual Society of Civil Servants of the State (MUFACE) was created, which introduced a co-payment model with a 30% contribution based on the medication packaging. The General Mutual Society of the Judiciary (MUGEJU) and the Social Institute of the Armed Forces (ISFAS) followed the MUFACE pharmaceutical co-payment system. However, over the years, both the National Health System and the rest of the Administrative Mutualism have been regulated by the same law to ensure that the patient's financial contribution is the same across all scales. Among the existing mutual societies in Spain, MUFACE encompasses the largest number of individuals.

The growth of public expenditure on prescribed pharmacy items has increased since the end of the last century until 2011, partly due to the increase in the number of pensioners, greater life expectancy, and an increase in pharmacological treatments due to the presence of more diseases. However, these factors alone do not fully explain the continuous reduction in the effective co-payment percentage (the total part of the retail price that is covered). In 2012, a change in the co-payment model was introduced, which is now determined based on an individual's income and is assigned a number according to their contribution: TSI 001, TSI 002, TSI 003, TSI 004, TSI 005, and TSI 006 (Administrative Mutualism). In this reform, certain populations were exempted from co-payments, including unemployed individuals not receiving subsidies and pensioners with low pensions, in contrast to the previous law where pensioners were exempt from any co-payment.

As previously mentioned, the Spanish healthcare system aims to be accessible and universal. Therefore, to address economic insolvency or social difficulties in purchasing medications, particularly for patients with chronic diseases or combined therapies, a pharmaceutical co-payment system for prescription medications has been created. This helps control medication costs and improves their responsible use. The social importance of disease control is that this system can serve as a means to prevent healthcare issues because the population becomes more aware of the medical services available. In the case of serious and mental illnesses, the co-payment system can enhance resources allocated to treat these conditions.

The Spanish pharmaceutical model is a unique social-health business controlled by the state. It has its own peculiarities in terms of the prices of medicines, particularly expensive medicines, and their use in hospitals.

Peculiarities of the Spanish pharmaceutical model:

Low investment in research and development (R&D): Spanish pharmaceutical companies are recommended to increase their investment in R&D, as this plays a crucial role in knowledge production and commercialization in the pharmaceutical sector. By increasing their investment in R&D, Spanish pharmaceutical companies can contribute to the development of new and innovative medicines, which can have a positive impact on the prices of medicines and their availability in the market [39].

State-controlled healthcare system: The Spanish healthcare system follows the principles of the Beveridge model, which is a state-controlled and financed healthcare system. This model emphasizes the provision of healthcare services by the state and ensures that healthcare is accessible to all citizens. The Spanish NHS healthcare system is one example of a state-controlled healthcare system [40]. However, the crisis caused by the COVID-19 pandemic has highlighted the failures of the Spanish healthcare system and its semi-federal model, which lacks coordination to effectively manage such crises [41]. This crisis has also raised concerns about the sustainability of the Spanish private healthcare system [42].

Pricing and reimbursement of medicines: The pricing and reimbursement of medicines by the Spanish National Health System (NHS) is based on a set of criteria included in the Royal Legislative Decree 1/2015 (RDL 1/2015). These criteria are used to make decisions regarding the inclusion of new drugs in the Spanish NHS and to determine their prices and reimbursement [43]. However, there are challenges and limitations in the current system, and a profound political change is required to ensure transparency, accountability, and efficiency in the pricing and reimbursement process [44].

Thorough evaluation process for the approval of pharmaceutical products: The Spanish pharmaceutical model also includes a thorough evaluation process by the Spanish Agency of Medicines and Medical Devices (AEMPS) for the approval of pharmaceutical products. This evaluation process includes the assessment of preclinical and clinical data, as well as the inspection and accreditation of the GMP Cell Production Facility and a Pharmacovigilance Plan, among other aspects, to ensure the quality, safety, and efficacy of the pharmaceutical product. [45] This rigorous evaluation process is similar to the requirements for centralized marketing authorization and contributes to the control of prices and the quality of medicines in the Spanish market.

Inadequate access to medicines affected by uncontrolled prices is a major concern in developing countries, including Spain. The lack of comprehensive data on medicine prices in Spain further exacerbates this issue. Therefore, there is a need for comprehensive data on medicine prices and availability to address this concern and ensure affordable access to essential medicines.

Objective

In general, the objective is describing the principles and characteristics of the Mediterranean pharmacy model, which is distinguished by providing universal healthcare regardless of socioeconomic status and ensuring that the pharmacist establishes a close relationship with the patient. Pharmaceutical care and guidance play a significant role in delivering high-quality healthcare services in conjunction with other healthcare professionals.

a. In more detail, the objectives of this chapter regarding the Mediterranean pharmacy and the need for its perpetuation in society despite the developments that will take place in the field of telepharmacy and telemedicine are:
b. Describe the Mediterranean model of pharmacy, emphasizing its focus on proximity with patients and providing personalized care.
c. Explain the role of the pharmacist in this model, including aspects like patient education, medication review, and offering guidance on milder health conditions.
d. Highlight the importance of a national healthcare system with universal coverage for achieving better health outcomes.
e. Discuss the role of pharmacists in mental health care, including offering treatment management, counselling, and supporting adherence.
f. Ensure Transparency and Efficiency in Drug Pricing and Reimbursement
g. Facilitate Access to Essential Medicines at Affordable Prices

h. Explain the role of pharmacists in supporting families dealing with neurodegenerative diseases, including providing guidance on diet and medication management (paragraph 19).
i. Analyze the co-payment system for prescription medications in Spain.
j. Improve the Coordination and Efficiency of the Spanish Healthcare System.

Materials and Methods

1. *Initial Search:*
   - A comprehensive search was conducted in the PubMed, Web of Science, and Scopus databases.
   - The following keywords were used:
     - "Spanish pharmacy"
     - "Spanish national health system"
     - "Interrelation between healthcare professionals in Spain"
     - "Mediterranean pharmacy model"
     - "Health monitoring in the pharmacy"
   - The keywords were combined using the Boolean operators AND and OR.
   - A total of 324 articles were retrieved.
2. *Duplicate Removal:*
   - Duplicates were removed from the different databases.
   - The removal of duplicates was manually verified to ensure accuracy.
   - A reduction to 184 unique articles was achieved.
3. *Date Filtering:*
   - Only articles published between January 1, 2020, and December 31, 2023, were selected.
   - The publication date of each article was verified.
   - A final collection of 71 articles was obtained.
4. *Abstract Assessment:*
   - A critical reading of the abstracts of the 71 selected articles was performed.
   - The thematic relevance of each abstract was assessed with respect to the systematic review.
   - 61 articles that met the pre-established relevance criteria were selected.
- *Methodological Quality Assessment:*
   - A specific methodology was applied to evaluate the methodological quality of the 61 articles.
   - Aspects such as study design, sample size, analysis methodology, and presentation of results were evaluated.
   - 43 articles that met the methodological quality criteria were selected.
5. *Search for Laws and Data from the Ministry of Health:*
   - An independent search for laws and official data from the Spanish Ministry of Health will be conducted.

- Government websites and official repositories of the Ministry of Health will be searched.
- Data relevant to the systematic review will be collected.

6. *Analysis and Synthesis of Information:*
   - The information collected in the 43 selected articles will be analyzed.
   - The research findings will be synthesized to answer the questions of the systematic review.

Discussion

The Spanish National Health System (SNS) and community apothecaries are two pillars of the Spanish healthcare system. The SNS is a universal system that provides comprehensive content to all citizens, anyhow of income or social status. This healthcare institutions are patient-centered and concentrated on furnishing substantiated pharmaceutical care. They're characterized by their propinquity, scientific and specialized rigor, commitment to society, emphasis on trust- grounded connections, and fidelity to pharmaceutical care. Also, the SNS is one of the most effective and indifferent healthcare systems in the world, furnishing high-quality care to all citizens. It's also largely accessible, with over 99 of the population living within 10 kilometers of a primary care center.

The SNS prioritizes forestallment, investing heavily in preventative healthcare programs similar as nonage vaccination and cancer webbing. This has helped to reduce the prevalence of preventable conditions in Spain. The SNS also emphasizes primary care, the first point of contact for utmost cases with the healthcare system. Primary care is essential for early discovery and treatment of conditions, as well as for the operation of habitual conditions. The SNS has a well- developed network of primary care centers staffed by good healthcare professionals. it is important to emphasize that Spanish hospitals are known for their high- quality care, equipped with the rearmost medical technology and staffed by educated and largely good healthcare professionals.

Community apothecaries play a vital part in the Spanish healthcare system, furnishing cases with accessible access to pharmaceutical care. druggists are frequently the first point of contact for cases with health- related questions and enterprises. They can give cases with advice and support on a wide range of health issues, including drug operation, complaint forestallment, and healthy life choices. Community apothecaries also develop close connections with their cases over time, which allows them to more understand their individual requirements and enterprises. This trust-grounded relationship is essential for furnishing substantiated pharmaceutical care. Pharmaceutical care is a comprehensive approach to drug operation that focuses on the individual case's requirements and issues. druggists play a vital part in pharmaceutical care by furnishing cases with information about their specifics, helping them to manage their specifics effectively, and covering their progress.

The Mediterranean pharmacy model proposes a health strategy based on wellness and patient care. Both the evolution of pharmaceutical technology and the Mediterranean diet have a positive impact on patients' health when combined in their individual lifestyle. Pharmacists play an important role as healthcare professionals and are a fundamental part of the healthcare system due to the support and guidance they provide to patients, enabling them to improve their lifestyle and adherence to treatment. Accuracy in dispensing medicines and the development of patient databases have also improved pharmaceutical care. Care is safer and more efficient because it promotes a holistic approach among many healthcare professionals such as nurses, doctors and others. The co-payment system for health services and the purchase of medicines aims to control the resources allocated, encourage the correct use of medicines and guarantee a public, free and universal health system for the population.

It is important to consider the uniqueness of the co-payment system and government control. This control encompasses the medicine as a common framework. The system is able to control the licenses it issues for the operation of medicines, it is the one that approves whether a medicine can be marketed, it also imposes reference prices for marketed formulations and it is the one that marks price reductions according to reference groups through the anatomical, therapeutic and chemical classification system or ATC. Pharmacies are subject to the prices that are set and with them profit margins are established on a non-linear percentage basis. 143.05 do not have the same profit margin of 27.9% as those priced below this value. The same is true for effects and accessories that do not have the margin of prescription drugs. However, it should be borne in mind that the system allows the marketing of over-the-counter medicines with higher profit margins, and which relieve the primary care system. Patients requiring non-steroidal anti-inflammatory drugs (paracetamol, ibuprofen, dexketoprofen or naproxen) have the option of not having to go to the doctor for a prescription and to purchase the product freely from the pharmacy. In these cases, pharmaceutical care is important, as the pharmacist must warn the patient of the risks, must instruct the patient on how to take the medicine and on considerations for its use, such as checking for interactions with other medicines or natural supplements.

The co-payment system makes possible a collaborative system where patients, whether they belong to a higher or lower social stratum, can have access to treatment that they can afford out of their income. The system is organised in such a way that people with higher incomes have a higher co-payment and there is a very low contribution from pensioners and there is even a range of people who are excluded from the co-payment. This means that the entire population is protected within a public system that cushions social vulnerability. In a future where it is forgotten or not considered to maintain a system where the pharmacy remains a point of health care where the public and private parts are mixed, all social protection will tend to disappear. A fully liberalized system such as that in the United States requires a private insurance structure that is able to bear the costs of the most expensive treatments.

In the future landscape, the evolution towards telepharmacy poses significant challenges to preserving the essence of Mediterranean pharmacy. As technology advances, there is a risk of losing the personalised care and continuous contact between pharmacists and patients that are fundamental elements of pharmaceutical care. The potential transition to drug delivery services could transform pharmacy into a commercial transaction rather than a health care service. With a new model in which telepharmacy, understood as a mere medicine delivery service, will eliminate a large part of the benefits of pharmacy models such as the Mediterranean. Close therapeutic monitoring and continuous contact between patients and pharmacists, the most accessible health professional there is, will be replaced by economic profitability. Pharmacists must defend their professionalism, conferred in part by their academic training, but also by their experience and the Hippocratic oath they take when they graduate. Patients value very highly the presence of this type of pharmacist, for whom no appointment is required. Technical and pharmacological advice is completely free and accessible. The idea of charging for the act of pharmaceutical care does not exist now, but in an environment where the pharmacy can become a delivery service, it will probably be an extra service to be paid for by the consumer.

In a future urban environment, pharmacies should remain under the current or a future modified regulation but without losing the protection of the Mediterranean pharmacy. The parameters for opening new premises can be varied, other levels of training or experience can be required, and even a mixed system can be envisaged in which a pharmacy would follow up patients at home. All this should be regulated and governed by parameterisation to ensure the quality of the services themselves. The new mechanisms can be integrated into the architecture of the new communities by means of monitoring systems, with studies of resistance and weaknesses. Among others, it is possible to integrate personalized care spaces with pharmacists within the new megalopolises that are being built in the countries of major economic powers such as the city of "The Line" in Saudi Arabia. For example, a non-existent figure may be created in future private health insurance where the pharmacist will play the same role as the doctors to whom teleconsultations are made through IoT platforms. And all this for the benefits that the pharmacy can provide telematically as a telepharmacy that can provide the same as the Mediterranean model but in the new social structures.

It is crucial that pharmacists uphold their professional role, emphasising not only their academic training but also their ethical commitment. The deep connection and trust built over time with patients are invaluable assets that must be preserved. As new ways of integrating telepharmacy in urban settings are explored, a balance must be found to ensure the quality and accessibility of pharmaceutical care. Careful regulation and parameterisation will be essential to safeguard the integrity of the pharmacy profession and maintain the vital contribution of pharmacies to public health in the future.

In addition, it is important to consider the potential economic impact on the patient-pharmacist relationship. In a telepharmacy scenario, where certain services could be considered additional and subject to fees, there is a challenge to maintain accessibility to pharmaceutical care for all social strata. The implementation of a fee-based system could lead to disparities in access, particularly affecting those on lower incomes. It is therefore essential that any evolution in the pharmacy model ensures equity and continuity of quality care for the entire population, thus preserving the integrity of a public, universal and accessible healthcare system in Spain and in other countries.

Conclusion

- The Mediterranean pharmacy model is highly valued by the general population and has gained further recognition since the onset of the COVID-19 pandemic. It is a system focused on improving the patient's well-being both physically and psychologically, which is essential in today's society where detachment, individualism, and loneliness are spreading almost uncontrollably.
- In the new social structures, it is important to evaluate whether telepharmacy, as a solely commercial endeavor, will generate social benefits or merely economic gains, potentially diminishing quality of life.

- In the cities of the future, if models like the Mediterranean are adopted, a growth system should be established that maintains harmony between the target population and existing healthcare facilities. It would be a good strategy to implement dynamic restructurings where governments promote the presence of pharmacies in remote or sparsely populated areas.
- Pharmacists play a crucial role as a link and connection between doctors, nurses, and patients. They explain treatments and methods of administration, with the responsibility to master pharmaceutical knowledge such as aerosol application systems, insulins, and other complex devices. Additionally, they should be didactic to convey knowledge to patients, adapting to their cognitive and sensory capabilities.
- It is very important to maintain the fragile balance between business and health care in the future social structures and mega-city projects that are being generated. It is a delicate balance where health, care and accessibility to health services for all citizens of the states must be prioritised above all else. The mechanism is resilient because it has lasted over time, through governments and socio-economic restructuring. It would be a serious loss if it were to be eliminated in favour of large multinational lobbies engaged in large-scale sales.

References

[1] M. E. F. Izquierdo, J. V. M. Sánchez, and I. M. M. Alcalá, Integración de sistemas y servicios socio sanitarios para la alfabetización y el empoderamiento del paciente en su autocuidado. ARANZADI/CIVITAS, 2023.

[2] M. Fernández Rodríguez, F. Martínez Martínez, D. Iñiguez-Pineda, M. Morales-Flores, M. D. Cabezas-López, and J. P. García Corpas, "Farmacias comunitarias de Ecuador y España. Aspectos legales," *Ars Pharmaceutica*, vol. 62, no. 2, pp. 163–174, Mar. 2021, doi: 10.30827/ars.v62i2.16704.

[3] M. A. Strand, N. A. DiPietro Mager, L. Hall, S. L. Martin, and D. F. Sarpong, "Pharmacy Contributions to Improved Population Health: Expanding the Public Health Roundtable," *Prev Chronic Dis*, vol. 17, p. 200350, Sep. 2020, doi: 10.5888/pcd17.200350.

[4] M. A. Gastelurrutia, M. J. Faus, and F. Martinez-Martinez, "Primary health care policy and vision for community pharmacy and pharmacists in Spain," *Pharm Pract* (Granada), vol. 18, no. 2, p. 1999, Jun. 2020, doi: 10.18549/PharmPract.2020.2.1999.

[5] J. Patel, N. Christofferson, and K. J. Goodlet, "Pharmacist-provided SARS-CoV-2 testing targeting a majority-Hispanic community during the early COVID-19 pandemic: Results of a patient perception survey," *Journal of the American Pharmacists Association*, vol. 62, no. 1, pp. 187–193, Jan. 2022, doi: 10.1016/j.japh.2021.08.015.

[6] M. Lillo-Crespo, J. Riquelme-Galindo, E. De Baetselier, B. Van Rompaey, and T. Dilles, "Understanding pharmaceutical care and nurse prescribing in Spain: A grounded theory approach through healthcare professionals' views and expectations," *PLoS One*, vol. 17, no. 1, p. e0260445, Jan. 2022, doi: 10.1371/journal.pone.0260445.

[7] A. M. Jové, A. Fernández, C. Hughes, M. Guillén-Solà, M. Rovira, and M. Rubio-Valera, "Perceptions of collaboration between general practitioners and community pharmacists: findings from a qualitative study based in Spain," *J Interprof Care,* vol. 28, no. 4, pp. 352–357, Jul. 2014, doi: 10.3109/13561820.2014.898621.

[8] N. Amador-Fernández, M. Á. Gastelurrutia, and V. García-Cárdenas, "Development of self-care in Spanish community pharmacies," *Exploratory Research in Clinical and Social Pharmacy*, vol. 12, p. 100337, Dec. 2023, doi: 10.1016/j.rcsop.2023.100337.

[9] E. Bernal-Delgado Bernal-Delgado, E., Garcia-Armesto, S., Oliva, J., Sanchez Martinez, F. I., Repullo, J. R., Pena-Longobardo, L. M., Ridao-Lopez, M., & Hernandez-Quevedo, C, "Spain: Health System Review.," *Health Syst Transit*, vol. 20, no. 2, pp. 1–179, May 2018.

[10] A. S. Benedicto, "Public Health in Spain," in *Public Health Policies in the European Union*, Routledge, 2018, pp. 149–167. doi: 10.4324/9780429446351-7.

[11] Ministerio de Sanidad, *"Informe Anual del Sistema Nacional de Salud 2020-2021,"* Centro de Publicaciones, Madrid, 2022.

[12] M. Rubio-Valera, T. Chen, and C. O'Reilly, "New Roles for Pharmacists in Community Mental Health Care: A Narrative Review," *Int J Environ Res Public Health,* vol. 11, no. 10, pp. 10967–10990, Oct. 2014, doi: 10.3390/ijerph111010967.

[13] C. Martínez-Martínez, V. Sánchez-Martínez, J. Ballester-Martínez, M. Richart-Martínez, and J. D. Ramos-Pichardo, "A qualitative emancipatory inquiry into relationships between people with mental disorders and health professionals," *J Psychiatr Ment Health Nurs*, vol. 28, no. 4, pp. 721–737, Aug. 2021, doi: 10.1111/jpm.12727.

[14] C. Crespo-Gonzalez, S. Dineen-Griffin, J. Rae, and R. A. Hill, "A qualitative exploration of mental health services provided in community pharmacies," *PLoS One*, vol. 17, no. 5, p. e0268259, May 2022, doi: 10.1371/journal.pone.0268259.

[15] S. Shams and H. L. Hattingh, "Evaluation of mental health training for community pharmacy staff members and consumers," *Journal of Pharmacy Practice and Research*, vol. 50, no. 2, pp. 160–165, Apr. 2020, doi: 10.1002/jppr.1634.

[16] A. O. Bamgboye, I. A. Hassan, Y. A. Adebisi, R. O. Farayola, and T. Uwizeyimana, "Towards improving community pharmacy-based mental health services in Nigeria," *J Pharm Policy Pract*, vol. 14, no. 1, p. 34, Dec. 2021, doi: 10.1186/s40545-021-00316-9.

[17] D. Sud, E. Laughton, R. McAskill, E. Bradley, and I. Maidment, "The role of pharmacy in the management of cardiometabolic risk, metabolic syndrome and related diseases in severe mental illness: a mixed-methods systematic literature review," *Syst Rev,* vol. 10, no. 1, p. 92, Mar. 2021, doi: 10.1186/s13643-021-01586-9.

[18] S. A. Saka, O. S. Akanbi, and U. I. H. Eze, "Perceptions of Nigerian final year undergraduate students of the adequacy of the pharmacy curriculum for mental health care," *Journal of Pharmacy Practice and Research,* vol. 50, no. 1, pp. 48–54, Feb. 2020, doi: 10.1002/jppr.1607.

[19] D. Keating, S. McWilliams, C. Hynes, A. Purcell, M. Clarke, and J. Strawbridge, "Patients and Caregivers Helping to Shape the Undergraduate Pharmacy Mental Health Curriculum," *Am J Pharm Educ,* vol. 83, no. 9, p. 7138, Nov. 2019, doi: 10.5688/ajpe7138.

[20] Aza, A., Gómez-Vela, M., Badia, M., Begoña Orgaz, M., González-Ortega, E., Vicario-Molina, I., & Montes-López, E., "Listening to families with a person with neurodegenerative disease talk about their quality of life: integrating quantitative and qualitative approaches.," *Health Qual Life Outcomes*, vol. 20, no. 1, p. 76, May 2022, doi: 10.1186/s12955-022-01977-z.

[21] Kępka, A., Ochocińska, A., Borzym-Kluczyk, M., Chojnowska, S., Skorupa, E., Przychodzeń, M., & Waszkiewicz, N., "Healthy Food Pyramid as Well as Physical and Mental Activity in the Prevention of Alzheimer's Disease," *Nutrients,* vol. 14, no. 8, p. 1534, Apr. 2022, doi: 10.3390/nu14081534.

[22] E. Basdeki, C. Salis, and M. Hagidimitriou, "The effects of Mediterranean diet and EVOO consumption in relation to human health," *Not Sci Biol,* vol. 12, no. 3, pp. 466–485, Sep. 2020, doi: 10.15835/nsb12310784.

[23] G. A. Franco, L. Interdonato, M. Cordaro, S. Cuzzocrea, and R. Di Paola, "Bioactive Compounds of the Mediterranean Diet as Nutritional Support to Fight Neurodegenerative Disease," *Int J Mol Sci,* vol. 24, no. 8, p. 7318, Apr. 2023, doi: 10.3390/ijms24087318.

[24] Iwata, H., Shibano, K., Okazaki, M., Fujimaki, K., Kobayashi, N., Fujimoto, K., Hayashi, N., Goto, T., & Yamaura, K., "Patient satisfaction with oral health check-ups at a community pharmacy and their effect on oral self-care habits and dental consultation behavior," *Drug Discov Ther,* vol. 14, no. 6, pp. 319–324, Dec. 2020, doi: 10.5582/ddt.2020.03098.

[25] Kizaki, H., Ota, T., Mashima, S., Nakamura, Y., Kiyokawa, S., Kominato, H., Satoh, H., Sawada, Y., & Hori, S., "Questionnaire survey investigation of the present status of dietetic consultation at

community pharmacies from the perspectives of registered dietitians and pharmacists," *BMC Health Serv Res,* vol. 21, no. 1, p. 935, Dec. 2021, doi: 10.1186/s12913-021-06959-3.

[26] R. Varghese, P. Sood, S. Salvi, J. Karsiya, and D. Kumar, "3D printing in the pharmaceutical sector: Advances and evidences," *Sensors International,* vol. 3, p. 100177, 2022, doi: 10.1016/j.sintl.2022.100177.

[27] Forsyth, P., Radley, A., Rushworth, G. F., Marra, F., Roberts, S., O'Hare, R., Duggan, C., & Maguire, B., "The Collaborative Care Model: Realizing healthcare values and increasing responsiveness in the pharmacy workforce," *Research in Social and Administrative Pharmacy*, vol. 19, no. 1, pp. 110–122, Jan. 2023, doi: 10.1016/j.sapharm.2022.08.016.

[28] F. Pereira, M. Bieri, M. del Rio Carral, M. M. Martins, and H. Verloo, "Collaborative medication management for older adults after hospital discharge: a qualitative descriptive study," *BMC Nurs*, vol. 21, no. 1, p. 284, Oct. 2022, doi: 10.1186/s12912-022-01061-3.

[29] C. Powell, J. Tomlinson, C. Quinn, and B. Fylan, "Interventions for self-management of medicines for community-dwelling people with dementia and mild cognitive impairment and their family carers: a systematic review," *Age Ageing*, vol. 51, no. 5, May 2022, doi: 10.1093/ageing/afac089.

[30] M. Kumai, K. Kumai, G. Kuroki, M. Shoji, K. Nakamura, and K. Meguro, "Disturbed medication management in older adults with good cognitive health and mild cognitive impairment associated with semantic memory impairment: The Wakuya Project," *Geriatr Gerontol Int,* vol. 23, no. 5, pp. 319–325, May 2023, doi: 10.1111/ggi.14563.

[31] O. Arikawe, H. Morrissey, and P. Ball, "Community pharmacy brief screening intervention to improve health outcomes for patients diagnosed with chronic diseases," *Journal of Advanced Pharmacy Education and Research*, vol. 12, no. 3, pp. 1–8, 2022, doi: 10.51847/bmamIaRVB8.

[32] A. Matchanova, D. P. Sheppard, L. D. Medina, E. E. Morgan, and S. P. Woods, "Health literacy mediates the effects of educational attainment on online pharmacy navigation skills in older adults with HIV disease," *Psychol Health,* vol. 38, no. 3, pp. 348–368, Mar. 2023, doi: 10.1080/08870446.2021.1960990.

[33] A. Bombarda, S. Bonfanti, and A. Gargantini, "*Developing Medical Devices from Abstract State Machines to Embedded Systems: A Smart Pill Box Case Study*," 2019, pp. 89–103. doi: 10.1007/978-3-030-29852-4_7.

[34] R. Turjamaa, S. Kapanen, and M. Kangasniemi, "How smart medication systems are used to support older people's drug regimens: A systematic literature review," *Geriatr Nurs* (Minneap), vol. 41, no. 6, pp. 677–684, Nov. 2020, doi: 10.1016/j.gerinurse.2020.02.005.

[35] By the 2019 American Geriatrics Society Beers Criteria® Update Expert Panel*, "American Geriatrics Society 2019 Updated AGS Beers Criteria® for Potentially Inappropriate Medication Use in Older Adults," *J Am Geriatr Soc,* vol. 67, no. 4, pp. 674–694, Apr. 2019, doi: 10.1111/jgs.15767.

[36] Crespo, T. S., Andrade, J. M. O., Lelis, D. de F., Ferreira, A. C., Souza, J. G. S., Martins, A. M. E. de B. L., & Santos, S. H. S., "Adherence to medication, physical activity and diet among older people living with diabetes mellitus: Correlation between cognitive function and health literacy," *IBRO Rep,* vol. 9, pp. 132–137, Dec. 2020, doi: 10.1016/j.ibror.2020.07.003.

[37] Kwon, H. S., Lee, D., Lee, M. H., Yu, S., Lim, J. S., Yu, K. H., Oh, M. S., Lee, J. S., Hong, K. S., Lee, E. J., Kang, D. W., & Kwon, S. U., "Post-stroke cognitive impairment as an independent predictor of ischemic stroke recurrence: PICASSO sub-study," *J Neurol,* vol. 267, no. 3, pp. 688–693, Mar. 2020, doi: 10.1007/s00415-019-09630-4.

[38] R. Mendes, S. Martins, and L. Fernandes, "Adherence to Medication, Physical Activity and Diet in Older Adults With Diabetes: Its Association With Cognition, Anxiety and Depression," *J Clin Med Res,* vol. 11, no. 8, pp. 583–592, 2019, doi: 10.14740/jocmr3894.

[39] T. García-Valderrama, J. Sanchez-Ortiz, and E. Mulero-Mendigorri, "Knowledge production and commercialization from R&D: the pharmaceutical sector," *Management Decision*, vol. 61, no. 13, pp. 222–247, Jul. 2023, doi: 10.1108/MD-05-2022-0567.

[40] P. I. Vidal-Carreras, J. J. Garcia-Sabater, and J. A. Marin-Garcia, "Applying Value Stream Mapping to Improve the Delivery of Patient Care in the Oncology Day Hospital," *Int J Environ Res Public Health*, vol. 19, no. 7, p. 4265, Apr. 2022, doi: 10.3390/ijerph19074265.

[41] A. Sánchez-Bayón, E. González-Arnedo, and Á. Andreu-Escario, "Spanish Healthcare Sector Management in the COVID-19 Crisis Under the Perspective of Austrian Economics and New-Institutional Economics," *Front Public Health*, vol. 10, Mar. 2022, doi: 10.3389/fpubh.2022.801525.

[42] M. del C. Valls Martínez, J. M. Santos-Jaén, R. F. Valls-Úbeda, and R. Soriano Román, "COVID-19 and Public Health Spending; Effects on the Economic Sustainability of the Spanish Private Healthcare System," *Int J Environ Res Public Health*, vol. 20, no. 2, p. 1585, Jan. 2023, doi: 10.3390/ijerph 20021585.

[43] M. Á. Calleja and X. Badia, "Feasibility study to characterize price and reimbursement decision-making criteria for the inclusion of new drugs in the Spanish National Health System: the cefiderocol example," *Int J Technol Assess Health Care*, vol. 38, no. 1, p. e48, May 2022, doi: 10.1017/S0266462322000332.

[44] J. Oliva-Moreno, J. Puig-Junoy, M. Trapero-Bertran, D. Epstein, C. Pinyol, and J. A. Sacristán, "Economic Evaluation for Pricing and Reimbursement of New Drugs in Spain: Fable or Desideratum?," *Value in Health,* vol. 23, no. 1, pp. 25–31, Jan. 2020, doi: 10.1016/j.jval.2019.06.012.

[45] Sánchez-Guijo, F., Avendaño-Solá, C., Badimón, L., Bueren, J. A., Canals, J. M., Delgadillo, J., Delgado, J., Eguizábal, C., Fernández-Santos, M. E., García-Olmo, D., González-Aseguinolaza, G., Juan, M., Martín, F., Mata, R., Montserrat, N., Pérez-Martínez, A., Pérez-Simón, J. A., Prósper, F., Urbano-Ispizua, Á., Moraleda, J. M., "Role of Hospital Exemption in Europe: position paper from the Spanish Advanced Therapy Network (TERAV)," *Bone Marrow Transplant*, vol. 58, no. 6, pp. 727–728, Jun. 2023, doi: 10.1038/s41409-023-01962-0.

Chapter 11

The Effects of Electronic Light Equipment at Night on Children's Health

Cándida Filgueira Arias[1,*]
David Baeza Moyano[2]
and Roberto Alonso González-Lezcano[3]

[1]Department of Education, Faculty of Humanities and Communication Sciences, San Pablo-CEU University, CEU Universities Member of the Institute for Addiction Studies (IEA-CEU), Madrid, Spain
[2]Departamento Química y Bioquímica, Facultad de Farmacia, Universidad San Pablo-CEU, CEU Universities, Miembro Instituto de Estudios de las Adicciones (IEA-CEU) Urbanización Montepríncipe, Alcorcón, Madrid, Spain
[3]Departamento de Arquitectura y Diseño, Escuela Politécnica Superior, Universidad San Pablo-CEU, CEU Universities, Urbanización Montepríncipe, Alcorcón, Madrid, Spain
Universidad San Pablo-CEU, CEU Universities, Madrid, Spain

Abstract

Never before in human history have people had access to such a variety of light-emitting devices at night. There is a growing body of research on dependence on these devices and the potential adverse effects of their indiscriminate use, particularly in children. This paper will focus on the review of recent publications and studies related to unwanted effects on cognitive development, circadian rhythms, sleep disturbances, and overall health of children during their pre-school development. In just a few years, children all over the world have reduced the number of hours of sleep and broken their continuity. Due to the novelty and rapidity of this phenomenon, it is not possible to know exactly what the consequences on cognitive function and general health will be for children as they reach adulthood, but what has been published so far suggests that the unintended effects could be significant. There is an urgent need for more research on this issue and for health authorities and society in general to open the debate on limiting access to any kind of light-emitting equipment for children in the evening, especially in the early stages of their development.

Keywords: sleep duration, electronic equipment light, children's health, electronic equipment displays, health and well-being

---

* Corresponding Author's Email: candi.bib@ceu.es

In: Psycho-Environmental Variables That Ensure People's Well-Being and Health …
Editors: Roberto Alonso González Lezcano and Guadalupe Cantarero García
ISBN: 979-8-89530-831-8

© 2025 Nova Science Publishers, Inc.

Introduction

Cognitive development is an ongoing process essential for a child's adaptation to their environment, facilitating learning and skill acquisition. According to the American Academy of Pediatrics (AAP), it constitutes a fundamental tool to absorb knowledge, promote cognitive learning, and involves the assimilation and integration of previous structures (AAP, 2020).

For Piaget (cited by Hernández 2016), cognition is known as "the successive acquisition of increasingly complex logical structures that underlie the different tasks and situations that the subject is capable of solving as their development progresses" (p. 20).

Piaget's theory (1976), known as genetic epistemology, explores the origin and development of cognitive abilities based on biological, organic, and genetic foundations, emphasizing that individuals develop at their own pace. Likewise, he makes a description of cognitive development from the newborn phase, where reflex mechanisms predominate, to the adult stage characterized by conscious processes of regulated behavior. In the genetic development of the individual, periods of intellectual development are identified and differentiated, such as the sensory-motor period, the period of concrete operations and the period of formal operations. Piaget (1973) considers thinking and intelligence as cognitive processes that are based on a specific organic-biological substrate that develops in parallel with maturation and biological growth.

Based on our genetic makeup, Piaget (1973) insists, we respond to the environment in which we are immersed, but as the stimuli increase, decrease or there is an inappropriate variation in them, the expansion, decrease or deterioration of the stimuli will be processed.

Sensory stimulation in the first years of life creates significant learning, positively or negatively. Sensation has the great task of receiving information from the outside through the senses; perception, for its part, plays the role of carrying information to the brain, activating it to process the information, developing responses that will generate behaviors and behaviors in accordance with the environment it creates. In this order of ideas, sensory stimulation occurs thanks to the union of perception and the senses, thus creating a path for learning (Soler, 1992).

These findings highlight the need for experimental data quantifying the melatonin suppression response in young children. In this study, we address this gap in the literature by examining the magnitude of light-induced melatonin suppression to bright evening light in preschool children.

The scientific community is increasingly aware - although still not enough - of the complexity of the genesis of sleep problems and, therefore, of the correct neurocognitive development of children due to the bad habits developed by exposure to light emitted by electronic devices as a routine behavior before falling asleep (Rodriguez-Sacristán, 2015)

It is necessary to understand the psycho-bio-physiological processes that occur in children as a consequence of the exposure and capture of light through electronic devices at night as a habit or ritual that precedes falling asleep.

The Influence of Light During the Night on Children and Its Possible Influence on Sleep

Since the 1960s, there has been reflection on the importance of nighttime in brain development in childhood (Roffwarg, Muzio, & Dement, 1966). In the comments on the texts of Anders, Thoman and Holditch-Davis (Challamel, in Tremblay, Boivin and Peters (2006), the phenomenology of the various states of sleep and wakefulness and their phases of development are described, more specifically on the individualization of the different phases of non-REM sleep, ontogenesis of the sleep-wake rhythm, reaching the determination of the complex relationship that is established between the biological determinants of maturation of the sleep phases, nocturnal awakenings and daytime cognitive behavior, emotional and social development of the child. It is interesting to note how a significant correlation is detected between lack of sleep, parental stress, and parent-child relationships. Also, the social and emotional events experienced during the day may be determining factors in night sleep patterns. However, in the research of these authors, the importance of the development of circadian rhythms in the regulation of day/night rhythms is missing, because it does not depend on sleep or on the development of the brain, but also on many environmental factors and on parent-child relationships.

Findings from several studies examining changes in ocular characteristics across the lifespan have proposed a decline in circadian photoreception with age. For example, cross-sectional data show that young children have lenses that are more transparent and pupils that are larger than adults (Weale 1985; Yang et al. 2002; Charman 2003). At the age of 45 years, humans have approximately half the circadian photoreception of a 10-year-old child due to age-related yellowing of the lens and pupillary miosis (Turner and Mainster 2008).

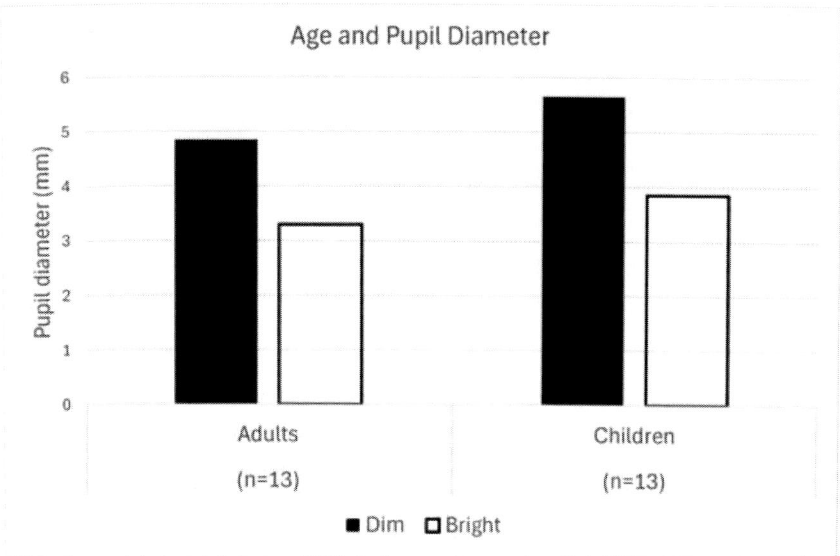

Figure 1. Age and Pupil Diameter. Source: (Higuchi, et al., 2014; MacLachian & Howard, 2002; Adhikari, et al., 2015).

A recent study that examined pupil size in a controlled environment of moderate bright light found that school-aged children had larger pupil diameters than their parents (Higuchi et al., 2014). These data suggest that greater lens transparency and larger pupil size facilitate increased retinal illumination, likely resulting in a stronger signal to the SCN in children than in adults. This greater sensitivity on the part of children may be due to the greater sensitivity of the pupil due to having more transparent lenses, so the reception of light by the retina is 10 times greater (Charman 2003; Turner and Mainster 2008) (Figure 1).

The research of these authors tells us that dilated pupils in dim or bright light are associated with greater melatonin suppression and melatonin suppression increases when the pupils are dilated pharmacologically.

In children, melanopsin is present in the human eye 8 weeks after conception. The pupillary reflex emerges 30-35 weeks. Intrinsically photosensitive retinal ganglion cells (ipRGCs) are light sensitive at one year of birth (Tarttelin et al, 2003). That is why the use of cyclical lighting in the neonatal intensive care unit leads to greater activity during the day, faster weight gain, less crying, shorter hospital stays, and less time with ventilation (Guyer et al., Vázquez-Ruiz et al., 2014).

The light received in the evening by preschool children plays an important role in their circadian balance. They have high suppression in a wide range of light intensities from 5 to 5000 lx 86.4% on average, being significantly lower in the range of 5-40 lux in which it is still 77%. Melatonin secretion in preschool children is very sensitive to light one hour before bedtime in a wide range of intensities. Children's nighttime lighting environments can alter the regular production of melatonin, contributing to delayed sleep onset and resistance to going to bed in early childhood. Exposure to light delays DLMO by approximately one hour. These results highlight the importance of reducing light levels in the home before bedtime to support healthy sleep and circadian rhythms in children (Hartstein, Behn, Akacem, Stack, Wright, & LeBourgeois, 2022).

The Ontogenetic Development of the Sleep-Wake Cycle

All of our body functions are influenced by the alternation of wakefulness and sleep, but we still do not know why we do sleep. The most accepted hypotheses about the biological functions of sleep can be grouped into the hypothesis of recovery and restoration, energy conservation and plasticity, memory and learning (Pedemonte and Velluti, 2007).

Prenatal brain development includes neuronal proliferation with subsequent cell migration, in addition to axonal, dendritic and synaptic development. This process begins early in the embryo and ends during adolescence with the culmination of the axonal myelination process (Kolb and Fantie, 1997). During the first three months of gestation, cell differentiation and the formation of the structures of the nervous system occur. The differentiation and growth of neurons occurs embryologically before the production of glial cells and appears to play an important role in stimulating the growth and proliferation of glia. Unlike neurons, glial cells continue to proliferate after birth.

The coupling of the fetus to the sleep-wake rhythm begins in utero, as a passive response to maternal secretion of melatonin. In infants and young children, light exposure controls the timing of melatonin secretion and, consequently, the timing of sleep. Circadian rhythms are fully developed in the first 6 months of life. The number of hours of darkness (less than 3 lux) to which the child is exposed can influence the duration of melatonin secretion and the number of hours the child sleeps. The child's propensity to sleep is influenced by the time at which he or she is awakened, the time exposed to artificial light and its intensity after dusk and before dawn, eating behaviors and schedules, the time of physical exercise, and the time at which that social relationships are carried out (Pin and Sampedro, 2018).

The amplitude of the circadian rhythm (that is, the difference between the peak and nadir of T^a, for example), is an estimate of the ability to oscillate each day from deep sleep to intense alertness. This amplitude of the circadian cycle is minimal at birth and reaches adult levels within the first year. The light perceived by the photosensitive ganglion cells of the retina is transformed into nervous impulses that reach the SCN, which, in turn, transmits day length information to the secondary oscillators (Pin and Sampedro, 2018).

It has been shown (Montes-Rodríguez, 2008; Portas, 2005) that newborns can assimilate auditory information during sleep. Adequate and regular sleep is essential for adequate subsequent psychomotor and cognitive development. Sleep, with all its stages, contributes to the organization of the information that has been obtained during wakefulness and learning improves when it is followed by a night of sleep. Slow sleep is closely related to brain plasticity, memory and learning. On the other hand, among the earliest signs of sleep deprivation, the following are observed: memory loss, difficulty in acquiring new knowledge, decreased motor skills and mood changes such as irritability (VV. AA, 2005).

Homeostatic mechanisms that tend to maintain an internal balance also intervene in the physiology of sleep. Among the internal synchronizers, the following stand out: melatonin secretion, cortisol secretion and body temperature. The more hours an individual spends sleeping, the less the need for sleep is (the regulation of sleep is similar to that of appetite and thirst, activities also controlled by the hypothalamus) (Pin and Sampedro, 2018).

Negative Impact Due to Exposure to the Light of Technological Media on Children's Neurodevelopment

The human circadian rhythm or clock, located in the suprachiasmatic nucleus (SCN) in the ventral region of the anterior hypothalamus above the optic chiasm (Silver & Schwartz, 2005), is conditioned by light and its properties as a determining and decisive factor such and as supported by the research of Czeisler et al., (1981), Ralph et al., (1990) and Duffy and Wright (2005). Advancing along this same line, Moore and Card (1985) and Johnson et al., (1988) specified that retinal photoreceptors, through the retinohypothalamic tract, are the channel through which external light/dark cycle information reaches the circadian clock. This information also influences the outputs of the biological clock, including the sleep-inducing hormone melatonin. (Gastel et al. 1998).

The genetic factors of the circadian rhythm are represented by a group of genes called CLOCK that are responsible for the activation and inhibition mechanism of the neurons of the suprachiasmatic nucleus. The mission of these genes is to encode the synthesis of cytosolic proteins TIM (timeless) and PER (period) that progressively accumulate in the cytoplasm of the cell. When these proteins reach a certain concentration, their properties change and are capable of migrating to the cell nucleus. This process takes around 12 hours. Once in the nucleus, these proteins bind to other specific RNA locations, acting as transcription inhibitors of the CLOCK genes themselves, gradually reducing the concentration of TIM and PER in the cytoplasm. They eventually lose their affinity for the RNA segment, allowing the cycle to restart. This complex molecular mechanism is regulated by transcription factors and epigenetic processes (Ko and Takahashi, 2006).

The evidence of the role that the circadian rhythm plays in the regulation of sleep has allowed us to create models to understand its homeostatic regulation: The multisynaptic pathway that originates in the SCN and ends in the pineal gland regulates the secretion of melatonin and initiates the process with efferent projections from the SCN itself to the paraventricular nucleus (PVN) (Kalsbeek et al., 2006; Moore and Klein, 1974); Teclemariam-Mesbah et al., 1999). It subsequently sends descending projections to the mediolateral cell column (IML) of the spinal cord and preganglionic sympathetic neurons project to the superior cervical ganglion (SCG). This synaptic pathway terminates with postganglionic sympathetic nerve fibers that project to the pineal gland (Borjigin et al., 1999). During the biological night, these postganglionic fibers release norepinephrine into the pineal gland, which stimulates melatonin secretion by binding to adrenergic receptors (Drijfhout et al., 1996a).

Light exposure during the biological night inhibits the release of norepinephrine and significantly suppresses melatonin secretion (Drijfhout et al., 1996b). These findings highlight the need for experimental studies to quantify melatonin suppression in children due to nocturnal exposure to light from electronic devices. This is of particular interest due to the increase and modification of their sleep initiation habits at night.

Current scientific literature supports evidence of the negative effects caused by exposure to light from technological devices before bedtime, resulting in an incorrect psychophysiological performance during the sleep period in children and, consequently, negatively affecting their correct neurocognitive development (Cespedes et al. al., 2014; Garrison et al., 2011.

Indeed, exposure to light and screen activity before going to bed alters sleep phases, affecting melatonin levels, increasing nocturnal awakenings (arousals), delaying the neurocognitive development of children, conditioning their correct psychophysiological evolution, their school performance (cognitive impairment, attention, concentration) and their behavior (Hartstein et al., 2022). The Common Sense (2020) census of media use in children ages zero to eight and media use in children from low-income households reveals that 49% of children ages 0 to 8 use screens an hour before bedtime. 30% of young children have short sleep and/or sleep behavior disorders. Its use is associated with delayed bedtime, shorter sleep, and more time to exit sleep latency (LeBourgeois, Hale, Chang, Akacem, Montgomery-Downs, Buxton, 2017).

The recommendation and trend in this sense is aimed at reducing routine habits and behaviors of exposure time to screen media and not necessarily that parents should keep children in absolute darkness before going to bed, but scientific evidence shows an irrefutable reality. To give an example, a tablet at full brightness, placed 30 cm from the eyes in a dark room, measures up to 100 lux. Children at an early age are very sensitive to exposure to light in the hour before before going to bed and lighting environment may play a crucial role in the development and maintenance of sleep behavioral problems through impacts the human timing system (Akacem et al., 2018).

Studies Carried Out in Preschool Children Related to the Use of Screens and Their Possible Influence (Dependence) on Sleep

There are a considerable number of studies currently conducted on the possible unwanted effects of the use of light-emitting screens by preschool children. A high level of screen use is associated with increased odds of developmental delay in preschool children. Children of these ages can be sedentary for up to 12 hours a day and there are currently few recommendations on the time they can spend in front of screens (Downing et al., 2017; Yu, Hsieh, Lin, Lee, Huang, & Chen, 2022).

Based on information from parents and caregivers of preschool children in the USA, a shortening of nighttime sleep was found if they used electronic equipment or watched television during the week at night, and an increase in nap time if they watched television in the morning during on the weekend (Moorman, and Harrison, 2019). In another study carried out with 402 mothers with an average age of 35 years with children aged 3 to 5 years, greater use of electronic devices was associated with a lower sleep pattern that could have implications for their cognitive development (Beyens and Nathanson, 2019).

In a study of 126,433 preschool children from 551 cities in China, excessive screen use (ESE) was associated with suspected increased developmental coordination disorder (DCD) if screens were used before going to bed (Geng, Wang, Huang, Xie, Williams, Baker, Du, & Hua, 2023).

Australian scientists report in their research that around 68% of children under 3 years of age use some type of electronic equipment with screens that emit light, which can have negative consequences on their health (Duch, Fisher, Ensari, & Harrington, 2013).

In a study carried out in Japan with children between 1 and 3 years old with a total of 74,525 participants, it was concluded that there was no shortening of sleep if they watched TV, while it did occur if electronic equipment was used. In 2022, a study conducted in Japan by Nishioka, Hasunuma, Okuda, Taniguchi, Fujino, Shimomura, Tanaka, Shima, and Takeshima, of 2,903 preschool children, 40% do not reach the recommended sleep duration. They associate each hour in front of electronic equipment with 11 minutes less sleep and it affects their circadian balance. Children who followed recommended screen time guidelines had longer sleep duration and better sleep habits (Lan, Chan, Yu, Chan, Wing, Li, & Au., 2020).

A systematic review of 53 studies chosen from around the world on children between 0 and 5 years old reveals a huge disparity in the correlations examined. They recommend focusing in future studies on sociocultural correlations, especially parental factors, economic and behavioral factors (Veldman, Altenburg, Chinapaw and Gubbels, 2023).

Conclusion

As mentioned in previous sections, we must keep in mind that sensory stimulation in the first years of children's lives generates significant learning that in turn will process responses that will shape behaviors and adaptations to the environment. Therefore, if the main channel of knowledge and learning does not meet the appropriate conditions, we will be deteriorating said knowledge and this will have an inexorable impact on their correct development and growth as an adult.

After the bibliographic review of the current scientific literature reflected in this chapter, it is evident that the misuse of technologies, specifically the screens of the various devices that exist today on the market and, especially at the time before of sleeping, has a negative impact on the sleep pattern, decreased quality and quantity, insomnia, circadian rhythm, etc.

Let us not forget that homeostatic mechanisms that tend to maintain internal balance also intervene in the physiology of sleep. Melatonin secretion, cortisol secretion and body temperature, as we well know, are internal synchronizers that are also affected. Biological nighttime light exposure inhibits the release of norepinephrine and significantly suppresses the secretion of melatonin, etc. In short, adequate and regular sleep is essential for correct subsequent psychomotor and cognitive development. It is necessary, therefore, to understand the psycho-bio-physiological processes that occur in children as a consequence of the exposure and capture of light through electronic devices at night as a habit or ritual that precedes falling asleep.

The scientific community is increasingly aware of the complexity of the genesis of sleep problems and, therefore, of the correct neurocognitive development of children due to bad habits developed by exposure to light emitted by electronic devices such as behavior-routine before falling asleep (Rodriguez-Sacristán, 2015).

The recommendation and trend in this sense is aimed at reducing routine habits and behaviors of exposure time to screen media. Scientific evidence shows an irrefutable reality.

References

Akacem, L. D., Wright, K. P. Jr., LeBourgeois, M. K., (2018), Sensitivity of the circadian system to evening bright light in preschool-age children, *Physiological Reports*, v. 6, n. 5 e13617 https://doi.org/10.14814/phy2.13617.

Beyens I, Nathanson AI., (2019). Electronic Media Use and Sleep Among Preschoolers: Evidence for Time-Shifted and Less Consolidated Sleep. *Health Commun.* May;34(5):537-544. doi: 10.1080/10410236.2017.1422102. Epub 2018 Jan 11. PMID: 29323943.

Borjigin, J., Li X., y Snyder S. H., (1999). The pineal gland and melatonin: molecular and pharmacologic regulation. *Annu. Rev. Pharmacol. Toxicol.* 39, pp.53-65.

Cespedes EM, Gillman MW, Kleinman K, Rifas-Shiman SL, Redline S, Taveras EM., (2014). Television viewing, bedroom television, and sleep duration from infancy to mid-childhood. *Pediatrics*, 133(5), pp. 163-71.

Challamel MJ. (2006) Estados de Vigilia y Desarrollo Psicosocial/Emocional. Comentarios sobre los textos de Anders, Thoman y Holditch-Davis. En: Tremblay RE, Boivin M, Peters RDeV, eds. Petit D, ed. tema. Enciclopedia sobre el Desarrollo de la Primera Infancia https://www.enciclopedia-infantes.com/conducta-del-sueno/segun-los-expertos/estados-de-vigilia-y-desarrollo-psicosocialemocional.

Charman WN. (2003), Age, lens transmittance, and the possible effects of light on melatonin suppression. *Ophthalmic Physiol Opt*. Mar;23(2):181-7. doi: 10.1046/j.1475-1313.2003.00105. x. PMID: 12641706.

Common Sense Media (2020). All rights reserved. Common Sense, associated names, associated trademarks, and logos are trademarks of Common Sense Media, a 501(c)(3) nonprofit organization. https://www.commonsensemedia.org/sites/default/files/research/report/2020-0-8-census-spanish-fact-sheet-lower-income-final2.pdf.

Czeisler, C. A., Richardson, G. S., Zimmerman, J. C., Moore-Ede M. C., y Weitzman, E. D., (1981). Dragging of human circadian rhythms by light-dark cycles: a reassessment. *Photochemistry. Photobiol.* 34, pp. 239-247.

Drijfhout, W. J., van der Linde A. G., Kooi S. E., Grol C. J., and Westerink B. H., (1996a). Norepinephrine release in the rat pineal gland: the input from the biological clock measured by in vivo microdialysis. *J. Neurochem*. 66, pp.748-75.

Drijfhout, W. J., van der Linde A. G., de Vries J. B., Grol C. J., and Westerink B. H., (1996b). Microdialysis reveals dynamics of coupling between noradrenaline release and melatonin secretion in conscious rats. *Neurosci. Lett.* 202, pp.185-188.

Downing et al., (2017). Do the correlates of screen time and sedentary time differ in preschool children? *BMC Public Health* 17:285 DOI 10.1186/s12889-017-4195-x.

Duch H, Fisher EM, Ensari I, Harrington A. (2013). Screen time use in children under 3 years old: a systematic review of correlates. *Int J Behav Nutr Phys Act*. Aug 23;10:102. doi: 10.1186/1479-5868-10-102. PMID: 23967799; PMCID: PMC3844496.

Duffy, J. F., and K. P. Jr. Wright. 2005. Dragging of the human circadian system by light. *J. Biol. Rhythms* 20, pp. 326-338.

Ebling, F. J. 1996. The role of glutamate in the photic regulation of the suprachiasmatic nucleus. *Prog. Neurobiol.* 50, pp. 109-132

Garrison MM, Liekweg K, Christakis DA. (2011). Media use and child sleep: the impact of content, timing, and environment. *Pediatrics*, 128(1), pp. 29-35.

Gastel, J. A., Roseboom, P. H., Rinaldi, P. A., Weller, J. L., y Klein, D. C., (1998). Melatonin production: proteasome proteolysis in the regulation of serotonin N-acetyltransferase. *Science* 279, pp. 1358-1360.

Geng S, Wang W, Huang L, Xie J, Williams GJ, Baker C, Du W, Hua J. (2023). Association between screen time and suspected developmental coordination disorder in preschoolers: A national population-based study in China. *Front Public Health.* Mar 27; 11:1152321. doi: 10.3389/fpubh.2023.1152321. PMID: 37050955; PMCID: PMC10083417.

Guyer C, Huber R, Fontijn J, Bucher HU, Nicolai H, Werner H, Molinari L, Latal B, Jenni OG. (2012) Cycled light exposure reduces fussing and crying in very preterm infants. *Pediatrics*. Jul;130(1): e145-51. doi: 10.1542/peds.2011-2671. Epub 2012 Jun 11. PMID: 22689866.

Hale L, y Guan S. (2015). Screen time and sleep among school-aged children and adolescents: a systematic literature review. *Sleep Med Rev*. 21, pp. 50-8.

Hartstein LE, Behn CD, Akacem LD, Stack N, Wright KP Jr, LeBourgeois MK. (2022) High sensitivity of melatonin suppression response to evening light in preschool-aged children. *J Pineal Res*. Mar;72(2):e12780. doi: 10.1111/jpi.12780. Epub 2022 Jan 8. Erratum in: J Pineal Res. 2023 Oct;75(3):e12903. PMID: 34997782; PMCID: PMC8933063

Hartstein, L. E, Behn, C. D., Akacem, L. D., Pila N., Wright K. P., LeBorugeois, M. K., (2022), High sensitivity of melatonin suppression response to evening light in preschool-aged children. *Journal of Pineal Research* v. 72, Issue 2 March. https://doi.org/10.1111/jpi.12780.

Johnson, R. F., R. Y. Moore, and L. P. y Morin, (1988). Loss of drag and anatomical plasticity after lesions of the hamster retinohypothalamic tract. *Brain Res.* 460, pp. 297-313.

Kalsbeek, A., Palm I. F., La Fleur S. E., Scheer F. A., Perreau-Lenz S., Ruiter M., et al. (2006). SCN outputs and the hypothalamic balance of life. *J. Biol. Rhythms* 21, pp. 458-469.

Ko, C. H. y Takahashi, J. S. (2006). Molecular components of the mammalian circadian clock, *Human Molecular Genetics*, 15(2), pp. R271-R277.

Kolb, B. y Fantie, B. (1997). Development of the child brain and behavior. En: Reynolds, C. R. y Fletcher-Janzen, E. (Eds.), (1997) *Handbook of Clinical Child Neuropsychology*. New York: Plenum Press.

Lan Q. Y, Chan K. C., Yu K. N., Chan N. Y., Wing Y. K., Li A. M., Au C. T. (2020). Sleep duration in preschool children and impact of screen time. *Sleep Med*. Dec;76:48-54. doi: 10.1016/j.sleep.2020.09.024. Epub 2020 Oct 1. PMID: 33091726.

LeBourgeois M. K. Hale L., Chang AM, Akacem LD, Montgomery-Downs HE, Buxton OM. (2017). *Medios digitales y sueño en la infancia y la adolescencia. Pediatría*. Noviembre; 140(Supl. 2): S92-S96. doi: 10.1542/peds.2016-1758J. PMID: 29093040; PMCID: PMC5658795.

Montes-Rodríguez CJ, Domínguez-Martín EA, Próspero-García O. (2008) Restauración neuronal o plasticidad sináptica a lo largo del ciclo sueño-vigilia *Rev Med UV*, Sup 2 8(1), pp. 71-77.

Moorman JD, Harrison K. (2019). Beyond Access and Exposure: Implications of Sneaky Media Use for Preschoolers' Sleep Behavior. *Health Commun.* May;34(5):529-536. doi: 10.1080/10410236.2017.1422103. Epub 2018 Jan 9. PMID: 29313720.

Moore, R. Y., y Card, J. P. (1985). Visual pathways and the entrainment of circadian rhythms. *Ann. N. Y. Acad.* 453, pp. 123-133.

Moore, R. Y., y Klein D. C., (1974). Visual pathways and the central neural control of a circadian rhythm in pineal serotonin N-acetyltransferase activity. *Brain Res.* 71, pp. 17-33.

Nishioka T, Hasunuma H, Okuda M, Taniguchi N, Fujino T, Shimomura H, Tanaka Y, Shima M, Takeshima Y, (2022). Japan Environment And Children's Study Group. Effects of Screen Viewing Time on Sleep Duration and Bedtime in Children Aged 1 and 3 Years: Japan Environment and Children's Study. *Int J Environ Res Public Health.* Mar 25;19(7):3914. doi: 10.3390/ijerph19073914. PMID: 35409594; PMCID: PMC8997461.

Pedemonte M., Velluti R. A., (2007), *Fisiología General del sueño. Máster en Sueño: Fisiología y Medicina* (1ª edición). Barcelona: Vigueras

Pin Arboledas, G., Sampedro Campos, M., (2018), Fisiología del sueño y sus trastornos. Ontogenia y evolución del sueño a lo largo de la etapa pediátrica. Relación del sueño con la alimentación. Clasificación de los problemas y trastornos del sueño. *Pediatr Integral*; XXII (8), pp. 358-371

Portas C. M. (2005). Cognitive aspects of sleep: perception, mentation, and dreaming. In Vellutti R.A, Parmegianni P. L, Eds. (2005). *The physiologic nature of slee*p. London: Imperial College Press, pp. 535-69.

Ralph, M. R., Foster,R.G. Davis,F.C. y Menaker, M. (1990). El núcleo supraquiasmático trasplantado determina el período circadiano. Science 247, pp. 975-978.

Rodríguez-Sacristán Cascajo, A. (2015). *Relación entre los trastornos del sueño y los hábitos en el dormir en la población infantil de Sevilla*. Universidad de Sevilla, Sevilla.

Roffwarg HP, Muzio JN, Dement WC. (1966). Ontogenetic development of the human sleep-dream cycle. *Science* ,152(3722):604-619.

Silver, R. y Schwartz, W. J. (2005). The suprachiasmatic nucleus is a functionally heterogeneous timekeeping organ. *Methods in Enzymology,* 393, pp. 451-465.

Teclemariam-Mesbah, R, Ter Horst G. J., Postema F., Wortel J., y Buijs R. M., (1999). Anatomical demonstration of the suprachiasmatic nucleus-pineal pathway. *J. Comp. Neurol.* 406, pp.171-182.

Vásquez-Ruiz S, Maya-Barrios JA, Torres-Narváez P, Vega-Martínez BR, Rojas-Granados A, Escobar C, Angeles-Castellanos M. (2014). A light/dark cycle in the NICU accelerates body weight gain and shortens time to discharge in preterm infants. *Early Hum Dev.*Sep; 90 (9): 535-40. doi: 10.1016/j.earlhumdev.2014.04.015. Epub 2014 May 13. PMID: 24831970.

Veldman SLC, Altenburg TM, Chinapaw MJM, Gubbels JS. (2023). Correlates of screen time in the early years (0-5 years): A systematic review. *Prev Med Rep.* Apr 19; 33:102214. doi: 10.1016/j.pmedr.2023.102214. PMID: 37223568; PMCID: PMC10201873.

VV. AA. (2005). Psychobiology and dreaming. In Kryger M. H, Roth T, Dement W. C, Eds. (2005), *Principles and practice of sleep medicine*. 4 ed. Philadelphia: Elsevier Saunders, pp. 519-87.

Xu H., Wen L. M., Hardy L. L, Rissel C. (2016), Associations of outdoor play and screen time with nocturnal sleep duration and pattern among young children. *Acta Paediatr.,* 105(3), pp. 297-303.

Yu Y. T., Hsieh T. L., Lin G. H., Lee S. C., Huang C. Y., Chen K. L. (2022). High levels of screen time were associated with increased probabilities of lagged development in 3-year-old children. *Acta Paediatr.* Sep;111(9):1736-1742. doi: 10.1111/apa.16373. Epub 2022 May 8. PMID: 35472250.

Chapter 12

The Next Generation of Biosensors for Telemedicine: The Evolution of Tattoos. Real-Time Monitoring Without the Need for Physical Medical-Pharmaceutical Devices

Guillermo Sáez Cruz[1]
Natalia García-Tenorio Fernández[1]
and Daniel Arranz-Paraíso[2,*]
[1]Universidad San Pablo CEU, Alcorcón, Madrid, Spain
[2]R&D Development Manager at Pinisan SL. C/Gran Canaria, Madrid, Spain

Abstract

The emergence of new materials has enabled technical advances for nanotechnology with which nanorobotic systems can be developed to micrometer-sized layers of autonomous nanomaterial that has the ability to collect and transmit information. Graphene is a recently discovered material attributed with various functionalities, such as energy storage capacity, lossless electrical transmission, heat dissipation, and bio-printing, among others. Pathologies usually have specific biomarkers that can be monitored through the patient's biological fluids, such as blood, serum, sweat, and urine. The measurement and monitoring of blood glucose is one of the most studied parameters due to the pathological implications of non-physiological levels of glucose. Among the pathologies, the most serious ones are those that affect the neurological level since it can even induce the death of patients in case of presenting severe hypoglycemia due to brain death from lack of energetic nutrients. Mental disorders are one of the pathologies that can be a risk factor for patients not adhering to pharmacological treatments. Lack of time control, states of lethargy, little initiative to improve, cognitive deterioration and physical impairments such as alteration of the extrapyramidal system that generates body tremors, are some of the causes of lack of adherence to treatments. The new era of telemedicine focuses on developing, among other control and monitoring instruments, biometric tattoos. These are intraepithelial impressions that do not require batteries or signal receivers or emitters to collect the necessary biometric data to diagnose or monitor patients. These biosensors can be made up of organic, inorganic compounds, graphene and nanowires that give them measurement capabilities, signal reception and data communication to external devices such as smartphones. Biometric tattoos can be considered medical devices being systems where disciplines such as engineering and pharmaceutical technology must be more involved both

* Corresponding Author's Email: daniel.paraiso@pinisan.com

In: Psycho-Environmental Variables That Ensure People's Well-Being and Health ...
Editors: Roberto Alonso González Lezcano and Guadalupe Cantarero García
ISBN: 979-8-89530-831-8
© 2025 Nova Science Publishers, Inc.

for development and for government and health regulations required by these new therapeutic advances.

Keywords: tattoos, glycaemia, blood parameters, monitoring, glycosometer, diabetes

Introduction

The monitoring of blood parameters makes it possible to control, detect and monitor the health status of animals and people. This allows instantaneous knowledge of the general state of health at the time of sampling. Among all measurable parameters, glucose is one of the most frequently analyzed worldwide to assess the status of both diabetic and non-diabetic patients. Glucose is essential to maintain brain function and therefore it is very important to maintain physiological levels of glucose. If glucose concentrations fall below physiological levels, an individual may lose consciousness and, in severe cases, die. If the levels are elevated above physiological levels, pathological processes can be generated that can also induce the death of the person or animal by damage to the blood capillaries inducing a poor vascularization of vital organs such as heart, kidneys and brain.

Managing diabetes, particularly in patients reliant on insulin, entails effective glycemic control. Regularly monitoring blood glucose levels is essential to calibrate insulin doses and uphold stable glycemic levels. However, the frequent necessity for glucose analysis through fingerstick testing can be burdensome for patients and may entail financial implications for the healthcare system. In this scientific article, we will investigate the average frequency of fingerstick testing for glucose analysis and insulin administration in insulin-dependent patients, as well as the associated costs incurred by the healthcare system.

Type I and Type II diabetes are two distinct forms of diabetes mellitus that have different etiologies and treatment approaches. Type I diabetes is an autoimmune disease characterized by the destruction of pancreatic beta cells, leading to an absolute deficiency of insulin production. On the other hand, Type II diabetes is a metabolic disorder characterized by insulin resistance and impaired insulin secretion [1].

Treatment for Type I diabetes primarily involves exogenous insulin administration to maintain blood glucose levels within the target range. This can be achieved through multiple daily injections or continuous subcutaneous insulin infusion using an insulin pump. Additionally, patients with Type I diabetes are advised to monitor their blood glucose levels regularly and adjust their insulin doses accordingly. Adherence to insulin therapy and blood glucose monitoring is crucial for achieving optimal glycemic control in Type I diabetes [1].

In contrast, the treatment approach for Type II diabetes is more diverse and includes lifestyle modifications, oral antidiabetic medications, and, in some cases, insulin therapy [2]. Lifestyle modifications, such as adopting a healthy diet and engaging in regular physical activity, are recommended as the first-line treatment for Type II diabetes. These lifestyle changes can help improve glycemic control and reduce the risk of complications [3]. However, medication adherence is a significant challenge in the management of Type II diabetes [4].

Adherence to the control of type I diabetes is a critical factor in achieving optimal glycemic control and preventing complications [5]. However, adherence can be challenging for many patients due to various psychosocial barriers. Fear, concern, and distress, exhaustion and burnout, poor financial support, communication challenges, and poor work conditions are some of the perceived psychosocial barriers to medication adherence identified in qualitative studies [6]. Additionally, factors such as forgetfulness, lack of access to healthcare providers, cost of medications, and injection site reactions have been associated with non-adherence to insulin therapy [7].

To address these barriers and improve adherence, various interventions have been explored. Brief interventions, such as psychoeducation, coping skills training, and stress management, have shown promise in improving diabetes-related outcomes and self-management [8]. Behavioral interventions delivered in group settings have also been associated with improvements in self-management and glycemic control. Furthermore, the use of medication reminders through smartphone apps has been identified as a potential strategy to improve adherence to medication regimens [9].

In addition to psychosocial barriers, factors such as knowledge about diabetes and its management play a significant role in adherence to treatment regimens. Studies have shown that higher knowledge levels about diabetes and its biochemical processes are associated with better glycemic control [10]. Educational programs that focus on improving knowledge and providing instruction on self-monitoring of blood glucose levels have been found to be effective in improving glycemic control [11]. Furthermore, involving caregivers in the management of type I diabetes in children has been shown to have a positive impact on adherence and glycemic control [12].

It is important to note that adherence to treatment regimens is not limited to medication adherence alone. Adherence to dietary recommendations and regular physical activity are also crucial for managing type I diabetes. Strategies such as tracking calories, counting carbohydrates, and choosing low glycemic index foods have been associated with better glycemic control in individuals with type I diabetes [13].

Several factors contribute to poor medication adherence in patients with Type II diabetes. Non-patient factors, such as lack of integrated care and clinical inertia among healthcare professionals, can hinder medication adherence. Patient demographic factors, including young age, low education level, and low-income level, have also been associated with poor adherence. Critical patient beliefs about their medications, such as perceived treatment inefficacy, and perceived patient burden regarding obtaining and taking their medications, such as treatment complexity and out-of-pocket costs, can also impact adherence [4].

Adherence to self-care behaviors, such as self-monitoring of blood glucose (SMBG), physical activity, medication adherence, and dietary management, is crucial for achieving optimal glycemic control in Type II diabetes. However, studies have shown that adherence to self-care practices is often suboptimal in patients with Type II diabetes. For example, a study conducted in Ethiopia found that most respondents did not perform SMBG. Similarly, another study conducted in Ethiopia reported poor glycemic control and low adherence to self-care practices among patients with Type II diabetes [3].

Illness perception, which refers to an individual's beliefs and understanding of their illness, has been found to be associated with medication adherence in patients with Type II diabetes. A study conducted in Iran showed a significant relationship between illness perception and medication adherence in patients with Type II diabetes. Similarly, another study conducted in Mexico found that knowledge about tools for diabetes self-management was poor, highlighting the importance of diabetes education in improving adherence to self-care behaviors [14].

Pharmacist interventions have been shown to improve therapeutic outcomes and medication adherence in patients with Type II diabetes. A study conducted in India demonstrated that pharmacist interventions led to significant reductions in HbA1c levels and improvements in self-reported medication adherence and self-care activities. Similarly, a systematic review of randomized controlled trials found that pharmacist interventions might potentially improve adherence to Type II diabetes medication [15].

To commence, it is imperative to acknowledge that the frequency of glucose analysis and insulin administration varies according to individual patient requirements, treatment plans, and insulin therapy type. Nevertheless, several studies provide insights into these aspects.

A study by Sunny et al. 2021 [16] examined the knowledge, attitudes, and practices of insulin administration among diabetic patients and their caregivers. While the study primarily focused on insulin therapy in general, it provided valuable information regarding the frequency of insulin administration. The findings indicated that the majority of diabetic patients require multiple daily insulin administrations, typically preceding meals. This implies that insulin-dependent patients may need to undergo multiple daily fingerstick tests for insulin administration.

Regarding glucose analysis, the frequency of fingerstick testing can also fluctuate. Traditional self-monitoring of blood glucose (SMBG) entails routine fingerstick tests to measure blood glucose levels. The American Association of Clinical Endocrinologists and American Diabetes Association Consensus Statement on Inpatient Glycemic Control by Moghissi et al. [17] underscores the significance of frequent glucose monitoring for hospitalized diabetes patients. While this statement concentrates on inpatient care, it underscores the need for regular glucose monitoring to attain glycemic control. The frequency of glucose analysis may hinge on factors such as the patient's glycemic control, treatment regimen, and healthcare provider's recommendations.

Nonetheless, advancements in technology have introduced alternative methods for glucose monitoring. For instance, the utilization of flash glucose monitoring systems (FGMS) has surged in popularity. FGMS enables continuous glucose monitoring without the requirement for frequent fingerstick tests. A study conducted by Liu et al. [18] explored the integration of FGMS with insulin pump therapy in the management of blood glucose levels in type 2 diabetes mellitus patients. The study observed that employing FGMS reduced the necessity for frequent fingerstick testing, offering a more convenient and less invasive approach to glucose monitoring.

In addition to glucose analysis and insulin administration, it is vital to consider the associated expenses. Insulin therapy and glucose monitoring can have financial implications for both patients and the healthcare system. A cost-effectiveness analysis by Ajjan et al. [19] assessed the utilization of FGMS in individuals with type 2 diabetes undergoing intensive insulin treatment. The study revealed that using FGMS incurred additional costs compared to traditional blood glucose monitoring. Nevertheless, it also demonstrated improved glycemic control and quality-adjusted life years, suggesting potential long-term cost savings linked to enhanced diabetes management.

The search for new FGMS systems that are more economical and easier to apply to the skin has led to the development of and interest in advancing the field of biometric tattoos. These tattoos are intended to be of a temporary type and can be small thin patches with microneedles that adhere to the skin in a similar way to the temporary tattoos of children or those that are applied for example to mark the type of ticket that has been purchased at the entrance of certain theme parks. The clinical evolution must include on the one hand the cost-benefit ratio as well as the patient's adherence to the treatment or to the battery of measures to which he must be submitted for the control of the disease he suffers from.

The origins of body tattoos can be traced back to preindustrial eras, where bodywork practices such as displaying tattoos and bodily adornments were cultural cues that signaled an individual's belonging to a specific social group [20]. Tattoos have been a part of human history for centuries and have held different meanings in various cultures. In some cultures, tattoos are deeply ingrained in society, acting as important symbols of personal identity and cultural history [21]. They have been used as a form of selfexpression, a way to communicate one's beliefs, values, and affiliations. Tattoos have also played a role in social rituals and rites of passage, reflecting key life events [21].

The meaning of tattoos varies across different cultures. For example, in the Ao Nagas and Konyak Nagas societies, tattoos are seen as important symbols of personal identity and cultural history [21]. Each tribe has its own set of patterns and symbolism to honor cultural contributions and storytelling traditions [21]. In the Bontoc Igorots of the Philippines, tattoos hold significant meaning, conveying symbolic meanings, especially among the male members of the tribe [22]. In South Korea, tattoos are associated with talismanic symbolic and status markers [23]. In the Catholic Croat culture, tattoos were believed to offer protection against the rule of the Ottoman Empire [24].

The evolution of tattooing techniques and practices has also changed throughout history. In modern times, tattooing has become more popular and accessible, with advancements in technology making the process more convenient [22]. Traditional tattooing methods have been replaced by modern tattoo machines, which allow for more precise and intricate designs [25]. However, traditional tattooing practices still exist in some cultures, preserving the artistry and symbolism of ancient tattooing techniques [22].

It is important to note that while tattoos have cultural and personal significance, they can also have medical implications. Tattoo associated cutaneous complications have been reported, including benign neoplasms, malignant tumors, and lymphoid conditions occurring within the tattoo [26]. There have also been associations between tattooing and the transmission of infectious diseases, such as hepatitis B and C [27,28]. Additionally, the removal of tattoos through laser procedures has become a common practice, offering a way for individuals to change or remove tattoos that no longer hold the same meaning or significance [29].

Tattoo inks contain a range of toxic compounds that can adversely affect human health. These harmful substances encompass heavy metals, polycyclic aromatic hydrocarbons (PAHs), primary aromatic amines (PAAs), and other hazardous chemicals [30–45].

Commonly found in tattoo inks, heavy metals like chromium, cadmium, lead, nickel, and cobalt can exert toxic effects on the body, potentially leading to allergic reactions, dermatitis, and even carcinogenic outcomes [30,35,38,39,43,45]. In particular, black tattoo inks containing PAHs have been pinpointed as genotoxic agents, capable of promoting tumor development in tattooed areas [35].

Beyond heavy metals and PAHs, additional harmful constituents like formaldehyde can be emitted from certain tattoo inks [34]. Formaldehyde, recognized as an irritant and allergen, can trigger dermatitis and other negative reactions [34]. Additionally, some tattoo inks contain azo pigments, substances classified as carcinogens [30].

The harmful attributes of tattoo inks extend not only to their chemical makeup but also to their physical properties. Exposure to sunlight can prompt photodegradation of tattoo inks, resulting in the formation of potentially toxic byproducts. This photolability is concerning, as it could lead to the release of harmful substances within the skin [36].Furthermore, the direct injection of tattoo inks into the skin can lead to pigment accumulation in the lymph nodes and other organs, potentially causing enduring health effects [32].

Crucially, the regulation of tattoo inks is currently inadequate. Unlike cosmetics or medical products, tattoo inks lack comprehensive regulations governing their composition and safety [33,41,42]. This regulatory gap permits the inclusion of potentially hazardous components in tattoo inks, thus jeopardizing human health. Moreover, the composition of tattoo inks can vary between brands and even within the same brand over time, posing challenges in assessing their safety [37].

Pain-free self-reading medical devices have revolutionized the field of healthcare by providing patients with the ability to monitor their health conditions in a convenient and non-invasive manner. Device continuous glucose monitoring system (CGM) [46]. CGM systems have been widely used for glucose monitoring in patients with diabetes [47]. These devices utilize sensors that are worn on the body and measure glucose levels in the interstitial fluid, providing real-time data on blood glucose levels [48].

The CGM systems have been shown to improve glycemic control and reduce the risk of hypoglycemia and hyperglycemia in patients with diabetes [47]. They provide valuable information on time in range (TIR), which is the time spent within the target glucose range, and hypoglycemic exposure, which measures the amount of time spent in low blood glucose level. These metrics are important for optimizing diabetes management and reducing the risk of complications. In addition to glucose monitoring, there are other pain-free self-reading medical devices available for various healthcare applications. For example, there are devices such as inhalers that can assess patients' adherence to prescribed inhaled medication [49]. These devices provide a simple and convenient way for patients to monitor their medication usage and ensure proper adherence to their treatment plans.

Another example is the sphygmomanometer, a device used to measure blood pressure. Digital sphygmomanometers are known for their ease of use, but their accuracy may be lower compared to mercury sphygmomanometers [50]. However, the use of digital sphygmomanometers is still widespread due to their convenience and availability. Furthermore, there are devices that can be used for cosmetic purposes, such as the Beautylizer Therapy Cosmospheres V, which is a non-invasive medical device used for gynoid lipodystrophy treatment [51]. This device has been shown to improve subcutaneous tissue morphology and reduce tissue hypoxia manifestations.

The accuracy and reliability of these pain-free self-reading medical devices are crucial for their effectiveness. Studies have been conducted to evaluate the accuracy of these devices, such as the Dexcom G6 Continuous Glucose Monitoring system, which has been shown to provide more comprehensive glycemic control data compared to intermittent point-of-care blood glucose monitoring [52]. The CGM systems has also been compared to self-monitoring of blood glucose in children with type I diabetes, and it has been found to be comparable in terms of glycemic control [53].

However, it is important to note that some individuals may experience adverse reactions to certain medical devices. For example, the CGM systems has been associated with allergic contact dermatitis caused by the allergen isobornyl acrylate [54,55].

Tattoos that have been developed are not permanent; there are also temporary ones that are applied and do not require subcutaneous injection of substances.

Glucose-meters with non-permanent tattoos are an emerging technology aimed at providing continuous and non-invasive glucose monitoring for individuals with diabetes. These devices use temporary tattoos applied to the skin, containing biosensors capable of measuring glucose levels in interstitial fluid [56,57]. These tattoos are designed to be flexible and body-compliant, allowing for comfortable and long-term wear. Glucose measurements are obtained through a process called reverse iontophoresis, involving the extraction of interstitial fluid from the skin using a low electrical current. The extracted fluid is then analyzed by the biosensors to determine the glucose concentration [56,57].

The development of glucose-meters based on tattoos has shown promising results in proof-of-concept studies. Bandodkar et al. demonstrated the feasibility of this technology by successfully monitoring glucose levels in interstitial fluid using a tattoo-based biosensor. The study highlighted the potential of these devices for non-invasive glycemic monitoring and efficient diabetes management [56,57]. Furthermore, the use of temporary tattoos for monitoring other analytes, such as sweat electrolytes and metabolites, has also been explored [58].

The integration of wearable sensors into tattoo-based platforms has opened up new possibilities for personalized healthcare and disease management. These devices can provide real-time monitoring of biomarkers indicative of human performance and physiological status. For example, Koh et al. developed a microfluidic system that directly harvested sweat from the pores to measure lactate, glucose, pH, and chloride. This demonstrates the versatility of tattoo-based sensors in monitoring various biomarkers and their potential applications in sports medicine and performance monitoring [59].

All-printed temporary tattoo glycosometer is an innovative glucose monitoring platform that has been designed for non-invasive tracking of blood glucose levels. This groundbreaking device employs a tattoo-like structure temporarily printed on the skin to extract interstitial fluid (ISF) and analyze glucose levels [60]. Multiple research groups have reported the development of the all-printed temporary tattoo glycosometer. Exist a proof-of-concept non-invasive glucose sensing platform based on an all-printed temporary tattoo. The system utilizes a low current density to extract ISF and achieves selective glucose sensing through a glucose oxidase-modified Prussian Blue transducer. This approach minimizes skin irritation and requires a low applied potential for glucose detection [60].

Additionally, Koklu et al. demonstrated the use of an all-printed flexible temporary tattoo for non-invasive glucose monitoring via ISF [61]. The tattoo sensor operates at a lower potential for amperometric detection of hydrogen peroxide (H2O2) using a conductive carbon-modified electrode with glucose oxidase (GOx) and Prussian Blue (PB). The reverse-iontophoresis electrodes employ minimal current density to extract and deliver ISF glucose to the sensing electrode [61].

Another all-printed temporary tattoo glycosometer combines reverse iontophoresis extraction of interstitial glucose with an enzyme-based amperometric biosensor. This flexible tattoo-based epidermal diagnostic device exhibits a linear response to physiologically relevant glucose levels with minimal interference from common coexisting electroactive species [62].

He et al. [63] developed a dermal biosensor that could be interpreted as a kind of temporary colorimetric tattoo using a microneedle patch. This biosensor is capable of multiplexed detection of health-related biomarkers such as uric acid, glucose, and body temperature. The patch is a minimally invasive product that avoids damaging blood vessels and nerves in the deep dermis, reducing bleeding and pain [63,64]. These dermal biosensors can be used to monitor metabolites in interstitial fluid, providing valuable information about an individual's health status. The dermal biosensors in this group use patterned microneedles on the skin. Microneedles are tiny needles with dimensions on the micrometer scale, typically ranging from 25 to 500 micrometers in length [65]. These microneedles can penetrate the outermost layer of the skin, known as the stratum corneum, without causing significant pain or bleeding. The patterned microneedles of the tattoo sensor are designed to deliver specific reagents or capture molecules to the desired depth in the skin, ensuring accurate and reliable detection of biomarkers [63].

Objective

1. The objective of this chapter is to conduct a search for new advances in the measurement of blood parameters that will indicate the health status of patients without the need for painful or harmful techniques that are used to perform blood tests. Another objectives are:
   - Exploring strategies to improve adherence in type I diabetes: psychoeducation, behavioral interventions, and medication reminders to improve adherence.
   - Emphasizing the importance of dietary modifications and physical activity: adherence to a healthy lifestyle plays a crucial role in managing type I diabetes alongside medication.
   - Investigating factors contributing to poor adherence in type II diabetes: non-patient factors such as lack of integrated care and patient demographics. Critical patient beliefs and perceived treatment burden can also impact adherence.
   - Highlighting the role of self-care behaviors in type II diabetes: Self-monitoring of blood glucose, dietary management, and physical activity are crucial for optimal glycemic control. Exploring the potential of novel monitoring methods: continuous glucose monitoring (CGM) systems as a less invasive alternative to fingerstick testing.
2. Additional objectives:
   - Analyze the cost implications of insulin therapy, glucose monitoring, and emerging technologies like CGM.
   - Evaluate the safety and efficacy of biometric tattoos for continuous glucose monitoring.
   - Discuss the evolution of tattooing practices and the associated health risks.
   - Explore the potential of pain-free, self-reading medical devices for various health applications.
   - Highlight the development of temporary tattoo-based glucose meters for non-invasive monitoring.
   - Discuss the integration of wearable sensors into tattoo platforms for personalized healthcare management.

Material and Methods

1. *Initial Search:*
    - A comprehensive search was performed in the PubMed, Web of Science, and Scopus databases.
    - The following keywords were used:
        - "biosensor tattoos"
        - "type I, type II diabetes"
        - "treatment, monitorization, cost diabetes"
        - "tattoos and cultures"
        - "novel blood glucose level monitoring system without needles"
    - Keywords were combined using the Boolean operators "AND" and "OR..
    - A total of 98 articles were retrieved.
2. *Duplicate Removal:*
    - Duplicates were removed from the different databases.
    - The removal of duplicates was manually verified to ensure accuracy.
    - A reduction to 84 unique articles was achieved.
3. *Date Filtering:*
    - Only articles published between January 1, 2020 and December 31, 2023 were selected.
    - The publication date of each article was verified.
    - A final collection of 69 articles was obtained.
4. *Abstract Assessment:*
    - A critical reading of the abstracts of the 69 selected articles was performed.
    - The thematic relevance of each abstract was assessed with respect to the systematic review.
    - 67 articles that met the pre-established relevance criteria were selected.
5. *Methodological Quality Assessment:*
    - A specific methodology was applied to evaluate the methodological quality of the 61 articles.
    - Aspects such as study design, sample size, analysis methodology, and presentation of results were evaluated.
    - 65 articles that met the methodological quality criteria were selected.
6. *Analysis and Synthesis of Information:*
    - The information collected in the 65 selected articles will be analyzed.
    - The research findings will be synthesized to answer the questions of the systematic review.

Discussion

In a world increasingly driven by technology, advances in healthcare are paving the way to address critical health challenges. As previously discussed, new medical research efforts are focusing on integrating biosensors into temporary tattoos, promising a revolution in how people manage chronic diseases, particularly diabetes. These "biosensor tattoos" represent a significant evolution in telemedicine and offer considerable advantages for enhancing adherence to control and treatment of this condition.

Diabetes is a complex metabolic disorder that affects millions of people worldwide. One of the most pressing challenges in managing diabetes, whether it's Type 1 or Type 2, is the need for strict control of blood glucose levels. Consistent adherence to a glucose monitoring and treatment regimen is essential to avoid severe complications and maintain a good quality of life.

However, the reality is that many patients face significant difficulties in maintaining this adherence. Traditional glucose monitoring involves frequent finger-prick tests, which can be uncomfortable and, in some cases, lead to finger calluses due to repeated punctures. Psychosocial barriers also play a significant role in non-adherence. Factors such as fear of needles, concerns about glucose level fluctuations, and stress related to disease management can demotivate patients. Moreover, financial limitations, lack of access to healthcare providers, and inadequate support can further hinder treatment adherence.

It is in this context that biosensor tattoos emerge as a promising solution. These tattoos, similar to temporary tattoos commonly used in popular culture, function as advanced biomedical sensors that enable continuous, non-invasive monitoring of interstitial glucose levels—the fluid surrounding cells in body tissues. This brings about several advantages.

The primary advantage of biosensor tattoos lies in their ability to improve treatment adherence. Continuous and painless monitoring of glucose levels eliminates the need for finger-prick tests, which are often perceived as unpleasant and painful. Instead, patients can simply look at their biosensor tattoo to obtain real-time information about their glucose levels. This convenience and simplicity can have a significant impact on patients' motivation to maintain strict disease control. The removal of psychological barriers related to needle fear and pain can lead to greater treatment adherence. Patients may feel more empowered and in control of their health, which, in turn, can reduce the stress associated with diabetes management.

The second advantage is that traditional glucose monitoring provides snapshots at specific times of the day. Glucose levels can vary widely throughout the day and night, and spot tests may not capture these fluctuations resulting from fasting and eating cycles. Biosensor tattoos offer the advantage of continuous monitoring. These sensors can provide real-time data 24 hours a day, 7 days a week, allowing patients and their doctors to have a comprehensive and detailed picture of how they respond to treatment and how food, exercise, and other factors influence their glucose levels. This is essential for adjusting treatment plans and maintaining optimal disease control.

The third advantage lies in the reduced invasiveness of traditional testing methods. The comfort of biosensor tattoos is partly due to their non-invasive nature. The sensors in the tattoo use advanced methods, such as reverse iontophoresis, to extract interstitial fluid from the skin through low electrical currents and then analyze it to determine glucose concentration. This technology minimizes pain and reduces the risk of skin irritation, making it a much more comfortable option for continuous glucose monitoring.

As a fourth advantage, the integration of biosensor tattoo technology into the everyday lives of diabetes patients is straightforward. These tattoos are thin, flexible, and adhere comfortably to the skin, much like a common temporary tattoo. They can be worn discreetly and do not require additional monitoring devices or bulky equipment. The ease of use and seamless integration into a patient's daily routine can enhance treatment adherence. Patients do not have to worry about carrying additional monitoring equipment or undergoing uncomfortable procedures during the day. Additionally, artificial intelligence algorithms can analyze the collected data and provide specific recommendations for each patient. This may include suggestions on insulin administration, dietary changes, and adjustments to exercise routines, as well as estimating disease progression to create personalized plans that improve patients' quality of life while preventing collateral complications such as diabetic foot issues.

Another advantage is that while the initial implementation of biosensor tattoo technology may require an investment, it is expected that this technology will reduce long-term overall costs for both patients and healthcare systems. Early detection of changes in glucose levels and improved treatment adherence can prevent severe diabetes complications, such as cardiovascular diseases, kidney damage, and neuropathy. By avoiding these costly and potentially life-threatening complications, biosensor tattoos can contribute to a significant reduction in long-term healthcare costs. This can benefit both patients and healthcare institutions and insurance systems.

Although much of this discussion has focused on diabetes, biosensor tattoos have potential that goes far beyond this disease. These devices have the ability to measure a variety of biomarkers in the body, making them suitable for monitoring and treating other medical conditions. For example, biosensor tattoos could be used for continuous monitoring of blood pressure, blood oxygen concentration, medication levels in the body, cardiovascular disease markers, and much more. This would open the door to a more comprehensive and personalized approach to healthcare across various health conditions.

Despite all these advantages, biosensor tattoos are not without challenges and ethical considerations. It is important to address these issues to ensure that this technology is used effectively and ethically.

The first point is the accuracy of sensors in biosensor tattoos is critical for their utility in healthcare. Devices must be properly calibrated and validated to ensure they provide reliable and accurate measurements of biomarkers. Technical challenges in this regard must be rigorously addressed so that doctors and patients can trust the generated data. To achieve this, they must undergo a series of tests similar to those required for medications in accordance with the standards set by the International Council for Harmonisation of Technical Requirements for Pharmaceuticals for Human Use.

Like any device connected to the internet, biosensor tattoos may be vulnerable to cyberattacks. The connectivity of biosensor tattoos raises data privacy and security issues. Health data is highly sensitive and must be handled securely and in compliance with privacy regulations. Manufacturers of these devices must take measures to ensure that data is protected against cyber threats and unauthorized access.

Another drawback may be access to this technology, which may initially incur high costs and only be affordable for segments of the population with high purchasing power. As biosensor tattoos become more common, it is essential to ensure they are available and affordable for all people, regardless of their geographical location or financial situation. This is crucial to avoid exacerbating healthcare disparities.

Biosensor tattoos represent a revolutionary innovation in healthcare, with the potential to significantly enhance adherence to control and treatment of chronic diseases, such as diabetes. These devices offer convenience, precision, and continuous monitoring, allowing them to address critical challenges in diabetes management and other medical conditions.

As research and development continue to advance in this field, it is essential to address technical, ethical, and access challenges appropriately. If these challenges are overcome, we may be on the cusp of an entirely new era of personalized and effective healthcare, where patients can take a more active role in controlling their health and enjoy a better quality of life. With biosensor tattoos, the future of telemedicine appears bright and full of promise.

Conclusion

- Temporary tattoos embedded with glucose sensors represent a promising innovation for continuous, non-invasive glucose monitoring in individuals with diabetes.
- These temporary tattoos use biosensors and monitoring technology to extract interstitial fluid and measure glucose levels in the skin.
- Flexible, body-compliant biometric tattoos offer a comfortable, long-term alternative for glucose monitoring, eliminating the need for frequent fingerstick tests.
- In addition to glucose, these tattoos can be extended to measure other medically relevant biomarkers, making them a versatile tool for health monitoring.
- Biometric tattoo technology has proven effective in proof-of-concept studies, providing real-time data and contributing to more effective diabetes management.
- Temporary tattoos with sensors represent an advancement in convenience and comfort for medical monitoring, avoiding invasive and painful procedures.
- While biometric tattoos have great potential, it is crucial to consider safety and regulatory aspects, ensuring that the inks and electronic components are safe for human use.
- These devices could be valuable for monitoring chronic medical conditions and health tracking in the future, opening new possibilities in personalized healthcare.
- Temporary tattoos with sensors can contribute to increased patient engagement in their own care, as they offer a more comfortable and less invasive way to monitor their health.
- Ongoing research and development in the field of biometric tattoos have the potential to revolutionize how health is monitored and managed, offering a more accessible and convenient option for patients.

References

[1] Zhou, A. Y., Taylor, B. E., Barber, K. G., Lee, C. A., Taylor, Z. R. R., Howell, S. J., & Taylor, P. R. (2023). *Anti-IL17A Halts the Onset of Diabetic Retinopathy in Type I and II Diabetic Mice. International Journal of Molecular Sciences*, 24(2), 1347. https://doi.org/10.3390/ijms24021347.

[2] Gebermariam, A. D., Tiruneh, S. A., Ayele, A. A., Tegegn, H. G., Ayele, B. A., & Engidaw, M. (2020). *Level of glycemic control and its associated factors among type II diabetic patients in debre tabor general hospital, northwest Ethiopia. Metabolism Open*, 8, 100056. https://doi.org/10.1016/j.metop.2020.100056.

[3] Gemeda, S. T., & Woldemariam, Z. B. (2022). *Assessment of self-care practice amongst patients with type II diabetes attending Adama Hospital Medical College, Ethiopia. BMC Endocrine Disorders*, 22(1), 132. https://doi.org/10.1186/s12902-022-01049-9.

[4] Polonsky, W., & Henry, R. (2016). *Poor medication adherence in type 2 diabetes: recognizing the scope of the problem and its key contributors. Patient Preference and Adherence*, Volume 10, 1299–1307. https://doi.org/10.2147/ PPA.S106821.

[5] Hood, K. K., Peterson, C. M., Rohan, J. M., & Drotar, D. (2009). *Association Between Adherence and Glycemic Control in Pediatric Type 1 Diabetes: A Meta-analysis. Pediatrics*, 124(6), e1171–e1179. https://doi.org/10.1542/ peds.2009-0207.

[6] Mostafavi, F., Alavijeh, F. Z., Salahshouri, A., & Mahaki, B. (2021). *The psychosocial barriers to medication adherence of patients with type 2 diabetes: a qualitative study. BioPsychoSocial Medicine*, 15(1), 1. https://doi.org/10.1186/s13030-020-00202-x.

[7] Fayyaz, F., Aghamahdi, F., Noorian, S., Tabatabaei-Malazy, O., & Qorbani, M. (2022). *Associated factors to insulin adherence in type 1 diabetes in Tehran and Karaj, Iran. Journal of Diabetes & Metabolic Disorders*, 21(2), 1591–1597. https://doi.org/10.1007/s40200-022-01105-0.

[8] Barry-Menkhaus, S. A., Wagner, D. V., & Riley, A. R. (2020). *Small Interventions for Big Change: Brief Strategies for Distress and Self-Management Amongst Youth with Type 1 Diabetes. Current Diabetes Reports*, 20(1), 3. https://doi.org/10.1007/s11892-020-1290-7.

[9] Jimenez, G., Lum, E., Huang, Z., Theng, Y. L., Boehm, B. O., & Car, J. (2020). *Reminders for medication adherence in Type 2 diabetes management apps. Journal of Pharmacy Practice and Research*, 50(1), 78–81. https://doi.org/10.1002/jppr.1595.

[10] Dagan, E., Dubovi, I., Levy, M., Zuckerman Levin, N., & Levy, S. T. (2019). *Adherence to diabetes care: Knowledge of biochemical processes has a high impact on glycaemic control among adolescents with type 1 diabetes. Journal of Advanced Nursing*, 75(11), 2701–2709. https://doi.org/10.1111/ jan.14098.

[11] Rusdiana, R., Savira, M., Widjaja, S. S., & Ardinata, D. (2020). *The Effect of Health Education on Control Glycemic at Type 2 Diabetes Mellitus Patients. Open Access Macedonian Journal of Medical Sciences*, 8(E), 133–137. https://doi.org/10.3889/oamjms.2020.3371.

[12] Nassar, S., ELbahnasawy, H., Elnagar, S., & Elfeshawy, R. (2022). *Effect of Mothers' Care Adherence on Control of type 1 Diabetes Mellitus Among their Children. Menoufia Nursing Journal*, 7(2), 385–400. https://doi.org/10.21608/menj.2022.276315.

[13] Sauder, K. A., Stafford, J. M., The, N. S., Mayer-Davis, E. J., Thomas, J., Lawrence, J. M., Kim, G., Siegel, K. R., Jensen, E. T., Shah, A. S., D'Agostino Jr, R. B., & Dabelea, D. (2020). *Dietary strategies to manage diabetes and glycemic control in youth and young adults with youth-onset type 1 and type 2 diabetes: The search for diabetes in youth study. Pediatric Diabetes*, 21(7), 1093–1101. https://doi.org/10.1111/pedi.13091.

[14] Romo-Romo, A., Gómez-Velasco, D. V., Galán-Ramírez, G. A., Janka-Zires, M., Brito-Córdova, G. X., Gómez-Munguía, L., Sarmiento-Moreno, A. L., Gómez-Pérez, F. J., García-Ulloa, C., Hernández-Jiménez, S., Aguilar-Salinas, C. A., & Almeda-Valdés, P. (2021). *Diabetes education and self-care behaviors in patients with diabetes in Mexico. Revista Mexicana de Endocrinología, Metabolismo y Nutrición*, 8(4). https://doi.org/10.24875/ RME.20000115.

[15] Antoine, S. L., Pieper, D., Mathes, T., & Eikermann, M. (2014). *Improving the adherence of type 2 diabetes mellitus patients with pharmacy care: a systematic review of randomized controlled trials. BMC Endocrine Disorders*, 14(1), 53. https://doi.org/10.1186/1472-6823-14-53.

[16] Sunny, A., Mateti, U. V., Kellarai, A., Shetty, S., Rafikahmed, S. R., Sirimalla, S., & Madhusoodanan, A. (2021). *Knowledge, attitude, and practice on insulin administration among diabetic patients and their caregivers – Cross-sectional study. Clinical Epidemiology and Global Health*, 12, 100860. https://doi.org/10.1016/j.cegh.2021.100860.

[17] Moghissi, E. S., Korytkowski, M. T., DiNardo, M., Einhorn, D., Hellman, R., Hirsch, I. B., Inzucchi, S. E., Ismail-Beigi, F., Kirkman, M. S., & Umpierrez, G. E. (2009). *American Association of Clinical Endocrinologists and American Diabetes Association Consensus Statement on Inpatient Glycemic Control. Diabetes Care*, 32(6), 1119–1131. https://doi.org/10.2337/ dc09-9029.

[18] Liu, P., Zeng, T., Cai, L., Wang, J., & Xue, L. (2021). *Role of Flash Glucose Monitoring System Combined With Insulin Pump in Blood Glucose Treatment of Patients with Type 2 Diabetes Mellitus. Indian Journal of Pharmaceutical Sciences*, 83. https://doi.org/10.36468/pharmaceutical-sciences.spl.180.

[19] Ajjan, R., Bilir, S. P., Hellmund, R., & Souto, D. (2022). *Cost-Effectiveness Analysis of Flash Glucose Monitoring System for People with Type 2 Diabetes Receiving Intensive Insulin Treatment. Diabetes Therapy*, 13(11–12), 1933–1945. https://doi.org/10.1007/s13300-022-01325-w.

[20] Abrams, B., & Gardner, P. R. (2023). *Symbolic Objects in Contentious Politics. University of Michigan Press.* https://doi.org/10.3998/ mpub.11722857.

[21] Kavahru A, & Ndang C. (2023). *The Culture of Tattooing in Woman Society: The Ao Nagas and The Konyak Nagas. International Journal For Multidisciplinary Research*, 5(4). https://doi.org/10.36948/ijfmr.2023. v05i04.4325.

[22] Kisofen, A. M. (2022). Fatek (Tattoo): *An Ethnic Bontoc Marker in the Northern Philippines. International Journal of Research and Innovation in Social Science*, 06(07), 329–334. https://doi.org/10.47772/IJRISS.2022.6722.

[23] Vyshka, G., Elezi, F., Çomo, A., & Xhemali, B. (2022). *Occultism and playing with the dead: When rituals go wrong. Medico-Legal Journal*, 90(2), 90–93. https://doi.org/10.1177/00258172221081736.

[24] Barabas, T. (2023). *In(k)scribed Identities: A Sociological Analysis of Catholic Croat Tattoos. AM Journal of Art and Media Studies*, 18, 33–50. https://doi.org/10.25038/am.v0i18.297.

[25] Jumpo, S. A., & Bebit, M. P. bin. (2021). *The Depiction of Asian Tattoos in Popular Culture and the Mainstream media. Global Conference on Business and Social Sciences Proceeding*, 12(1), 12–12. https://doi.org/10.35609/gcbssproceeding.2021.12(12).

[26] Cohen, P. R. (2022). *Squamous Cell Carcinoma and Tattoo: A Man With a Tattoo-Associated Squamous Cell Carcinoma and Review of Benign Tumors, Lymphoid Conditions, and Malignant Neoplasms Occurring Within a Tattoo. Cureus*. https://doi.org/10.7759/cureus.21083.

[27] Kassaw, B., Abera, N., Legesse, T., Workineh, A., & Ambaw, G. (2022). *Sero-prevalence and associated factors of hepatitis B virus among pregnant women in Hawassa city public hospitals, Southern Ethiopia: Cross-sectional study design. SAGE Open Medicine*, 10, 205031212211407. https://doi.org/10.1177/20503121221140778.

[28] Sharma, P., Satija, M., Chaudhary, A., Singh, S., Sharma, S., Girdhar, S., Gupta, V., & Bansal, P. (2022). *Epidemiological correlates of hepatitis C infection- A case control analysis from a tertiary care hospital. Journal of Family Medicine and Primary Care*, 11(5), 2099. https://doi.org/10.4103/jfmpc.jfmpc_1965_21.

[29] Pincelli, G., Sena, M. M., & Pavani, C. (2022). *Nd:YAG Laser Tattoo Removal in Individuals With Skin Phototypes IV-VI: A Case Series. Journal of Lasers in Medical Sciences*, 13, e79. https://doi.org/10.34172/jlms.2022.79.

[30] Han, S. H., Jo, D. I., & Kim, S. H. (2020). *Staged excision of basal cell carcinoma arising from a tattooed eyebrow. Archives of Craniofacial Surgery*, 21(5), 315–318. https://doi.org/10.7181/acfs.2020.00346.

[31] Scalia, S., Bertoni, S., Dozzo, A., Rimessi, A., Pinton, P., Passerini, N., & Albertini, B. (2020). *Glyceryl Tristearate-Based Lipid Microparticles Loaded with the Tattoo Colorant, Acid Red 87: Colorant Retention Capacity in Excised Porcine Skin. Skin Pharmacology and Physiology*, 33(6), 323–330. https://doi.org/10.1159/000512643.

[32] Karadagli, S. S., Cansever, I., Armagan, G., & Sogut, O. (2023). *Are Some Metals in Tattoo Inks Harmful to Health? An Analytical Approach. Chemical Research in Toxicology*, 36(1), 104–111. https://doi.org/10.1021/ acs.chemrestox.2c00323.

[33] Andreou, E., Hatziantoniou, S., Rallis, E., & Kefala, V. (2021). *Safety of Tattoos and Permanent Make up (PMU) Colorants. Cosmetics*, 8(2), 47. https://doi.org/10.3390/cosmetics8020047.

[34] Liou, Y. L., Voller, L. M., Liszewski, W., Ericson, M. E., Siegel, P. D., & Warshaw, E. M. (2021). *Formaldehyde Release From Predispersed Tattoo Inks: Analysis Using the Chromotropic Acid Method. Dermatitis*, 32(5), 327–332. https://doi.org/10.1097/DER.0000000000000663.

[35] Leijs, M., Schaefer, H., Rübben, A., Cacchi, C., Rustemeyer, T., & van der Bent, S. (2021). *Cutaneous Malignancies in Tattoos, a Case Series of Six Patients. Current Oncology*, 28(6), 4721–4737. https://doi.org/10.3390/ curroncol28060398.

[36] Scalia, S., Dozzo, A., Magli, S., & Scarcella, G. (2020). *Incorporation in Lipid Microparticles of Acid Red 87, a Colorant Used in Tattoo Inks: Effect on Photodegradation Under Simulated Sunlight and*

Laser Radiation. Photochemistry and Photobiology, 96(5), 998–1004. https://doi.org/10.1111/php.13258.

[37] Devcic, J., Dussol, M., Collin-Faure, V., Pérard, J., Fenel, D., Schoehn, G., Carrière, M., Rabilloud, T., & Dalzon, B. (2022). *Immediate and Sustained Effects of Cobalt and Zinc-Containing Pigments on Macrophages. Frontiers in Immunology, 13, 865239*. https://doi.org/10.3389/fimmu.2022.865239.

[38] Karbowska, B., Rębiś, T., Zembrzuska, J., & Nadolska, K. (2020). *Thallium in color tattoo inks: risk associated with tattooing. Medycyna Pracy*. https://doi.org/10.13075/mp.5893.00934.

[39] Negi, S., Bala, L., Shukla, S., & Chopra, D. (2022). *Tattoo inks are toxicological risks to human health: A systematic review of their ingredients, fate inside skin, toxicity due to polycyclic aromatic hydrocarbons, primary aromatic amines, metals, and overview of regulatory frameworks. Toxicology and Industrial Health*, 38(7), 417–434. https://doi.org/10.1177/ 07482337221100870.

[40] Colboc, H., Bazin, D., Reguer, S., Lucas, I. T., Moguelet, P., Amode, R., Jouanneau, C., Soria, A., Chasset, F., Amsler, E., Pecquet, C., Aractingi, S., Bellot-Gurlet, L., Deschamps, L., Descamps, V., & Kluger, N. (2022). *Chemical characterization of inks in skin reactions to tattoo. Journal of Synchrotron Radiation*, 29(6), 1436–1445. https://doi.org/10.1107/ S1600577522008165.

[41] Sadura, F., Wróbel, M. S., & Karpienko, K. (2021). *Colored Tattoo Ink Screening Method with Optical Tissue Phantoms and Raman Spectroscopy. Materials*, 14(12), 3147. https://doi.org/10.3390/ma14123147.

[42] Karregat, J. J. J. P., Rustemeyer, T., van der Bent, S. A. S., Spiekstra, S. W., Thon, M., Fernandez Rivas, D., & Gibbs, S. (2021). *Assessment of cytotoxicity and sensitization potential of intradermally injected tattoo inks in reconstructed human skin. Contact Dermatitis*, 85(3), 324–339. https://doi.org/10.1111/cod.13908.

[43] Weiß, K. T., Schreiver, I., Siewert, K., Luch, A., Haslböck, B., Berneburg, M., & Bäumler, W. (2021). *Tattoos – more than just colored skin? Searching for tattoo allergens. JDDG: Journal Der Deutschen Dermatologischen Gesellschaft,* 19(5), 657–669. https://doi.org/10.1111/ ddg.14436.

[44] Colboc, H., Bazin, D., Moguelet, P., Reguer, S., Amode, R., Jouanneau, C., Lucas, I., Deschamps, L., Descamps, V., & Kluger, N. (2020). *Chemical composition and distribution of tattoo inks within tattoo-associated keratoacanthoma. Journal of the European Academy of Dermatology and Venereology*, 34(7). https://doi.org/10.1111/jdv.16220.

[45] Wang, X., Josefsson, L., Meschnark, S., Lind, M., Emmer, Å., Goessler, W., & Hedberg, Y. S. (2021). *Analytical survey of tattoo inks—A chemical and legal perspective with focus on sensitizing substances. Contact Dermatitis*, 85(3), 340–353. https://doi.org/10.1111/cod.13913.

[46] Svedman, C., Ulriksdotter, J., Lejding, T., Bruze, M., & Mowitz, M. (2021). *Changes in adhesive ingredients in continuous glucose monitoring systems may induce new contact allergy pattern. Contact Dermatitis*, 84(6), 439–446. https://doi.org/10.1111/cod.13781.

[47] Al Hayek, A. A., & Al Dawish, M. A. (2021). *Frequency of Diabetic Ketoacidosis in Patients with Type 1 Diabetes Using FreeStyle Libre: A Retrospective Chart Review. Advances in Therapy*, 38(6), 3314–3324. https://doi.org/10.1007/s12325-021-01765-z.

[48] Atar, M., Pirgon, Ö., & Çetin, G. (2021). *Allergic Reaction Following Implantation of a Blood Glucose Sensor. The Journal of Pediatric Academy*, 121–123. https://doi.org/10.51271/jpea-2021-0143.

[49] Toelle, B. G., Marks, G. B., & Dunn, S. M. (2020). *Validation of the inhaler adherence questionnaire. BMC Psychology*, 8(1), 95. https://doi.org/10.1186/s40359-020-00461-x.

[50] Irianto, B. G. I. G., Sumber, S., Al Haq, E. R., & Asghari, M. (2022). *Sphygmomanometer Sphygmomanometer with Led Bar Display to Improve the Blood Pressure Reading Accuracy. Jurnal Teknokes*, 15(3), 154–160. https://doi.org/10.35882/teknokes.v15i3.321.

[51] Pervykh, S., & Bychkova, N. (2022). *Effect of combined compression-vibration therapy using non-invasive Beautylizer Therapy Cosmospheres V on the subcutaneous tissue morphology in women with gynoid lipodystrophy (pilot study). Journal of Cosmetic Dermatology*, 21(10), 4631–4636. https://doi.org/10.1111/jocd.14874.

[52] Davis, G. M., Spanakis, E. K., Migdal, A. L., Singh, L. G., Albury, B., Urrutia, M. A., Zamudio-Coronado, K. W., Scott, W. H., Doerfler, R., Lizama, S., Satyarengga, M., Munir, K., Galindo, R. J., Vellanki, P., Cardona, S., Pasquel, F. J., Peng, L., & Umpierrez, G. E. (2021). *Accuracy of Dexcom G6*

Continuous Glucose Monitoring in Non–Critically Ill Hospitalized Patients With Diabetes. Diabetes Care, 44(7), 1641–1646. https://doi.org/10.2337/ dc20-2856.

[53] Styles, S., Wheeler, B., Boucsein, A., Crocket, H., de Lange, M., Signal, D., Wiltshire, E., Cunningham, V., Lala, A., Cutfield, W., de Bock, M., Serlachius, A., & Jefferies, C. (2021). *A comparison of FreeStyle Libre 2 to self-monitoring of blood glucose in children with type 1 diabetes and sub-optimal glycaemic control: a 12-week randomised controlled trial protocol. Journal of Diabetes & Metabolic Disorders*, 20(2), 2093–2101. https://doi.org/10.1007/s40200-021-00907-y.

[54] Oppel, E., Kamann, S., Heinemann, L., Klein, A., Reichl, F., & Högg, C. (2020). *Freestyle libre 2: The new isobornyl acrylate free generation. Contact Dermatitis*, 83(5), 429–431. https://doi.org/ 10.1111/cod.13638.

[55] Pyl, J., Dendooven, E., Van Eekelen, I., den Brinker, M., Dotremont, H., France, A., Foubert, K., Pieters, L., Lambert, J., De Block, C., & Aerts, O. (2020). *Prevalence and Prevention of Contact Dermatitis Caused by FreeStyle Libre: A Monocentric Experience. Diabetes Care*, 43(4), 918–920. https://doi.org/10.2337/dc19-1354.

[56] Bandodkar, A. J., Jia, W., Yardımcı, C., Wang, X., Ramirez, J., & Wang, J. (2015). *Tattoo-Based Noninvasive Glucose Monitoring: A Proof-of-Concept Study. Analytical Chemistry*, 87(1), 394–398. https://doi.org/10.1021/ac504300n.

[57] He, F., Li, K., Lv, X., Zeng, Q., Zhu, Y., Li, X., & Deng, Y. (2022). *Flexible biochemical sensors for point-of-care management of diseases: a review. Microchimica Acta*, 189(10), 380. https://doi.org/10.1007/s00604-022-05469-1.

[58] Guk, K., Han, G., Lim, J., Jeong, K., Kang, T., Lim, E.-K., & Jung, J. (2019). *Evolution of Wearable Devices with Real-Time Disease Monitoring for Personalized Healthcare. Nanomaterials*, 9(6), 813. https://doi.org/10.3390/nano9060813.

[59] Seshadri, D. R., Li, R. T., Voos, J. E., Rowbottom, J. R., Alfes, C. M., Zorman, C. A., & Drummond, C. K. (2019). *Wearable sensors for monitoring the physiological and biochemical profile of the athlete. Npj Digital Medicine*, 2(1), 72. https://doi.org/10.1038/s41746-019-0150-9.

[60] Juska, V. B., & Pemble, M. E. (2020). *A Critical Review of Electrochemical Glucose Sensing: Evolution of Biosensor Platforms Based on Advanced Nanosystems. Sensors*, 20(21), 6013. https://doi.org/ 10.3390/s20216013.

[61] Koklu, A., Ohayon, D., Wustoni, S., Druet, V., Saleh, A., & Inal, S. (2022). *Organic Bioelectronic Devices for Metabolite Sensing. Chemical Reviews*, 122(4), 4581–4635. https://doi.org/10.1021/ acs.chemrev.1c00395.

[62] Bandodkar, A. J., Jia, W., Yardımcı, C., Wang, X., Ramirez, J., & Wang, J. (2015). *Tattoo-Based Noninvasive Glucose Monitoring: A Proof-of-Concept Study. Analytical Chemistry*, 87(1), 394–398. https://doi.org/10.1021/ac504300n.

[63] He, R., Liu, H., Fang, T., Niu, Y., Zhang, H., Han, F., Gao, B., Li, F., & Xu, F. (2021). *A Colorimetric Dermal Tattoo Biosensor Fabricated by Microneedle Patch for Multiplexed Detection of Health-Related Biomarkers. Advanced Science*, 8(24). https://doi.org/10.1002/advs.202103030.

[64] Yetisen, A. K., Moreddu, R., Seifi, S., Jiang, N., Vega, K., Dong, X., Dong, J., Butt, H., Jakobi, M., Elsner, M., & Koch, A. W. (2019). *Dermal Tattoo Biosensors for Colorimetric Metabolite Detection. Angewandte Chemie International Edition*, 58(31), 10506–10513. https://doi.org/10.1002/ anie.201904416.

[65] Zhou, Q., Li, H., Liao, Z., Gao, B., & He, B. (2023). *Bridging the Gap between Invasive and Noninvasive Medical Care: Emerging Microneedle Approaches. Analytical Chemistry*, 95(1), 515–534. https://doi.org/10.1021/ acs.analchem.2c01895.

Chapter 13

The Triz Methodology for the Design of a Water Saving System in a Household Toilet

Omar Eduardo Sánchez Estrada*
Mario Gerson Urbina Pérez
and Raymundo Ocaña Delgado
Autonomous University of México State, Toluca de Lerdo, México

Abstract

Over the years, renowned scientists have developed creative theories, linked different discoveries, and applied creative inventions; However, results remain questionable. Genrich Altshuler, an expert scholar on patents, created the TRIZ Methodology or Theory of Inventive Problem Solving, (Altshuller & Altov, 1996), which has scientifically proved its scopes, based on the study of more than two million patents in different countries (Shirwaiker & Okudan, 2011). According to Carvalho and Back (2001), the TRIZ methodology interconnects different methods and algorithms to identify, decompose, and solve problems innovatively across various fields. Under such criteria, unmeasurable water usage and waste in cities, due to different companies, the state and population, is increasing day after day. Therefore, this research work has the objective to define design technical-conceptual criteria and usage of technical contradictions established in the TRIZ method in order to promote and facilitate prefiguration of water saving systems in housing.

Keywords: industrial design, triz methodology, water saving system

Introduction

Throughout the years, science and technology have revolutionized the problem-solving approach in different fields and levels, and invention comes from these concepts as a challenging activity for scientists, considered as a turning point to discover hidden answers to determined uncertainties. In the 1940s, it was believed that inventors carried out their creative

* Corresponding Author's Email: omarseuaem@yahoo.com.mx

In: Psycho-Environmental Variables That Ensure People's Well-Being and Health …
Editors: Roberto Alonso González Lezcano and Guadalupe Cantarero García
ISBN: 979-8-89530-831-8
© 2025 Nova Science Publishers, Inc.

process fortuitously, driven merely by their state of mind at the time, to materialize inventions and advance science and technology. (Rodriguez et al., 2015). Teti and D'Addona (2011) state that the application of the TRIZ method allows innovation through analysis and resolution of contradictions. This methodology is integrated by different methods, tools and algorithms, which take into account the evolution of socio-technical systems and levels of invention (li et al., 2012). In addition, it facilitates the categorization and modeling of problems, by means of concepts and tools aligned to systematic approaches and generic criteria, and it is also feasible to understand possible future product or service trends (Sivan and Kanthavel, 2004).

TRIZ can be considered as the integration of conceptual and technical tools for understanding and solving problems assertively (Gadd, 2011). It is worth highlighting the concept of contradictions, which arise when two needs that integrate simple and complex technical problems that occur in a product or process are in conflict; however, both of them are the key to problem solving (Lopez, 1999). According to the method, another relevant concept is that of ideality, and this is recognized as the natural tendency of all technical systems based on a developing evolution process, and it is represented as the sum of the total useful functions of a system divided by the sum of the total harmful effects (Altshuller et al., 1996).

Currently, organizations in business, management, and technology systems are conducting studies to find solutions through functional analysis, a tool that identifies functions and characteristics within management and technological systems while protecting the business system. This work shows the errors, damages, unnecessary functions, excessive cost of components and the definition of the proposed system (Sklyarova et al., 2020).

Meanwhile, the global water shortage has created a concern for inhabitants of all regions in the world; collection and storage systems are an alternative to subsequently treat water already used in toilets and in different areas in a household. According to the World Health Organization (WHO) (2017), by the year 2100, millions of people will not have access to water service. It is noteworthy that poor management of the resource, technical capacities and economic factors in developing countries are components that aggravate the problem (Thiam et al., 2021). On the other hand, researchers work for the saving and reuse of this valuable resource, in countries such as China, waterfalls, ecological wetland waterscapes and artificial lakes among others have been developed, the projects promote a good circulation and utilization of rainwater (Xie et al., 2021). Although planning the ecological landscape is a valuable starting point, such action proposes to set the places where the different multilayer plants will be located, those with lower layer that grow under the shade of light and do not consume as much water, as well as the way in which plants and foliage are placed reduces the force of rain when precipitating, managing to reduce surface runoff (he, 2021).

Consequently, TRIZ has motivated companies such as Toyota to develop the methodology in the Research and Development department; Samsumg and its work together with Russian companies have achieved 50 patents in just 12 months and have obtained savings over 100 million dollars (Purchasecontrol, 2020). Based on the theory, it is possible to combine solutions for contradictions and procedures for creativity, imagination, creativity and associative thinking, that is, different areas of the psyche (Mi Dahlgaard-Park, S, 2006). Furthermore, it was found that the theory can be applied in most decision-making processes, as well as in organizational management, which allows project leaders to leave behind the intuition and improvisation of technical-practical solutions, this has driven the search for thought-leading executives in order to make the right decisions in a timely manner (Wang, Zhang & Zhang,

2015). All of the above have the potential to be reinterpreted for their application in water saving systems in a household toilet.

The use of TRIZ with a focus on system development expands the possibility of managing, using and reusing the vital liquid efficiently in different living spaces. Everything starts with a specific problem, which is disarticulated to obtain more relevant aspects of it, which turns it into an abstract problem that can be solved through a pre-established solution for such abstract approach; finally, the solution must be defined as a specific solution to address the specific original problem. Thus, a water saving system developed through the resolution of technical contradictions in a complex system favors a better prognosis regarding depletion of the valuable resource (Butt, 1997). TRIZ as a set of tools for the creative process not only opens the possibility of approaching problems logically and systematically towards the conceptualization of any system, it also accelerates initiatives to commercialize it in any region of the world.

Therefore, shortage and good management of water resources represents one of the most important challenges for scientists in the world. The inability to manage water resources technically and financially, especially in developing countries, represents a major problem in terms of health, employment and environmental care. It is worth noting that the World Health Organization estimates that 2.1 billion people around the world do not have a drinking water service (UN, 2017). In addition, 97 percent of this resource found on the planet is contained in the oceans, which makes it difficult to use for domestic, industrial or agricultural consumption and use. Only 3 percent is fresh water, while no agreements have emerged among countries that are considered economic and technological world powers to plan, develop and implement projects (viable, feasible and desirable) to save the water consumed in household toilets, mainly in countries with higher poverty rates (Fuenfschilling & Truffer, 2016).

Hence, the main objective of this research focuses on defining the design criteria through the TRIZ method based on the understanding of abiotic, biotic and socioeconomic systems, the organization in a harmonious balance of materials, the integration of technological requirements and the configuration of responses to biological needs or psychological effects related to form, color, volume or space.

Previous Analysis

For the TRIZ method development, the concept defined as contradictions is a key to identify a conflict among needs of a product, which are in contradiction in the origin of every technical problem, in their conception they must be analyzed and associated to solve specific requirements, such contradictions are classified as technical, physical and human: (a) technical contradiction, it occurs when solution proposals are made concerning the improvement of some attributes or functions of a useful object, artifact, instrument or system, which are affected automatically; (b) physical contradiction, it arises when the same physical element or component presents two contradictory conditions; and (c) human contradiction, it occurs when users resist or simply block a possible change (Rantanen & Domb, 2010). From their simplest structure, problems generally integrate different contradictions, resulting from technical, physical or human problems. The use of the contradiction matrix simplifies analysis by structuring different types of problems through the division of two parameters within the same category. It should be emphasized that Altshuller assumed that there are universal principles for innovation, which accelerates creativity and technological progress. Thus, the principles of invention can be a practical guide to resolve contradictions in any water-saving system in a household toilet. Table 1 describes the 39 technological systems parameters, and Table 2 the 40 invention principles developed by Altshuller.

Therefore, designing water-saving systems in households and other areas has been a concern for centuries. The processes and systems proposed over time have also faced different contradictions, for example, increasing water flow in an "X" water stream, naturally enhances the amount of material to be used to contain water, the TRIZ method as an analysis and systematization tool streamlines the solution of the problem (Sivan & Kanthavel 2013). Figure 1 exemplifies Altshuller's contradiction matrix in water-saving systems for a household.

Table 1. Altshuller parameters of technological systems

1 Weight of a moving object	11 Tension, pressure	21 Power	31 Effects of damages collateral
2 Weight of an object stationary	12 Form	22 Loss of energy	32 Manufacturability or ease of manufacturing
3 Length of an object mobile	13 Stability of the object.	23 Loss of material	33 Convenience of use.
4 Length of an object stationary	14 Resistance	24 Loss of information	34 Ease of repair
5 Area of a moving object	15 Durability of an object mobile	25 Waste of time	35 Adaptability
6 Area of an object stationary	16 Durability of an object stationary	26 Amount of Substance or matter	36 Complexity of device or object
7 Volume of an object mobile	17 Temperature	27 Reliability	37 Complexity of control
8 Volume of an object stationary	18 Brilliance	28 Accuracy in measurement	38 Level of automation
9. Velocity	19 Energy expended by the object mobile	29 Accuracy in manufacture	39 Productivity
10. Strength	20 Energy expended by the object stationary	30 External damage that affects an object	

Source: (Altshuller, 1996).

Table 2. 40 principles of Altshuller's invention

1 Segmentation	2 Extraction	3 Local quality	4 Asymmetry
5 Combination	6 Universality	7 Nesting	8 Anti-weight
9 Preliminary anti-action	10 Preliminary action	11 Beforehand cushioning	12 Equipotentiality
13 Investment	14 Sphericity	15 Dynamics	16. Partial actions, on clutches or excessive
17 Move to a new dimension	18 Vibrations mechanical	19 Periodic Action	20. Continuity of useful action
21 Pass quickly	22 Convert damage into benefit.	23 Feedback	24 Intermediaries
25 Self-service	26 Copying	27 Cheap short-lived objects	28 Mechanics substitution
29 Use of systems hydraulic or pneumatic	30 Flexible membranes or thin films	31 Use of Porous Materials	32 Color changes
33 Homogeneity	34 Rejection and regeneration of parts	35 Transformation of states chemical or physical	36 Transitions of Phase
37 Thermal Expansion	38 Accelerated oxidations	39 Inert environments	40 Materials compounds

Source: (Altshuller, 1996).

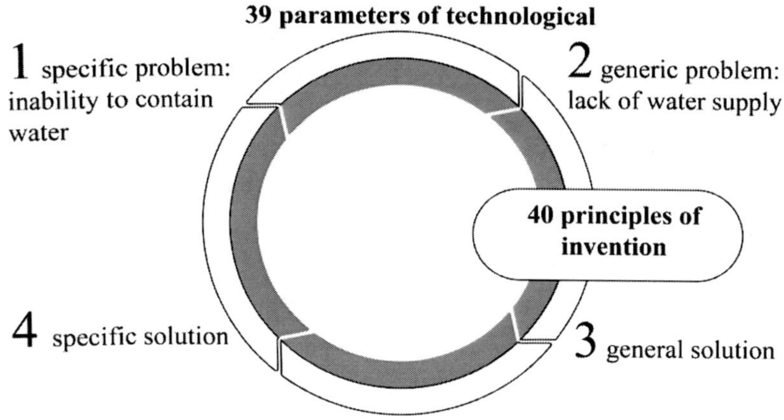

Figure 1. Matrix of Contradictions.

Functional Analysis (Creativity)

Water saving is not a priority in the supply systems of household toilets, the operation that occurs in every toilet equipment is identified from interaction characteristics in each one of them, that is to say, generally there is no interconnection in all the furniture, which breaks the idea of saving and managing water. So, there is a need in the supply systems design and it is precisely that an interconnected system could work to address contradictions from the TRIZ method (Table 3) and (Table 4).

Within water saving systems in toilets there are different errors related to contradictions (technical, physical and human), which are described below:

Table 3. Identified contradictions

Techniques	Physics	Human
Irregular supply	Water leaks in different components	Irresponsabilidad
Lack of water recovery	Low quality materials	Different activities
Interconnected systems	Component incompatibility	Lack of communication between users
Water contamination	Deficient valves	Lack of knowledge
Lag in function	Poor configuration of the conventional system	Resistance to change

Table 4. Damage, unnecessary functions and excessive cost

Damage	Unnecessary functions	Excessive cost
Pipeline	Waste of water	W.C, sink and shower
Toilet furniture	Low quality materials	Recovery systems
Containers	Component incompatibility	Heating and lighting systems
Watering can	Deficient valves	Ecological education
Sewer system	Poor system	Construction

Creative Thinking for System Design

Solving problems creatively starts from identifying the need, going through the categorization of factors such as creativity, sustainability, user, context, investment, etc. This shows how complex it can be to consolidate creative thinking. Planners, designers, engineers or scientists do not share a common definition for creativity, which leads to some uncertainty in the face of problems with permanent evolution; however, it does not mean that it is not addressed on a daily basis, regardless of its conceptual multidimensionality, which refers to a high level of analysis, synthesis, interpretation and techniques, but it is still far from consensus (Williams, Ostwald & Askland, 2010). Therefore, finding a concept is required to accelerate the cognitive process and to reconfigure ways to solve specific problems (Kim et al. 2007).

Creativity for design related to problem definition, conceptualization, functionality, ergonomics, aesthetics, sustainability and originality are factors that modify the manufacturing, use, disuse, disassembly and life cycle of projects. Creativity has been defined as the ability to create an appropriate and innovative product (Lubart, 1994; Sternberg & Lubart, 1996; Amabile, 1997; Sternberg, 2001). Teachers and researchers specializing in the field seek to transfer knowledge and agree upon them to generate ideas and determine their effectiveness, based on the functional analysis of systems and multidimensionality of problems to be solved, without omitting the quality and level of originality (Shroyer, Lovins, Turns, Cardella, & Atman, 2018), such a process accelerates identifying creativity evaluation indicators (Demirkan & Afacan 2012). For Altshueller, creative thinking: a) eliminates contradictions through creative solutions; b) creative solutions are defined by a limited number of methods to eliminate contradictions; and c) it is feasible to develop effective tactics to find meaning among different types of contradictions. Randomness for creative problem solving is not acceptable, but is governed by systematization.

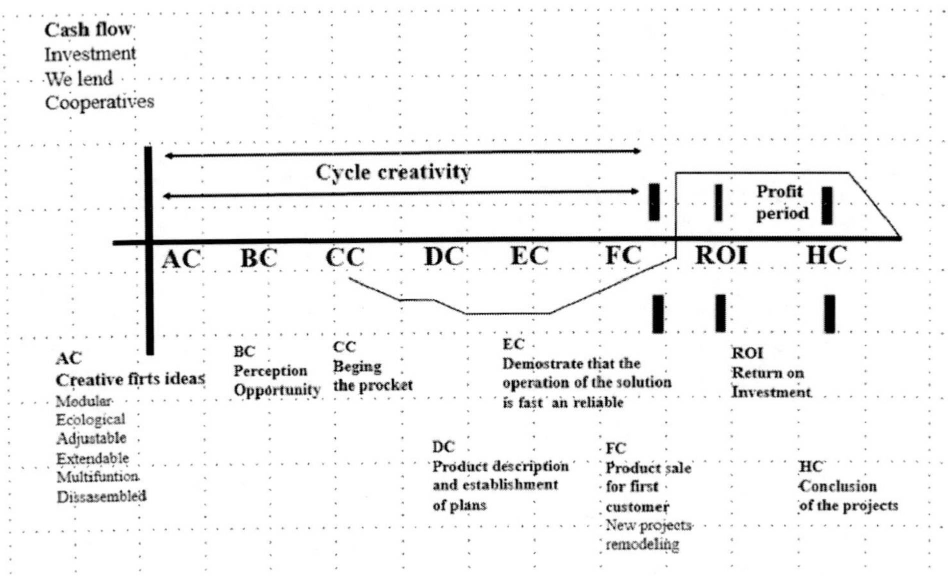

Figure 2. Cycle creativity, Source: (Adapted from. Ekmekci & Koksal, (2015), Triz methodology and an application example for product development. 195(Suppl. C), 2689-2698.

Altshuller defines two types of problems: those of known solution and those of unknown solution, the former referring to those shown in books, magazines, internet, scientific articles, and the latter, defined as creative problems. Figure 2 presents the creativity cycle for the solution of creative problems in water saving systems in household toilets.

Design Theory

Technical, physical or human problems must be approached from codification and categorization of their components. From design practice it is important to build a user profile to identify the different use sequences that occur in the interactions between objects or systems of objects and people, as well as to work with the trinomial (object-person-environment). This enables decomposition of systems into their different parts and facilitates the identification of different contradictions. If we consider that design is based on the construction of shape, ergonomics, aesthetics and sustainability, among other factors, it may be more practical to systematize problems. It should be noted that each of these concepts integrates an important number of factors, which are logically intertwined and make design to be efficient in its multiple sections.

Shape Construction

Every idea developed starts from a conceptual beginning, which means that everything created, developed or manufactured must consider the basic principle of construction that will be given according to the purpose, conditions, method or technique to carry it out. For designers it is easy to identify that a structural shape starts from mental configuration given to something, that is, it seeks to prefigure ideas from different approaches and strategies, for example, geometry seeks linearity, symmetry, axiality, modularity or just organic structure. This supports the analysis of objects or systems of objects, since it will be simpler to identify characteristics or functions determined by each useful object.

Ergonomics

Every object that goes through the design process in some way has been manufactured with the idea of facilitating interactions, whether manual, semi-automatic or automatic, working from preventive, corrective, dynamic or static ergonomics, to determine the best performance in different intervals of use and to improve quality of life. Each use sequence that occurs among primary users (those who will be in permanent contact with the object) and secondary users (those who have incidental contact with the product), salespeople, transporters, packers, etc., is considered to address factors related to the surroundings: environmental, lighting, thermal and acoustic, among others. This science supports defragmentation of components according to their use, safety, comfort and dimensions. Therefore, ergonomics not only facilitates identification of interactions, but it also reveals possible technical, physical and human contradictions that may arise in different systems.

Aesthetics

Object condition well-valued by consumers, if an object or system is beautiful, pleasant, identifiable, balanced and congruent in its shapes, it will surely facilitate identification of human contradictions, which is basic to apply the TRIZ method, because perception and adaptability of people with objects or systems, show different conditions of use, function, maintenance and reuse.

Sustainability

The main objective of this article is to define conceptual parameters for the project beginning, going through the theoretical-practical characteristics of use, function, structure, interaction, identification and communication of the object, based on the useful object that will be ecologically bearable, economically viable and socially equitable, together with transversality of cultural, political and state requirements. Therefore, development of innovative packaging with low environmental impact will promote the construction of a new, more sustainable material culture. At present, this factor is of paramount importance, since ideation, as the first phase of design, must consider objects that are ecologically bearable, economically viable and socially, politically and culturally equitable. Manufacturing with energy savings, reduction of operations and optimization of production phases, not only reveals the most common contradictions in different systems, but also the waste and excessive use of resources to produce objects. Thus, disassembly as a primary action in sustainable design should also be worked on in the first phase of ideation, and with it determine whether it will be a destructive disassembly or not, to carry out recycling, remanufacturing or reuse through implementation of the four evaluation characteristics:

- *Identification easiness:* speed to identify the parts and disassemble them, ease to recognize location and joining systems.
- *Accessibility:* determining the ease with which disassembly tools can access the attachment point and item to be disassembled.
- *Ease of detachment:* properties of a component joining element to separate from another or from the rest of the product.
- *Ease of handling:* easiness of handling that components have throughout the disassembly process (Figure 3).

The main objective of the Design for Disassembly (DFD) is to choose phases and sequences as chains of actions that will occur one after the other (Srinivasan et al., 1997), the graph called "nodes and meshes" is simple disassembly, where the physical parts are represented as nodes and the existing connections between the parts as meshes. It should be noted that disassembly allows the designer to locate technical contradictions that are not so visible (Figure 4).

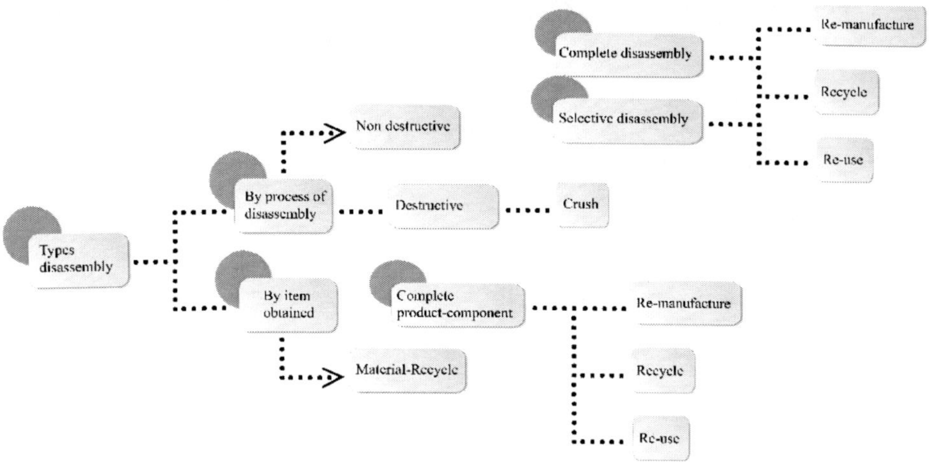

Source: (Srinivasan et al., 1997; Greedel & Allenby, 1995).

Figure 3. Overall programme structure.

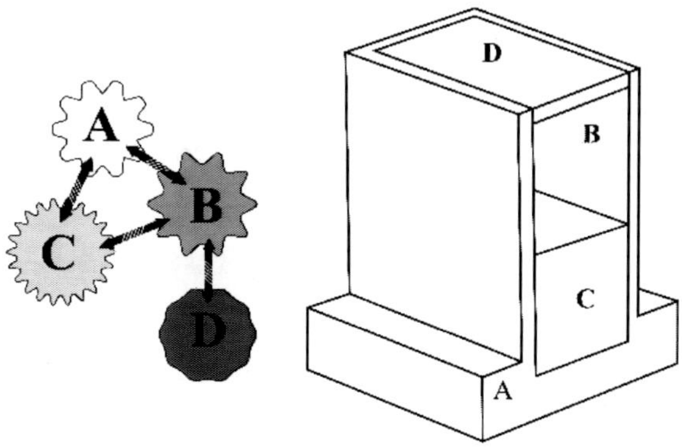

Source: (Cappelli et al., 2007).

Figure 4. Connection diagram "nodes and meshes."

Material Selection

For developing sustainable projects, the aim is to select materials with low environmental impact, based on a rigorous analysis of the product's life cycle, disassembly by phases, elimination of any possible use of toxic materials, gas emissions from the adhesives, chemical compounds and coatings used for finishing, (Calkins, 2008). In addition, it is also necessary to consider psychosocial factors associated with: a) ecological thinking; b) defense of sustainability theories; and c) fostering values and habits for the construction of a new sustainable integral culture. It is worth mentioning that selection of materials is based on: a) initial conceptualization of the project; b) design by phases; c) manufacture and assembly; d) availability and replacement; e) preservation of shape at different temperatures; and f) resistance to corrosion and wear. Thus, design interconnects possible solutions through physical, chemical, mechanical, thermal, electrical and manufacturing parameters (Gonzalez &

Meza, 2004). The following is suggested for selecting materials with low environmental impact (Table 5) and (Figure 5).

Simple Application of Inventive Problem-Solving Theory

Table 5. Simple TRIZ app

Technical Contradiction	Physical contradiction	Altshuller parameters	Inventive principles
Variable to be improved (Adaptability) Benefit (Multifunction) Variable That is affected (Durability)	Physical variable that is improved (Function) Physical variable that is affected (Durability of an object stationary)	Identified parameter (35) Adaptability Identified parameter (14) Resistance	Principle of inventiveness identified (35, 3, 32, 6)

Source: (Own elaboration).

	Variable that is affected → / Variable to be improved ↓	Tension or pressure	Shape	Stability of the composition of the object	Resistance	Durability o fan object
		11	12	13	14	15
35	Adaptability				35, 3, 32, 6	
36	Complexity of a mechanism				2, 13, 28	

Figure 5. Source: The matrix of contradictions proposes the inventive principles that according to Altshuller should be used in the solution of the contradiction (35/3/32/6).

Conclusion

Creativity development in various fields has significantly lagged in reconfiguring and addressing specific problems. The Theory of Inventive Problem Solving (TRIZ) not only fragments and systematizes problems, but offers a wide scope for addressing problems of high impact and benefit, related to the development of material culture. Understanding technical, physical, and human contradictions enables the interconnection of different solutions to various problems while accelerating technological advancements. However, it also enhances the critical and productive thinking of developers and professionals across disciplines. Under these terms, design must be technically and theoretically aligned to the methodology concepts and parameters to fully exploit creating multidimensional objects that meet the requirements for which they were manufactured, in addition to questioning the paradigms related to product development, weakening the value system that integrates economy, production and quality of life. In addition to the above, there is a need to address problems related to natural resources, their exploitation and the impact it leaves on the planet.

References

Altshuller, G., Al'tov, G., & Altov, H. (1996). *And suddenly the inventor appeared: TRIZ, the theory of inventive problem solving*. Technical Innovation Center, Inc.

Amabile, T. M. (1997). *Entrepreneurial creativity through motivational synergy*. Journal of Creative Behavior, 31(1), 18-26.

Butts, K. H. (1997). *The strategic importance of water. The US Army War College Quarterly: Parameters, 27*(1), 1.

Calkins, M. (2008). *Materials for sustainable sites: a complete guide to the evaluation, selection, and use of sustainable construction materials*. John Wiley & Sons.

Cappelli, F., Delogu, M., Pierini, M., & Schiavone, F. (2007). *Design for disassembly: a methodology for identifying the optimal disassembly sequence*. Journal of Engineering Design, 18(6), 563-575. Retrevied from https://doi.org/10.1080/09544820601013019.

CARVALHO, MD, & Back, N. (2001, September). Use of the fundamental concepts of TRIZ and the method of inventive principles in product development. In *Brazilian Congress of Product Development management* (Vol. 3).

Demirkan, H., & Afacan, Y. (2012). *Assessing creativity in design education: Analysis of creativity factors in the first-year design studio*. Design Studies, 33(3), 262-278. Retrieved from https://doi.org/10.1016/j.destud.2011.11.005.

Ekmekci, I., & Koksal, M. (2015). *Triz methodology and an application example for product development.* Procedia-Social and Behavioral Sciences, 195(Suppl. C), 2689-2698. Retrevied from https://doi.org/10.1016/j.sbspro.2015.06.481.

Fuenfschilling, L., & Truffer, B. (2016). The interplay of institutions, actors and technologies in socio-technical systems—An analysis of transformations in the Australian urban water sector. *Technological Forecasting and Social Change, 103*, 298-312.

Gadd, K. (2011). *TRIZ for engineers: enabling inventive problem solving*. John wiley & sons.

González, H. Á., & Mesa, DH (2004). The importance of the method in the selection of materials. *Scientia et technica , 10* (24), 175-180.

Graedel, T. E., & Allenby, B. R. (1995). Matrix approaches to abridged life cycle assessment. *Environmental Science & Technology, 29*(3), 134A-139A.

He, J. (2021). Planning and design of water-saving green plant landscape under human intervention after a great earthquake. *Arabian Journal of Geosciences, 14*(23), 1-10.

Kim, M. H., Kim, Y. S., Lee, H. S., & Park, J. A. (2007). *An underlying cognitive aspect of design creativity: Limited Commitment Mode control strategy.* Design Studies, 28(6), 585-604. Retrieved from https://doi.org/10.1016/j.destud.2007.04.006.

Li, Z., Tate, D., Lane, C., & Adams, C. (2012). A framework for automatic TRIZ level of invention estimation of patents using natural language processing, knowledge-transfer and patent citation metrics. *Computer-aided design, 44*(10), 987-1010.

López, E. (1999) *La metodología TRIZ y su impacto en la innovación industrial en México.*

Lubart, T. I. (1994). *Creativity*. In R. J. Sternberg (Ed), Handbook of Perception and Cognition: Thinking and problem solving. (1st. ed., pp. 289-332). Academic Press.

Mendes, G., Arroyo-Rodríguez, V., Almeida, W. R., Pinto, S. R. R., Pillar, V. D., & Tabarelli, M. (2016). Plant trait distribution and the spatial reorganization of tree assemblages in a fragmented tropical forest landscape. *Plant Ecology*, *217*(1), 31-42.

Mi Dahlgaard-Park, S. (Ed.). (2006). Inventive thinking through TRIZ: a practical guide. *The TQM Magazine*, *18*(3), 312-314.

Purchasecontrol (2020). *¿Can The TRIZ Method Help Improve Your Company?*. https://www.purchasecontrol.com/blog/triz-method/.

Rodríguez, J. L. M., Machado, A. S., & Robaina, R. (2015). Design of cylindrical spur gears using TRIZ. *ITEGAM-JETIA*, *1*(3).

Rantanen, K., & Domb, E. (2010). *TRIZ simplificado: Nuevas aplicaciones de resolución de problemas para ingenieros y profesionales de la fabricación.* Prensa CRC.

Sivan, H., & Kanthavel, K. (2013). TRIZ: A Perfect Tool for Process Innovation by Tackling Engineering contradictions. *IOSR J. Mech. Civ. Eng*, 21-26.

Shirwaiker, R. A., & Okudan, G. E. (2011). Contributions of TRIZ and axiomatic design to leanness in design: an investigation. *Procedia Engineering*, *9*, 730-735.

Sklyarova, O. A., Musaelyan, A. K., Bukhov, N. V., Medvedeva, L. S., & Bidzhieva, A. S. (2020). Application of TRIZ Technique in the Organizations' Activity. *International Journal of Economics & Business Administration (IJEBA)*, *8*(4), 563-571.

Srinivasan, H., Shyamsundar, N., & Gadh, R. (1997). *A framework for virtual disassembly analysis.* Journal of Intelligent Manufacturing, 8(4), 277-295. Retrieved from https://doi.org/10.1023/A:1018537611535.

Sternberg, R. J., & Lubart, T. I. (1996). *Investing in creativity*. American psychologist, 51(7), 677-688. Retrevied from https://doi.org/10.1037/0003-066X.51.7.677.

Teti, R., & D'Addona, D. (2011). TRIZ based tool management in supply networks. *Procedia Engineering*, *9*, 680-687.

Thiam, D. R., Dinar, A., & Ntuli, H. (2021). Promotion of residential water conservation measures in South Africa: the role of water-saving equipment. *Environmental Economics and Policy Studies*, *23*(1), 173-210.

Wang, M., Zhang, D., & Zhang, L. (2015). Introduction of TRIZ theory for the conflict-solving in the building energy and environment management system innovation. *Procedia Engineering*, *121*, 2232-2239.

Williams, A., Ostwald, M. J., & Askland, H. H. (2010). *Creativity, design and education: Theories, positions and challenges.* Australian Learning & Teaching Council.

World Health Organization (WHO). (2017). United Nations Children's Fund (UNICEF). *Progress on drinking water, sanitation and hygiene*, 140.

Xie, Q., Lee, C., Lu, Z., & Yuan, X. (2021). Interactions with artificial water features: a scoping review of health-related outcomes. *Landscape and Urban Planning*, *215*, 104191.

Shroyer, K., Lovins, T., Turns, J., Cardella, M. E., & Atman, C. J. (2018). *Timescales and ideaspace: An examination of idea generation in design practice.* Design Studies, 57, 9-36. Retrevied from https://doi.org/10.1016/j.destud.2018.03.004.

Sklyarova, O. A., Musaelyan, A. K., Bukhov, N. V., Medvedeva, L. S., & Bidzhieva, A. S. (2020). Application of TRIZ Technique in the Organizations' Activity. *International Journal of Economics & Business Administration (IJEBA),* 8(4), 563-571.

Biographical Sketches

Omar Eduardo Sánchez Estrada

Affiliation:

Autonomous University of Mexico State, UAEM Valle de Chalco University Center, Industrial Design

Education:

- 1998-2002 Graduate in Industrial Design, Metropolitan Autonomous University
- 2005-2007 Master in Industrial Design, National Autonomous University of Mexico
- 2014-2016 Doctor in Education, International Graduate Center, A.C Tabasco
- 2014-2016 Doctor in Education, International Graduate Center, A.C Tabasco
- 2018-2019 Posdoctoral Degree in higher education educational systems, Center for Advanced Studies for Teacher Development

Business Address:
Pablo Cidoza 3, Texcoco, State of México, México.

Research and Professional Experience:
Full-Time Research Professor, UAEM Valle de Chalco since 2009.

Professional Appointments:
Member of the Degree Committee, Member of the Curricular Committee of the Industrial Design, member of the Researchers Network for Sustainable Industrial Design Education, Academic coordinator of the degree in industrial design (2009-2013), 2 Published books, 50 published articles, 70 presentations and technical support 4 research projects, Research and Advanced Studies Coordinator (2016-2018), International Mobility Manager (2018-2023)

Honors:
Honorific mention, scholoarship of honor to academic excellence. Master in Industrial Design (2005, 2007).

Publications from the Last 3 Years:

1. Barragán-Ocaña, A., Merritt, H., Sánchez-Estrada, O. E., Méndez-Becerril, J. L., & del Pilar Longar-Blanco, M. (2023). Biorefinery and sustainability to produce biofuels and value-added products: A trends analysis based on network and patent analysis. *Plos one*, 18(1), e0279659.
2. Sánchez Estrada, O. E., Attention to Accident to accidents, victims and Sustainable *Industrial Design*, CENID,2022
3. Estrada, O. E. S., Aragon, J. D. R., & Pérez, M. G. U. (2021). Triz Model Approach for Conceptualizing Household Furniture With a Disassembling Design. In *Handbook of Research on Methodologies for Design and Production Practices in Interior Architecture* (pp. 201-217). IGI Global.
4. Sánchez Estrada, O. E., Urbina Pérez, M. G., & Pérez González, K. G. (2020). Reflections on the creative process, analysis of strategic models for the development of creative thinking in the Industrial Designer.
5. Sánchez Estrada, O., Rojas Aragón, J., Pérez Gonzalez, K., & Urbina Pérez, M. (2021, February). Teachers and students of industrial design from the UAEM Valle de Chalco University Center, educational adaptations for terminal degree projects in the face of COVID-19. In *Proceedings INNODOCT/20. International Conference on Innovation,*

Documentation and Education (pp. 729-739). Editorial Universitat Politècnica de València.

Mario Gerson Urbina Pérez

Affiliation:
Autonomous University of Mexico State, UAEM Valle de Chalco University Center, Industrial Design

Education:

- 1992-1997 Industrial Designer, Faculty of Architecture and Design (UAEM), Toluca Mexico Date: Sept
- 1999 Specialist in Strategic Design of Industrial Products, UAEM. 1998-1999
- 2017 Doctoral student in educational systems and environments UDG

Business Address:
Ignacio Lopez Rayón 242, Col. San Buenaventura, 50110, Toluca México.

Research and Professional Experience:
In addition to having the opportunity to live and do postgraduate studies abroad, he has gained experience working in one of the most important research centers in the world in the field of polymers, such as the "Giulio Natta" R&D center. from Ferrara, Italy.

Professional Appointments:
Definitive full-time Professor-Researcher for the Autonomous University of the State of Mexico, Industrial Designer, Specialist in Strategic Design of Industrial Products and Projects.

In charge of multiple areas within this university, but mainly dealing with the development of applied research and training of human resources. As a result of this line, multiple research projects and their respective products have been generated: presentations, patents, articles, book chapters. reports and degree modalities such as thesis, dissertation, work experience report and essays, Specialist and pioneer of distance education using platforms such as Microsoft Teams, Facebook live, Seduca, Sakai, etc.

Honors:
Laudatory Note 2013, 2016 (UAEMex)

Publications from the Last 3 Years:

1. The strengths and weaknesses of virtual/digital environments in health crises;
2. COVID-19 case study in Mexico and solution proposal by Industrial Design.
3. ED.Universitat politécnica de Valencia (2021). ISSN: 2695-8554. https://riunet.upv.es/handle/10251/161668.

4. Interface to develop research projects in Industrial Design: proposal for applied research on mobile devices. Ed.Universitat Politécnica de Valencia (2021) ISBN: 978-84-9048-873-7. https://riunet.upv.es/handle/10251/161668.

Raymundo Ocaña Delgado

Affiliation:

Autonomous University of Mexico State, UAEM Zumpango University Center,Industrial Design

Education:

- 1987-1992 Graduate in Industrial Design, Autonomous University of the State of México.1998-1999 Specialist in Strategic Design of Industrial Products, UAEM.
- 2001-2004 Master in Education, Franco Mexicana University.2009-2011 Doctor in Education, Open University of Tlaxcala.

Business Address:

Plazuela San Juan 12, Zumpango, State of México, México.

Research and Professional Experience:

Full-Time Research Professor, UAEM Zumpango since 2001.

Professional Appointments:

Member of the Institutional Quality Committee, Member of the Curricular Committee of the Faculty of Architecture and Design, and member of the Institutional Curricular Innovation Network of the UAEM; advisor of 35 degree projects, 45 published articles, 60presentations and collaborator in 4 research projects. And, Academic Coordinator of the degree in Industrial Design (1996-2005), Academic Deputy Director (2005-2013) and Director (2016-2020), the latter in the UAEM Zumpango campus.

Honors:

Recognition in the Program for Teacher Professional Development (PRODEP) Profile since 2005.

Publications from the Last 3 Years:

1. Ocaña, Delgado R. & Rodríguez, Leonel A.M. (2023) *The sketch, a basic designtool.* México: UAEMex.
2. Ocaña, D., Rodríguez, L., Leonel R., Estevez, V. (2023) Assertiveness as a Factor in School Dropout During the COVID-19 Pandemic. In Costa, E.,Pedrini, J. (Ed.), *A comunicação e os contextos comunicativos 3.* (AteneaEditora., DOI: https://doi.org/10.22533/at.ed.933231707).

3. Ocaña, D. R., Rodríguez, L., González, B. (2022) Interaction of Graphic Designand Public Administration. In Zarur, Cortez (Ed.) *Diseño Gráfico: enfoquesde formación y campo laboral en Administración Pública.* (1ra. ed., pp. 47-59) UAEMex.
4. Soto, R., Ocaña, D., Rodríguez, L., Sánchez, E. (2022) Creativity and the industrial designer… an essential skill. In Corrent, N. (Ed.) *Ciências sociais aplicadas: Estado, organizações e desenvolvimento regional 2* (AteneaEditora., https://doi.org/10.22533/at.ed.45722041014).
5. Ocaña, D., Rodríguez, L., Urbina, P., Sánchez, E. (2021) Enrollment in industrial design at CU UAEM Zumpango, analysis of its behavior 1987-2020 at first admission. In Puppim, R. (Ed.) *Design: contribuições significativas para o desenvolvimento sustentável.* (Atenea Editora., https://doi.org/10.22533/at.ed.9282114102).

Chapter 14

Improving the Quality of Life for People with Visual Disabilities: A Smart City Approach with Artificial Intelligence, GPS, Computer Vision, and Tactile and Auditory Assistance Technologies

Sandra Arranz Paraíso[1,*]
Miguel Ángel de Miguel Paraíso[2]
and Daniel Arranz-Paraíso[3]
[1]Universidad Autónoma de Madrid, Spain
[2]Rey Juan Carlos University, Madrid, Spain
[3]R&D Development Manager at Pinisan SL. C/Gran Canaria, Madrid, Spain

Abstract

Visual impairments affect a significant portion of the global population, reducing their quality of life. The development of smart applications for individuals with visual disabilities contributes to enhancing their quality of life and independence. Collaborative efforts between computer science and other scientific disciplines have led to the advancement of intelligent healthcare applications, smart homes, assistive technology, and technologies for haptic and auditory interaction. These apps leverage technologies such as GPS, computer vision, and real-time semantic segmentation to provide real-time navigation, obstacle avoidance, and spatial awareness. They also promote equal access to healthcare services and enable individuals with visual disabilities to participate in educational and occupational activities. Smart lifestyle applications promote the social participation of individuals with visual disabilities by improving accessibility to social networks and event planning. Artificial intelligence can enhance environmental understanding, navigation, and personalized educational support. However, to fully harness the potential benefits of these applications, it is essential to address challenges related to accessibility, awareness, and the competencies of all stakeholders in society. Finally, evaluating the performance of existing applications is crucial to achieve true inclusion and equal access for all citizens. In this chapter, we focus on the role of Smart City applications for individuals with visual disabilities.

* Corresponding Author's Email: sandra.paraiso@uam.es

In: Psycho-Environmental Variables That Ensure People's Well-Being and Health …
Editors: Roberto Alonso González Lezcano and Guadalupe Cantarero García
ISBN: 979-8-89530-831-8
© 2025 Nova Science Publishers, Inc.

Keywords: visual impairments, smart city apps, accessibility, collaborative technologies, artificial intelligence.

Introduction

Determining the precise count of individuals affected by visual impairments on a global scale presents a complex challenge, given that multiple eye conditions can coexist in each person [1] estimated that 161 million people globally had visual impairments, including 37 million who were blind and 124 million with less severe visual disabilities. However, they didn't include visual impairments caused by uncorrected refractive errors like myopia, hyperopia, or astigmatism, despite being the leading cause of visual disability worldwide [2].

In the World Report on Vision published by the World Health Organization (WHO) [3] in 2019, they provide a global estimation of individuals affected by certain eye diseases that can cause visual impairment, indicating the presence of 2.6 billion (CI, 1.97–3.43) people of all ages with myopia in 2020, 312 million (95%, CI, 265 million to 369 million) aged under 19 years with myopia in 2015, 76 million (95%, CI), 51.9–111.7) people (40 to 80 years of age) with glaucoma in 2020, 2.5 million people of all ages with trachomatous trichiasis in 2019, 1.8 billion (CI, 1.7–2.0) people of all ages with presbyopia in 2015, 146 million adults with diabetic retinopathy, and 195.6 million (95% CI 140–261) people aged 30 to 97 years with age-related macular degeneration in 2020. However, as previously indicated, these figures can't be summed up to estimate prevalence in the population as individuals may have multiple pathologies.

Additionally, the report notes that at least 1 billion people have a visual impairment that could have been prevented or remains unresolved, specifically 123.7 million with unaddressed refractive error, 65.2 million with cataracts, 6.9 million with glaucoma, 4.2 million with corneal opacities, 3 million with Diabetic Retinopathy, 2 million with Trachoma, and 826 million with unaddressed presbyopia. Despite the challenge of pinpointing an exact figure, it's evident that a significant percentage of the global population suffers from some form of visual disability. Moreover, both population growth and aging have increased the number of individuals affected by moderate to severe visual impairment and blindness [4], predicting a rise in the prevalence of the visually impaired.

Beyond its prevalence, it is crucial to highlight that visual disabilities significantly impact people's quality of life, reducing scores across environmental, physical, social, and psychological domains [5]. It's observed that the severity of visual disabilities is associated with a lower quality of life compared to individuals with normal vision [6,7].

Visual disabilities affect various aspects of psychosocial well-being, such as loneliness, depressive disorders, anxiety, and quality of life [7–15]. Several studies have shown that individuals with visual disabilities are at a higher risk of developing mental health issues such as isolation, substance use disorders, anxiety, and stress (see [12, 16–20]).

Moreover, visual disability has been identified as a predictor of suicide in the elderly, underscoring its significant impact on mental health [21]. Research has also indicated a higher prevalence of psychological distress in individuals with visual disabilities compared to those with normal vision. Hence, it's essential to enhance the overall well-being of affected individuals by adapting society to the specific needs of the visually impaired.

The United Nations estimated in 2018 that 68% of the population would reside in urban areas by 2050, implying a significant portion of these individuals may experience some form of visual disability. Thus, it's important to strive to enhance their quality of life by adapting society to their needs. Smart City apps serve as a highly useful tool in this regard, providing increased independence and security by improving mobility and access to information [22–24].

Objectives

The chapter aims to provide a comprehensive understanding of the current landscape of smart applications for individuals with visual impairments, evaluate their impact, and suggest pathways for future research and development to further enhance the quality of life and independence of visually impaired individuals in Smart Cities. To accomplish this, the study will:

- investigate the prevalence and impact of visual impairments on the quality of life of individuals globally, considering various eye conditions and their societal implications.
- explore the role of smart applications in improving the quality of life, independence, and social inclusion of individuals with visual disabilities within the context of Smart Cities.
- examine the collaborative efforts between computer science and other scientific disciplines in developing intelligent healthcare applications, smart homes, assistive technology, and technologies for haptic and auditory interaction to address the specific needs of individuals with visual impairments.
- assess the effectiveness and usability of existing smart navigation, transportation, healthcare, socialization, and education applications for individuals with visual disabilities, focusing on accessibility, awareness, and user satisfaction.
- identify innovative ideas, developments, challenges, and trends in the field of smart applications aimed at enhancing the quality of life for visually impaired individuals, including advancements in assistive devices, mobile applications, and IoT solutions.
- propose recommendations for future research directions and technological advancements to address existing challenges and improve the inclusivity and effectiveness of smart applications for individuals with visual disabilities in Smart Cities.

Smart City APPS for the Visually Impaired People

Ensuring that visually impaired individuals have access to services and resources on an equal footing is crucial, providing them with personalized assistance. Fortunately, numerous mobile applications currently exist, combining information from urban environments collected through various sensors and active citizen participation. These applications address the specific needs of people with disabilities in smart cities [25]. They primarily focus on enhancing quality of life, intelligent transportation, and healthcare [26].

Smart Navigation and Transportation Applications

Fortunately, navigating urban environments is becoming increasingly accessible for individuals with visual disabilities, thanks to interdisciplinary collaborations that have led to the development of smart navigation and transportation applications.

Smart navigation and transportation applications can offer real-time navigation, assisting individuals with visual impairments in navigating urban environments [27]. Numerous mobile applications have been developed to aid visually impaired individuals in their daily activities [28]. These applications make use of technologies such as GPS and advancements in computer vision, along with real-time semantic segmentation [29–33]. This not only facilitates the navigation of visually impaired individuals but also assists in obstacle avoidance, enhancing their understanding of the environment. Fortunately, many smart transportation applications can be used on conventional devices like mobile phones [34]. For example, one of the most widely used navigation apps, Google Maps, can be employed by people with visual disabilities, as it provides voice guidance [35]. There are other applications such as Dot Walker, which uses GPS to provide real-time alerts and navigation instructions, and Nearby Explorer, which offers information about landmarks, businesses, or public transport stops.

For guiding individuals with complete blindness, more sophisticated applications exist, such as the Navigation Assistance System for Visually Impaired People (NAVI), which guides people with specific sound instructions to assist those with visual disabilities in indoor environments. Using a consumer RGB-D camera, it is capable of detecting the main structural elements of the environment [31]. Another example is Visual Localizer, which, through global optimization techniques and convolutional neural networks (ConvNets) descriptors, provides GNSS location outdoors for visually impaired pedestrians [32]. Mobile robots, employing real-time obstacle detection and avoidance algorithms, serve as a viable option for visually impaired individuals to move freely and safely, avoiding obstacles in their path [36].

Using GPS and integrated with Bluetooth beacons to facilitate indoor navigation, the "BlindSquare" app [37] provides auditory instructions about street crossings, points of interest, or public transport stops, enhancing autonomy and spatial awareness during travel. Another GPS-based application is Georgiephone, designed for Android smartphones to assist visually impaired individuals in accessing local bus information through a voice interface. It locates and guides the user to the nearest bus stop, narrating stop names during the journey so the user knows where to alight [38].

Combining sensors, infrared, and GPS, the smart cane Sonar Stick enables individuals to detect obstacles and provides real-time information, contributing to their safety and facilitating movement [39–43]. Other indoor and outdoor navigation systems, such as "Drishti," offer precise and practical indoor navigation, adapting to environmental changes with dynamic routing and addressing [44].

NavCog, on the other hand, is a smartphone navigation system designed to assist visually impaired or blind individuals in navigating urban environments, both indoors and outdoors, especially in complex and unfamiliar settings [45], utilizing BLE beacons. Additionally, virtual audio displays inform about the spatial layout of events outside the visual field, allowing the identification of environmental elements and performing 'visual search' tasks through another sensory modality to compensate for visual system limitations [46].

Smart Healthcare APPS

The development of Smart healthcare apps tailored to visually impaired individuals enable telemedical care, thereby enhancing the quality of life for all members of society. Smart homes, assistive technology, and the development of technologies for haptic and auditory interaction play a significant role in this. Additionally, IoT-based healthcare monitoring systems have great potential to improve the quality of life for people with visual disabilities [47].

Smart homes [48,49], equipped with devices automating various functions such as lighting, heating, and security, enable personalized tracking of each inhabitant, intervening remotely when necessary. For example, if a person falls at home, sensors detect the sound, and subsequently, emergency services can be contacted, remotely monitoring vital signs through monitoring devices. This is just one example, with various applications like medication adherence tracking and monitoring activity levels.

Telemedicine has advanced significantly through research in haptic perception. Tactile feedback simulates the sense of touch, allowing healthcare professionals to practice procedures in a realistic and safe environment, even performing interventions from thousands of kilometers away [50]. This enhances the user experience in telemedicine applications, providing a more realistic interaction during remote consultations, thereby improving virtual healthcare provision [51]. Professionals also view the implementation of telemedicine positively [52], promoting accessibility and reducing healthcare inequalities.

Health applications facilitating auditory interaction are crucial, especially in telemedicine and remote monitoring, enabling virtual appointments and guidance on potential treatment plans. Speech recognition and natural language processing contribute to developing technologies for visually impaired individuals. For instance, [53] presented a smart healthcare system based on speech recognition, offering an effective solution for people with visual disabilities.

In navigating healthcare environments like clinics or hospitals, orientation and mobility applications for visually impaired individuals, as well as in other settings, become essential [54–56]. Auditory and haptic signals are crucial for guided navigation [57], commonly providing voice-guided navigation, accessible settings, and text-to-speech or speech-to-text conversion.

Assistive technology involves systems and devices enhancing the functional abilities, independence, and quality of life for people with disabilities. Communication devices and sensory aids improve visually impaired individuals' accessibility to healthcare, including magnifiers and screen readers making medical records accessible.

It is noteworthy that assistive technology has evolved to involve active participation from people with disabilities in designing and developing these technologies, promoting their engagement and contributing to their improvement [58]. The aim is to ensure that Smart healthcare apps foster patients' independence and provide them the opportunity to make informed decisions about their health.

Smart APPS for Socialization and Education

Socially and educationally, the quality of life and education for individuals with visual disabilities improves thanks to smart apps. Academic performance of students with visual disabilities enhances when utilizing adapted platforms for relevant tasks and gaining access to audiobooks [59, 60]. For instance, distance education portals prove beneficial for individuals with visual disabilities [61].

One example of these applications is OneStep Reader, formerly known as KNFB Reader (see [62]), which provides personalized feedback through voice comments. Seeing AI, on the other hand, leverages AI technologies to enhance environmental recognition through reading or spoken description. Another system aimed at improving the quality of life for individuals with severe blindness is the Aira assistive technology system. This system uses smart glasses and a mobile app to connect visually impaired users with trained agents who provide real-time visual assistance [63]. Following a similar concept, though without the use of smart glasses, BeSpecular [64] allows users with visual disabilities to take a photo of an object or text and send it to sight volunteers for quick assistance and descriptions.

To fully harness the potential benefits of smart applications for individuals with visual disabilities, addressing challenges related to accessibility, awareness, and teacher competencies is crucial. Therefore, it is important for educators to be trained and incorporate such technologies into their classes, overcoming underutilization of assistive technology and enhancing professional competencies [28, 65].

The Role of Artificial Intelligence in Smart City APPS for the Visually Impaired People

Artificial intelligence holds the potential to significantly enhance intelligent applications aimed at promoting the quality of life, independence, and safety of individuals with visual disabilities.

Examples of this include advanced artificial intelligence algorithms that efficiently detect obstacles [66] and generate descriptions of visual scenes, enabling individuals with visual disabilities to better understand their surroundings and navigate more effectively [67]. The evolution of visual scene description owes itself to neural network algorithms trained on selected datasets, such as MS-COCO [68].

Concerning safety, portable artificial intelligence-based systems have been designed, among other applications, to assist visually impaired individuals in crossing pedestrian crossings (see [69]). In terms of navigation, the routes of visually impaired individuals can be optimized through real-time data analysis. Moreover, artificial intelligence enables individuals with visual disabilities to identify objects [70]. For instance, smart glasses have been developed to aid visually impaired individuals by providing real-time information about their surroundings.

In the field of education, artificial intelligence virtual assistance can be utilized to support students with visual disabilities. By offering personalized and adaptive learning experiences, AI virtual assistants can help these students overcome educational barriers and improve their academic outcomes [71]. This is crucial for ensuring equal access to education and fostering equal opportunities.

In conclusion, artificial intelligence has the potential to significantly enhance intelligent applications that improve the quality of life for individuals with visual disabilities.

Usability Evaluation of Smart City APPS for the Visually Impaired People

Through the collaborative efforts of multiple disciplines alongside computer science, significant social benefits can be achieved by embedding personalized and accessible services for people with disabilities in smart cities, thereby improving their quality of life. Numerous Smart City Apps have been developed so far, and it is a continuously growing field of research and development.

However, the most crucial aspect is not the sheer quantity of tools but rather that the existing ones genuinely serve their intended purpose. Therefore, it is fundamental to assess the performance of these applications and determine whether the new smart cities genuinely ensure the inclusion of all citizens, ensuring equal access to all resources [72]. One way to evaluate the inclusion level of individuals with disabilities is through DIETool (Disability Inclusion Evaluation). Only through a comprehensive evaluation can we understand how to enhance Smart City Apps to bring about societal change, allowing all individuals to coexist in an environment where the stimuli they can perceive are sufficient for a good quality of life. For example, not all transportation technologies have undergone sufficient technological development to ensure that all individuals can benefit from their use [73]. It is essential, therefore, to verify that technological developments fulfill their purpose to continue improving them if they fall short.

Discussion

Determining the exact number of individuals affected by visual impairments globally is challenging due to the coexistence of multiple visual conditions in each person. However, a significant percentage of the global population suffers from visual disabilities, and these disabilities have a significant impact on people's quality of life. Adapting society to the specific needs of the visually impaired is crucial to enhance their overall well-being.

Smart apps for individuals with visual disabilities, combined with artificial intelligence, enhance their quality of life and independence. They do so by inclusively adapting various aspects of everyday life, including education and employment, socialization, transportation, and health.

The collaborative efforts of computer science and other scientific disciplines have led to the development of smart navigation and transportation applications that assist individuals with visual disabilities in navigating urban environments. These applications utilize technologies such as GPS, computer vision, and real-time semantic segmentation to provide real-time navigation, obstacle avoidance, and spatial awareness, enhancing the autonomy and safety of visually impaired individuals.

The development of smart healthcare apps, smart homes, assistive technology, and technologies for haptic and auditory interaction is crucial in providing visually impaired individuals with equal access to healthcare services, improving their quality of life, and promoting their independence.

Thanks to features such as text-to-speech capabilities, screen readers, and accessible interfaces, visually impaired individuals can listen to the content of texts. This is crucial for students to access educational materials, participate in classroom activities, and complete tasks. At the educational level, reducing barriers is crucial as it is the best way to empower students with visual disabilities to fully engage in their education and pursue academic goals, maximizing their capabilities. It is not only relevant in the educational field but also in the workplace, where it is essential to create a resume, access job search applications on equal terms, and participate in job interviews on an equal footing. Therefore, smart apps promote inclusion and equal opportunities for individuals with visual disabilities in both the workplace and education. However, addressing challenges related to accessibility, awareness, and digital literacy is crucial for fully harnessing the benefits of these applications.

Smart lifestyle applications also facilitate the social participation of individuals with visual disabilities by promoting accessibility to social networks through audio-based communication tools and adapted resources that allow for event planning. Thus, through assistive technology, individuals with visual disabilities can connect with others, participate in social activities, and access information about community events on equal terms. This technology promotes social inclusion and helps combat the isolation often experienced by individuals with visual disabilities.

Moreover, artificial intelligence has the potential to greatly improve the lives of individuals with visual disabilities by enhancing their understanding of their surroundings, assisting with navigation, and providing personalized educational support.

In conclusion, Smart City apps for individuals with visual disabilities offer valuable support in various aspects of everyday life. These applications leverage assistive technology and mobile apps to improve education, employment, and social participation for individuals with visual disabilities. By providing accessible features and resources, these applications empower individuals with visual disabilities to overcome obstacles, achieve their goals, and lead satisfying lives. Nonetheless, it is crucial to assess the performance of existing applications and ensure that they genuinely serve their intended purpose to achieve true inclusion and equal access for all citizens.

Innovate Ideas, Developments, Direction, Challenges or Trends in the Field of Smart APPS That Enhance the Quality of Life for Visually Impaired People

Numerous advancements have been made in recent years in the field of Smart City apps for the visually impaired people, leading to multiple innovative ideas aimed at enhancing the quality of life and overall well-being of individuals with visual disabilities.

Among the assistive devices and technologies, for instance, smart glasses tailored to the daily needs of users with moderate to severe visual impairment have been developed [74]. Additionally, smart clothing using IoT technology, such as NFC, has been designed to assist individuals with visual disabilities in dressing [75].

Mobile applications also enhance the quality of life for people with visual disabilities. For example, there are interactive mobile applications that provide access to audiobooks [59]. These applications enable individuals with visual disabilities to access a wide range of cultural and educational resources, promoting inclusion, independence, and equal opportunities.

Furthermore, Internet of Things (IoT) technology has opened new possibilities, with the development of mobile device based IoT solutions to assist users with visual disabilities [41]. These solutions leverage the interconnectivity of smart devices and applications to provide support and enhance the daily lives of people with visual disabilities.

However, despite these advances, challenges persist and need to be addressed as user satisfaction is not fully met [76], and there is still much work to be done in terms of inclusivity. Continuous innovation is required to ensure that the needs of people with visual disabilities are effectively met.

In conclusion, although there have been significant advancements and innovative ideas that improve the quality of life for individuals with visual disabilities, such as the development of assistive devices, mobile applications, and IoT solutions, challenges still exist that must be addressed.

Conclusion

This chapter summarizes relevant findings on the topic but is not a systematic review.

References

[1] Dandona L, Dandona R. What is the global burden of visual impairment? *BMC Medicine*. 2006;4(1):1-10.

[2] Hashemi H, Khabazkhoob M, Saatchi M, Ostadimoghaddam H, Yekta A. Visual impairment and blindness in a population-based study of Mashhad, Iran. *Journal of Current Ophthalmology*. 2018;30(2):161-168.

[3] World Health Organization. *World report on vision*. Geneva: World Health Organization; 2019.

[4] Ramke J, Gilbert CE. Universal eye health: are we getting closer? *The Lancet Global Health*. 2017;5(9):e843-e844.

[5] Amedo AO, Adade S, Koomson NY, Osae EA. Influence of visual impairment on the quality of life: a survey of patients reporting at the low vision centre of the eastern regional hospital of Ghana. *Journal of Ophthalmic Science*. 2016;1(1):1-7.

[6] Park Y, Shin JA, Yang SW, Yim HW, Kim HS, Park YH; Epidemiologic Survey Committee of the Korean Ophthalmologic Society. The relationship between visual impairment and health-related quality of life in Korean adults: The Korea national health and nutrition examination survey (2008–2012). *PLoS One*. 2015;10(7):e0132779.

[7] Yibekal BT, Alemu DS, Anbesse DH, Alemayehu AM, Alimaw YA. Vision-related quality of life among adult patients with visual impairment at University of Gondar, Northwest Ethiopia. *Journal of Ophthalmology*. 2020;2020:7-13.

[8] Nyman SR, Gosney MA, Victor CR. Psychosocial impact of visual impairment in working-age adults. *British Journal of Ophthalmology*. 2010;94(11):1427-1431.

[9] Vignesh D, Gupta N, Kalaivani M, Goswami AK, Nongkynrih B, Gupta SK. Prevalence of visual impairment and its association with vision-related quality of life among elderly persons in a resettlement colony of Delhi. *Journal of Family Medicine and Primary Care*. 2019;8(4):1432-1436.

[10] Murphy CC, Hughes EH, Frost NA, Dick AD. Quality of life and visual function in patients with intermediate uveitis. *British Journal of Ophthalmology*. 2005;89(9):1161-1165.

[11] Chia E-M, Mitchell P, Ojaimi E, Rochtchina E, Wang JJ. Assessment of vision-related quality of life in an older population subsample: The Blue Mountains Eye Study. *Ophthalmic Epidemiology*. 2006;13(6):371-377.

[12] Stevelink SAM, Fear NT. Psychosocial impact of visual impairment and coping strategies in female ex-Service personnel. *BMJ Military Health*. 2016;162(2):129-133.

[13] Jackson SE, Hackett RA, Pardhan S, Smith L, Steptoe A. Association of perceived discrimination with emotional well-being in older adults with visual impairment. *JAMA Ophthalmology*. 2019;137(7):825-832.

[14] Adigun K, Oluleye TS, Ladipo MMA, Olowookere SA. Quality of life in patients with visual impairment in Ibadan: a clinical study in primary care. *Journal of Multidisciplinary Healthcare*. 2014;7:173-178.

[15] Wu S-Y, Nemesure B, Hennis A, Leske MC. Visual acuity impairment and vision-related quality of life: the Barbados Eye Studies. *British Journal of Visual Impairment*. 2009;27(1):9-24.

[16] Boadi-Kusi SB, Asamoah S, Zaabaar E, Hammond F, Ackom CK. Psychological factors associated with visual impairment. *Journal of Visual Impairment & Blindness*. 2023;117(3):233-245.

[17] Choi HG, Lee MJ, Lee S-M. Visual impairment and risk of depression: A longitudinal follow-up study using a national sample cohort. *Scientific Reports*. 2018;8(1):2083.

[18] Han BH, Leddy JF, Lopez FA, Palamar JJ. Prevalence of psychoactive substance use among middle-aged and older adults with visual impairment in the US. *JAMA Ophthalmology*. 2022;140(1):94-95.

[19] Margrain TH, Nollett C, Shearn J, Stanford M, Edwards RT, Ryan B, et al. The Depression in Visual Impairment Trial (DEPVIT): trial design and protocol. *BMC Psychiatry*. 2012;12(1):1-8.

[20] Onyebueke GC, Okeke S, Asimadu IN. Burden and severity of depression in Nigeria: Relationship and association with visual impairment. *Open Journal of Psychiatry*. 2022;12(4):311-320.

[21] Munaw MB, Tegegn MT. Visual impairment and psychological distress among adults attending the University of Gondar tertiary eye care and training center, Northwest Ethiopia: A comparative cross-sectional study. *PLoS One*. 2022;17(3):e0264113.

[22] Nasralla MM, Rehman IU, Sobnath D, Paiva S. Computer vision and deep learning-enabled UAVs: proposed use cases for visually impaired people in a smart city. In: *Computer Analysis of Images and Patterns: CAIP 2019 International Workshops*. Springer; 2019. p. 91-99.

[23] Tu Y-F, Hwang G-J, Lai C-L. Facilitating learning by the visually impaired: development and usability evaluation of a specially designed ubiquitous library. *The Electronic Library*. 2021;39(2):169-185.

[24] Wu E, Sahagun J, Sun Y. An Object Detection Navigator to Assist the Visually Impaired using Artificial Intelligence and Computer Vision. *CS & IT Conference Proceedings*. 2021;11(9):91-107.

[25] Aguilera U, Peña O, Belmonte O, López-de-Ipiña D. Citizen-centric data services for smarter cities. *Future Generation Computer Systems*. 2017;76:234-247.

[26] Zhang B, Peng G, Xing F, Chen S. Mobile Applications in China's Smart Cities: State-of-the-Art and Lessons Learned. *Journal of Global Information Management*. 2021;29(6):1-18.

[27] Min B-C, Saxena S, Steinfeld A, Dias MB. Incorporating information from trusted sources to enhance urban navigation for blind travelers. In: *2015 IEEE International Conference on Robotics and Automation (ICRA)*. IEEE; 2015. p. 4511-4518.

[28] Griffin-Shirley N, Banda DR, Ajuwon PM, Cheon J, Lee J, Park HR, et al. A survey on the use of mobile applications for people who are visually impaired. *Journal of Visual Impairment & Blindness*. 2017;111(4):307-323.

[29] Kuriakose B, Shrestha R, Sandnes FE. Tools and technologies for blind and visually impaired navigation support: a review. *IETE Technical Review*. 2022;39(1):3-18.

[30] Yang K, Wang K, Bergasa LM, Romera E, Hu W, Sun D, et al. Unifying terrain awareness for the visually impaired through real-time semantic segmentation. *Sensors*. 2018;18(5):1506.

[31] Aladren A, López-Nicolás G, Puig L, Guerrero JJ. Navigation assistance for the visually impaired using RGB-D sensor with range expansion. *IEEE Systems Journal*. 2014;10(3):922-932.

[32] Lin S, Cheng R, Wang K, Yang K. Visual localizer: Outdoor localization based on convnet descriptor and global optimization for visually impaired pedestrians. *Sensors*. 2018;18(8):2476.

[33] Chen Z, Liu X, Kojima M, Huang Q, Arai T. A wearable navigation device for visually impaired people based on the real-time semantic visual slam system. *Sensors*. 2021;21(4):1536.

[34] Hakobyan L, Lumsden J, O'Sullivan D, Bartlett H. Mobile assistive technologies for the visually impaired. *Survey of Ophthalmology*. 2013;58(6):513-528.

[35] Isazade V. Advancement in navigation technologies and their potential for the visually impaired: a comprehensive review. *Spatial Information Research*. 2023;31(6):743-754.

[36] Vashisth T, Khareta R, Bhati N, Samsani VC, Sharma S. A low cost and enhanced assistive environment for people with vision loss. In: *Intelligent Computing Methodologies: 18th International Conference, ICIC 2022*. Springer; 2022. p. 245-255.

[37] MIPsoft Oy. BlindSquare [Mobile application software]. Version 8.0. App Store; 2012. Available from: https://apps.apple.com/us/app/blindsquare/id500557255

[38] Mourato P, Lima H, Luna C, Rocha T, Ferraz F. Analysis and proposed improvements in the support for the visually impaired in the use of public transportation. *Advances in Transportation Studies*. 2020;Special Issue:1-12.

[39] Furlan CA, Su V. Sonar walking stick. Senior Project, California Polytechnic State University; 2014. Available from: https://digitalcommons.calpoly.edu/eesp/255/

[40] Nada AA, Fakhr MA, Seddik AF. Assistive infrared sensor based smart stick for blind people. In: *2015 Science and Information Conference (SAI)*. IEEE; 2015. p. 1149-1154.

[41] Abdel-Jaber H, Albazar H, Abdel-Wahab A, Amir M El, Alqahtani A, Alobaid M. Mobile Based IoT Solution for Helping Visual Impairment Users. *Advances in Internet of Things*. 2021;11(4):141-152.

[42] Mahajan R, Kumar A, Shankar P. An integrated ultrasonic sensor based smart cane for assisting the visually impaired. *International Journal of Advanced Research in Computer Science*. 2017;8(5):1-6.

[43] Chandra RA, Fadlillah U, Wibowo P, Saputra FTN, Sulasyono RR. Blind People Stick Tracking Using Android Smartphone and GPS Technology. *Khazanah Informatika: Jurnal Ilmu Komputer dan Informatika*. 2022;8(1):18-24.

[44] Ran L, Helal S, Moore S. Drishti: an integrated indoor/outdoor blind navigation system and service. In: *Proceedings of the Second IEEE Annual Conference on Pervasive Computing and Communications*. IEEE; 2004. p. 23-30.

[45] Ahmetovic D, Gleason C, Kitani KM, Takagi H, Asakawa C. NavCog: turn-by-turn smartphone navigation assistant for people with visual impairments or blindness. In: *Proceedings of the 18th International ACM SIGACCESS Conference on Computers and Accessibility*. ACM; 2016. p. 1-2.

[46] Colombo M, Dolhasz A, Hockman J, Harvey C. Psychometric Mapping of Audio Features to Perceived Physical Characteristics of Virtual Objects. In: *2021 IEEE Conference on Virtual Reality and 3D User Interfaces Abstracts and Workshops (VRW)*. IEEE; 2021. p. 1-4.

[47] Abdulmalek S, Nasir A, Jabbar WA, Almuhaya MAM, Bairagi AK, Khan MA-M, et al. IoT-based healthcare-monitoring system towards improving quality of life: A review. *Sensors*. 2022;22(5):1993.

[48] Amiribesheli M, Benmansour A, Bouchachia A. A review of smart homes in healthcare. *Journal of Ambient Intelligence and Humanized Computing*. 2015;6(4):495-517.

[49] Majumder S, Aghayi E, Noferesti M, Memarzadeh-Tehran H, Mondal T, Pang Z, et al. Smart homes for elderly healthcare—Recent advances and research challenges. *Sensors*. 2017;17(11):2496.

[50] Bhaskar S, Bradley S, Chattu VK, Adisesh A, Nurtazina A, Kyrykbayeva S, et al. Telemedicine as the new outpatient clinic gone digital: position paper from the pandemic health system REsilience PROGRAM (REPROGRAM) international consortium (Part 2). *Frontiers in Public Health*. 2020;8:410.

[51] Haleem A, Javaid M, Singh RP, Suman R. Telemedicine for healthcare: Capabilities, features, barriers, and applications. *Sensors International*. 2021;2:100117.

[52] Assaye BT, Belachew M, Worku A, Birhanu S, Sisay A, Kassaw M, et al. Perception towards the implementation of telemedicine during COVID-19 pandemic: a cross-sectional study. *BMC Health Services Research*. 2023;23(1):967.

[53] Ismail A, Abdlerazek S, El-Henawy I. Development of smart healthcare system based on speech recognition using support vector machine and dynamic time warping. *Sustainability*. 2020;12(6):2403.

[54] Paratore MT, Leporini B. Exploiting the haptic and audio channels to improve orientation and mobility apps for the visually impaired. *Universal Access in the Information Society*. 2023;22(4):1-11.

[55] Papadopoulos K, Koustriava E, Koukourikos P, Kartasidou L, Barouti M, Varveris A, et al. Comparison of three orientation and mobility aids for individuals with blindness: Verbal description, audio-tactile map and audio-haptic map. *Assistive Technology*. 2017;29(1):1-7.

[56] Messaoudi MD, Menelas B-AJ, Mcheick H. Review of Navigation Assistive Tools and Technologies for the Visually Impaired. *Sensors*. 2022;22(20):7888.

[57] Huang YY, Moll J, Sallnäs EL, Sundblad Y. Auditory feedback in haptic collaborative interfaces. *International Journal of Human-Computer Studies*. 2012;70(4):257-270.

[58] Reyes-Cruz G, Fischer JE, Reeves S. Reframing disability as competency: Unpacking everyday technology practices of people with visual impairments. In: *Proceedings of the 2020 CHI Conference on Human Factors in Computing Systems*. ACM; 2020. p. 1-13.

[59] Meenakshi A, Sundar S, Nancy S. An Interactive Mobile Application for the Visually Impaired to Have Access to Listening Audio Books with Handy Books Portal. *International Journal of Interactive Mobile Technologies*. 2015;9(1):64-66.

[60] Siddiqua N, Parveen N, Ansari H. An Experimental Study to Identify the Effect of Assistive Technology on Academic Achievement of Visually Impaired Students. *Pakistan Social Sciences Review*. 2022;6(2):866-879.

[61] Yurtay N, Yurtay Y, Adak MF. An education portal for visually impaired. *Procedia-Social and Behavioral Sciences*. 2015;171:1097-1105.

[62] Chypak Y, Morozov Y. Audio reading assistant for visually impaired people. *Advances in Cyber-Physical Systems*. 2023;8(2):81-88.

[63] Nguyen BJ, Kim Y, Park K, Chen AJ, Chen S, Fossan DV, et al. Improvement in patient-reported quality of life outcomes in severely visually impaired individuals using the Aira assistive technology system. *Translational Vision Science & Technology*. 2018;7(2):30.

[64] BeSpecular Team. BeSpecular [Mobile application software]. Version 2.0. BeSpecular; 2016. Available from: https://www.bespecular.com/

[65] Zhou L, Parker AT, Smith DW, Griffin-Shirley N. Assistive technology for students with visual impairments: Challenges and needs in teachers' preparation programs and practice. *Journal of Visual Impairment & Blindness*. 2011;105(4):197-210.

[66] Masud U, Saeed T, Malaikah HM, Islam FU, Abbas G. Smart assistive system for visually impaired people obstruction avoidance through object detection and classification. *IEEE Access*. 2022;10:13428-13441.

[67] Faurina R, Jelita A, Vatresia A, Agustian I. Image captioning to aid blind and visually impaired outdoor navigation. *IAES International Journal of Artificial Intelligence*. 2023;12(3):1104-1117.

[68] Dognin P, Melnyk I, Mroueh Y, Padhi I, Rigotti M, Ross J, et al. Image captioning as an assistive technology: lessons learned from VizWiz 2020 challenge. *Journal of Artificial Intelligence Research*. 2022;73:437-459.

[69] de Freitas MP, Piai VA, Farias RH, Fernandes AMR, de Moraes Rossetto AG, Leithardt VRQ. Artificial intelligence of things applied to assistive technology: a systematic literature review. *Sensors*. 2022;22(22):8531.

[70] Chang W-J, Chen L-B, Hsu C-H, Chen J-H, Yang T-C, Lin C-P. MedGlasses: A wearable smart-glasses-based drug pill recognition system using deep learning for visually impaired chronic patients. *IEEE Access*. 2020;8:17013-17024.

[71] Mina PNR, Solon IM, Sanchez FR, Delante TK, Villegas JK, Basay FJ, et al. Leveraging Education through Artificial Intelligence Virtual Assistance: A Case Study of Visually Impaired Learners. *International Journal of Educational Innovation and Research*. 2023;2(1):10-22.

[72] Rebernik N, Szajczyk M, Bahillo A, Marušić BG. Measuring disability inclusion performance in cities using disability inclusion evaluation tool (DIETool). *Sustainability*. 2020;12(4):1378.

[73] Sochor J, Nikitas A. Vulnerable users' perceptions of transport technologies. *Proceedings of the Institution of Civil Engineers-Urban Design and Planning*. 2016;169(3):154-162.

[74] Ruffieux S, Hwang C, Junod V, Caldara R, Lalanne D, Ruffieux N. Tailoring assistive smart glasses according to pathologies of visually impaired individuals: an exploratory investigation on social needs and difficulties experienced by visually impaired individuals. *Universal Access in the Information Society*. 2023;22(2):463-475.

[75] Alabduljabbar R. An IoT smart clothing system for the visually impaired using NFC technology. *International Journal of Sensor Networks*. 2022;38(1):46-57.

[76] Busaeed S, Mehmood R, Katib I, Corchado JM. LidSonic for Visually Impaired: Green Machine Learning-Based Assistive Smart Glasses with Smart App and Arduino. *Electronics*. 2022;11(7):1076.

Chapter 15

Sustainability as a Communication Strategy: A Case Study of the Inditex Group (Zara)*

Beatriz Guerrero González-Valerio[1,†]
and Belén Ramírez Barredo[2,‡]
[1]Universidad San Pablo-CEU, CEU Universities, Madrid, Spain
[2]Universidad Complutense de Madrid, Madrid, Spain

Abstract

This chapter aims to examine the so-called "fast fashion" industry, as well as the challenges it will face in the coming years, using the Inditex Group as a case study based on its most prominent brand, Zara. The main objective is to examine the true implications of the group´s sustainability claims. To this end, the study takes a dual approach: first, to analyse the design and communication of the group's sustainability policy; second to evaluate consistency between communicated initiatives and current implementation.

Keywords: fashion, fast fashion, sustainability, challenges, communication

Introduction

The term "sustainable development" was defined in 1987 by the World Commission on Environment and Development, established in 1982 to design a global programme for environmental change. This led to the emergence of "Our Common Future Report," also known as the Brundtland Commission Report, named after the Norwegian prime minister. In that report, the Commission determined that sustainable development can be described as development that "meets the needs of the present generation without compromising the ability of future generations to meet their own needs as well" (World Commission on Environment, 1987, pg. 59).

---

* This research has been carried out within the framework of the consolidated GIR ICOIDI, with funding obtained from the San Pablo CEU University.
† Corresponding Author's Email: beguergo@ceu.es
‡ Corresponding Author's Email: bramirezb@ucm.es

In: Psycho-Environmental Variables That Ensure People's Well-Being and Health …
Editors: Roberto Alonso González Lezcano and Guadalupe Cantarero García
ISBN: 979-8-89530-831-8
© 2025 Nova Science Publishers, Inc.

A few years later, at the United Nations Conference in Rio de Janeiro in 1992, also known as the Earth Summit, world leaders adopted Agenda 21, a series of specific action plans designed to achieve sustainable development during the 21st century. Ten years later in 2002, the World Summit on Sustainable Development (WSSD) was held in South Africa, where the Johannesburg Plan of Implementation was adopted. As pointed out by Professor Carrera, all these reports speak of development rather than growth. In the words of Carrera, "Development is a qualitative improvement that involves passing through various stages, while growth is a physical accumulation (2017, pg. 23).

In the 21st century, the term "sustainable development" has taken on different shades of meaning. At the same time, the concern for sustainability has gradually increased in the fashion industry. In fact, at the United Nations Environment Assembly in Nairobi, Kenya in 2019, the United Nations Sustainable Fashion Alliance was born. This organisation issued a press release on the impact of fast fashion, highlighting some revealing facts: the fashion industry is the second largest worldwide consumer of water; it generates approximately 20% of all global wastewater; finally, it releases half a million tons of synthetic microfibers into the ocean each year. Another significant finding highlighted that 60% more clothes are purchased today than 15 years ago, yet each garment is kept for only half the time (United Nations Sustainable Fashion Alliance 2019).

The media have been very active in alerting and informing the public about this disturbing situation. Their actions, along with that of other pressure groups, especially NGOs, has helped raise awareness about the impact of fast fashion. Some of these groups and their bold campaigns include the following: "Detox" by Greenpeace; "Clean Clothes" by SETEM, which involves 17 countries in Europe; and "Whomademyclothes," by Fashion Revolution; and documentaries such as "The true cost," or "Before the flood" (Zambrano, 2018, pg. 7). All of this has led to increased awareness of the damage caused by this sector, whose main participants include governments, large textile companies, and consumers. Moreover, this situation has led to increased awareness regarding the finite nature of natural resources and the need to reduce their overexploitation in order to avoid potentially irreversible effects.

On the other hand, the available research suggests that a transformation is taking place regarding the lifestyle of end consumers, especially the younger generations. Among other changes, sustainability has become an important factor in their purchase decisions. Phenomena such as climate change, water scarcity, and population growth have intensified the focus on sustainability in just a few years, both in terms of product and manufacturing processes.

Thus, in recent years fast fashion companies have gone from being highly praised for democratising fashion to being viewed with suspicion due to the negative impact of their production processes, both ecologically and socially. As a result, faced with the increasing demand for environmental sustainability, fast fashion companies have adopted a series of measures. However, in some cases they are only trying to polish their image without making significant changes to their production methods. Some companies have limited themselves to making small changes that have allowed them to wear the label "sustainable," yet they have taken advantage of consumer misinformation in order to make products that appear to be 100% green, when in reality they are not (Fernandez, 2019, pg. 13). In this regard, it is important to bear in mind that "a garment goes through an average of one hundred people from raw material to sale, which is why it is so difficult to carry out a follow-up" (Riezu, 2021, pg. 32).

Analytical Framework

The fashion industry is a $1.3 trillion global market that employs more than 300 million people worldwide. Therefore, we can see that it represents a significant economic force. This is a highly competitive market that has been subjected to continuous changes in recent years, including economic insecurity and political instability, among others, which have increased market uncertainty (Gazzola et al., 2020, pg. 2).

From the end of the last century, the industry itself has witnessed a new phenomenon, which is the tremendous growth of "fast fashion." "*The New York Times* used the expression for the first time at the end of 1989 when Zara opened a shop in New York City" (Gazzola et al., 2020, pg. 3). Since that time, there has been a gradual change in the way fast fashion is perceived. In fact, in a recent interview with the *Financial Times*, the CEO of Inditex, Marta Ortega, made the following affirmation: "We do not see ourselves as part of the world that people call fast fashion" (Ellison, 2023).

Fast fashion is a model of textile production that focuses on producing garments that follow the latest trends at a reduced price, and in a short period of time (Martín, 2019, pg. 146). This business model relies on short-lived textile products, where companies "are constantly competing to meet demand in the shortest possible time" (Cristófol et al, 2021, pg. 20). For example, in 2001 Zara already had 507 shops worldwide. At that time, it took between five and six weeks for the company's garments to be designed and reach the point of sale, while traditional brands needed six months (Thomas, 2019, p. 48). Thus, we can see how speed and production capacity are the hallmarks of this consumer model that focuses on a rapid response, which has evolved from predicting future trends to the use of real-time information, thereby aligning itself with the needs and desires of the consumer. In this way, the buyer has been lured into adopting a new type of behaviour guided by the familiar phrase, "See now, buy now."

"This business model has been consolidated in the market in recent years through large retail companies such as Inditex, H&M and Primark, among others. However, it is a model that generates a huge amount of pollution throughout the entire process, from the collection and treatment of raw materials, to the final moment when a garment is thrown in the rubbish by the consumer" (Fernández, 2019, pg. 6). This has had a major impact on the industry, and the situation has been exacerbated by problems such as water consumption, the discharge of hazardous chemicals, and the emission of polluting gases. At the same time, the frenetic pace of production to which fast fashion companies are subjected forces them to relocate production to countries where labour costs and laws are less rigid, increasing the potential for labour exploitation.

As an alternative to this model, sustainable fashion promotes slowing down production and prioritizing quality over quantity. "Sustainable fashion tries to cause the least possible damage to the planet and the workers who produce the garments; it also tries to reduce the consumption volume and use organic materials and substances that are not harmful to the environment" (Zambrano, 2018, p. 7).

At the present time, the problem is that a large number of companies are using the term *sustainable* to describe themselves, but in their own way, so the term often ends up being vague and unclear as to what it refers. "In fact, the term sustainability, in relation to the fashion industry, has become almost an empty concept and growly difficult to define" (Sitaro, 2020, pg. 4). This strategy in which some brands try to give the impression of being sustainable and environmentally friendly by using words associated with sustainability, yet with commercial intentions, is known as *greenwashing*. As this technique is often strongly punished by consumers, these companies should bear in mind that "sustainability does not have the same impact on buyers when used as a one-off sales or marketing tactic; instead, it is successful in the long term when the company shows that sustainable values are part of its statement of purpose" (Cristófol et al, 2021, pg. 20).

According to experts in the field, sustainable fashion places emphasis on a number of key issues such as viable manufacturing, the use of environmentally-friendly materials, ecological distribution and points of sale, and raising consumer awareness (Sitaro, 2020, pg. 7).

At this point, it should be clarified that sustainability encompasses three areas: environmental, social, and economic. In other words, a company must be environmentally sound and socially fair, but economically profitable as well (Carrera, 2017, p. 24). Sustainable fashion considers all the agents and stages involved in the creation of a garment, including environmentally friendly cultivation, manufacturing processes and distribution, and respect for workers' rights. In a broad sense, it could be said that sustainable fashion makes a commitment to the community to be responsible.

In recent years, sustainability has become a key asset for textile companies worldwide. The annual reports of various Spanish companies, such as Inditex, Mango, and Tendam, highlight the progress made by these firms in this area. One that stands out is the collaborative and strategic alliances with associations and non-profit organisations that support causes aimed at developing third world countries, conserving ecosystems and biodiversity, supporting humanitarian work, and more. For example, in January of 2023, seven multinational companies in the textile industry joined forces to set up the first Collective Extended Producer Responsibility System (CEPRS), which was the first in Spain in this sector. The companies include H&M, Inditex, Decathlon, Ikea, Mango, Kiabi and Tendam. The aim of this association is to manage textile and footwear waste generated in the Spanish market in order to boost textile recycling in Spain and move toward a circular economy (Museo del Traje, 2023).

The greatest challenge facing the textile industry is using the least amount of resources possible in producing a garment, including crops, water, and toxic by-products, thereby extending the product lifespan of textiles. When the life of a garment has finished, the goal is to reinsert these clothes into the textile chain in order to bring them into the circular economy (Carrera, 2017, pg. 32). The labour conditions of the workers who produce the garments must also be kept in mind. All of the foregoing indicates that these products should be reconceived, as well as their production process, distribution, use, and destiny at the end of their lifespan.

It should also be noted that all the actors in this scenario need to take an active role, especially consumers. As customers, we can start by being aware that "for every three garments produced, only one is sold" (Riezu, 2021, p. 65). In our role as consumers, the main tools we can use are the following: the first is official certifications, although a multitude of certifications exist and each one is based on different criteria; the second is to consider the reputation and precedents of the brand (Riezu, 2021, pg. 48).

However, this usually implies an increase in production costs, and a higher retail price as a result. This is why sustainable fashion has been criticised in some cases for being elitist, as its price often makes it unaffordable for most people.

Among the areas that need to be addressed in order to produce more sustainable fashion are the following: technological challenges, transparency, and social welfare.

1. Technological challenges include the following:

Eco-efficiency - using the smallest amount of resources to produce a garment. This includes using technology capable of consuming the minimum amount of resources, including the necessary raw materials, water, and energy.

The textile production cycle also needs to be shortened, or in other words, from natural fibres to retail, as this is currently very long and costly (Carrera, 2017).

Carbon footprint: this is mainly a result of offshoring production to take advantage of working conditions in other countries, as well as the increase in traffic of maritime and air transport, which increase the carbon footprint.

Renewable raw materials: the use of natural fibres or renewable raw materials such as cotton or hemp is recommended.

Reduce consumption by extending the lifespan of textile products. This can be done in three ways:

1. By improving the quality of products and/or enhancing the treatment of tissues to extend their lifespan.
2. Secondly, by promoting the second-hand clothing trade.
3. And lastly, by facilitating recycling. This can be done in several ways, one of which is to use mono-component textile products, as these are more easily recyclable than those that are multi-component, and to manufacture from recycled textile fibres such as cotton or recycled polyester.

Two other important aspects that need to be addressed are transparency and social welfare.

2. Transparency is necessary at each stage of the manufacturing process; in other words, there needs to be more information about the origin of the products (suppliers and conditions under which the clothes have been manufactured), and the quality of the materials used. Consumers expect transparency throughout the entire value chain.
3. Social welfare is the final challenge. This refers to taking into account work conditions, such as working hours, suitable wages, healthy and safe standards, and ending child labour exploitation, especially in developing countries where most fashion workers are concentrated.

Method

The main objective of this chapter is to examine the so-called “fast fashion” industry and the challenges it will face in the coming years in terms of sustainability, as well as the policies of communicating the actions they carry out. By using the Inditex group as a case study, two specific objectives have been drawn from the main objective. The first is to study the design and communication of the group’s sustainability policy. The second is to establish the level of consistency between what is communicated and what is actually carried out. It should be kept in mind that “what makes consumers choose one brand over another in the sustainable fashion market depends on the image projected to consumers through a company’s actions, in addition to the consistency between these actions and the ethics and values they promote" (Fernández, 2019, pg. 31).

With regard to the sample selection, Zara was chosen because not only is it the leading Spanish fashion company, it is also a worldwide benchmark with more than 1,800 shops in 96 countries (Lipsky-Karasz, 2021). In the Inditex group, Zara is the flagship brand (Alonso, 2000, p. 157). It was the first brand when Amancio Ortega laid the groundwork for the company in 1963. Today, Zara generates the highest turnover for the group. "Zara has been evolving and adapting to new markets and emerging social networks over the last twenty-five years, as well as to customer styles, new generations of buyers, and technological innovation (Ramírez, Guerrero, et al., 2023).

This research adopts a qualitative approach, employing an inductive methodology to study the phenomenon holistically. On the one hand, the focus of this study is mainly theoretical, as it involves a review of the existing literature and academic research related to the fashion sector, specifically the fast fashion industry, sustainable fashion, and the Inditex group.

This research is also of an exploratory nature, which is based on the information published on the website of the Inditex group, and it mainly analyses what is published in the website section dedicated to sustainability, but also the information contained in the Overview of the Year 2021 published by the group in its annual report. As this group communicates its sustainability policies by using its corporate website as the main channel for transmission, an analysis of the website has been carried out as well, which is based on its corporate values and position with regard to sustainability.

As for the limitations of this research, we are aware that a large part of the information on the sustainability actions of the Inditex group comes from only one source, which is information that the Inditex group itself makes public, both on its website and in its yearly report. The main limitation is that we have relied mainly on their point of view and the data they have provided. Another limitation is related to the extent to which this information reaches consumers, as they are the ones who make the purchase decisions. We suggest that this topic could be explore further in a separate study.

The present analysis has been conducted based on a series of parameters that we have established as priorities, starting with the areas that fast fashion companies could address with regard to ethics, social responsibility, and sustainability. To this end, we have relied on various authors, including Enric Carrera (2019), who highlights the future challenges of this industry in his article "*Los retos sostenibilistas del sector textil*" [the sustainability challenges of the textile sector], focusing on the technological challenges above all.

Results

> "Inditex recognizes that sustainability is more than just a concept; it is a comprehensive approach for work and decision-making. Through #Boostyourpower, the company trains its employees and raises their awareness in this area" (*El Economista*, 2022).

In the second half of the 1990s, the Inditex group transformed the clothing industry, establishing itself as one of the pioneers in the design, production and distribution of all types of garments for mass consumption (Alonso, 2000, pg. 170). From those years to the present day, concern and awareness of sustainability has been increasing, and it has become clear that the fashion industry is the second most polluting sector, and therefore one of the most destructive to the environment. In response to this scenario, brands and designers have been developing more responsible manufacturing processes. Accordingly, since 2001 Inditex has been immersed in an ambitious sustainability strategy that is comprehensive, carrying out a wide range of initiatives in all phases of the value chain, from product design to shop management. Like other companies, the Inditex group has made sustainable development an essential part of its strategy.

We can see from its website that the Inditex group is founded on four basic principles: 1) Commitment to fashion; 2) Shopping experience; 3) Teamwork; 4) and Implementation of responsible practices in all phases of the value chain, from product design to shop management. Thus, we can see that among the four principles, the fourth refers specifically to "introducing responsible practices."

Its website also states that its model is divided into five sections: 1) Customer focus; 2) Brand experience; 3) Design; 4) Production process; 5) and Logistics. As discussed below, of these five areas, three of them refer to sustainability. With regard to the first section, "Customer focus," the buyer is clearly in the spotlight of this business model. Moreover, the ideas of "efficiency and more sustainable processes" are introduced in each of the phases of its activity. Furthermore, within these five sections, the integrated inventory management system (IIMS) is highlighted, which allows for a reduction of surplus and mitigation of the carbon footprint. With regard to the third section, "Design," the belief that "responsible fashion starts at the drawing board" is emphasised, which is why the designers themselves carefully consider the materials and processes used. Along the same lines, in her book entitled "*La moda justa*" [fair fashion], Marta Riezu points out that "the fabrics a designer chooses say a lot about his or her brand" (2021, p. 47). Finally, regarding the section called "Production Processes," the concept of high standards based on a commitment to ethics is mentioned. Likewise, the statement is also made that manufacturers who produce the end product are located in areas close to the headquarters (Spain, Portugal, Morocco, and Turkey), thereby reducing energy consumption and the carbon footprint as well. In addition to proximity, they also point out that flexible manufacturing allows for shorter production runs, resulting in more responsible fabrication. Based on all of the above, we can see that the Inditex group's presentation on its official website includes statements and practices that directly refer to its ethics, commitment, and social responsibility.

Continuing with the analysis of the Inditex group's corporate website, on the top menu is a tab for "Sustainability," which in turn is divided into 7 sections as follows: 1) Overview is a general presentation; 2) Roadmap details the main objectives in terms of sustainability; 3) A New Cycle explains that through its platform known as "Sustainability Innovation Hub," it focuses on the search for new materials and processes, working together with start-ups and innovation accelerators; 4) Production is where the company explains its "Compliance Programme," thereby putting the focus on the worker; 5) Distribution; 6) Moving beyond; and 7) Reporting."

The Inditex group relies on the argument of social change and does so with a positive tone. According to the "Roadmap" section, the effects of climate change, excessive human intervention in the natural world, and the scarcity of natural resources are issues that affect us all. Faced with this scenario, the group trusts in the power of fashion to make a transformation with a collective effort. Since 2001, when the group started its comprehensive sustainability strategy, they have been carrying out a wide range of initiatives at all stages of the value chain, from product design to shop management. These include the use of innovative raw materials, the reduction of emissions, the efficient use of water and energy, the use of recycled paper bags, and the possibility of depositing garments for recycling.

Inditex aims to position itself as change agent, spearheading innovation in the fashion industry. It is committed to its leadership role in transforming the sector through innovation. This is due to the company's belief that innovation is part of its corporate culture, and one of its cornerstones as well.

Consistent with what other companies in the sector are doing, the Inditex group has also published its sustainability objectives. The most noteworthy are highlighted as follows:

The two major targets that were set for 2022 included the following: firstly, 100% renewable energy consumption in all of its own facilities, including the head office, distribution centres, factories, and shops; secondly, more than 50% of its items were to have the "Join Life" label. This label is used by the group to identify articles that are made from the most sustainable raw materials, as well as production processes with maximum sustainability (Martínez, 2020). The targets set for 2023 include the following: firstly, 100% of the cotton used, along with 100% of the man-made cellulosic fibres, will come from more sustainable sources; secondly, viscose will become more sustainable. Another objective is "Zero Waste" in all of its own facilities, including the corporate headquarters, distribution centres, factories, and shops. With regard to plastic, the objective is to eliminate 100% of all single-use plastics for all its customers. Finally, another goal is to collect all parcel materials in order to recycle or reuse them in the supply chain. This action is known as "Green to Pack."

By 2025, the group aims to achieve three other major objectives: firstly, 100% of the polyester used will have to come from more sustainable sources; secondly, 100% of the linen will need to come from high-quality sources; and thirdly, there will be a 25% reduction of water consumption in the supply chain. By 2030, three additional goals have been set: 1) five million hectares will be protected, restored, regenerated, or managed in alternative ways in order to enhance biodiversity; 2) reduce the company's emissions by more than 50%, including its own operations and supply chain; 3) use only raw materials that have a lower impact on the environment, including fibres that are newly created, recycled, or that come from organic or regenerative agriculture. Finally, by 2040, the goal is to reach zero net emissions, bringing the achievement of this target forward by ten years, as it was previously planned for 2050. Moreover, this will reduce the group's carbon footprint by at least 90% compared to 2018.

Discussion

The present research has involved an in-depth study of sustainability communication in the sector known as "fast fashion," by specifically focusing on the company known as Zara. The information gathered, along with an analysis of both the corporate website and its Overview of the Year 2021, have made it possible to address the objectives initially proposed in the research.

The first goal was to study the design of the Inditex group's sustainability communication policy, along with the content of the policy itself. It was found that Zara places considerable importance on sustainability (Lipsky-Karasz, 2021), and that they are working hard "to promote a sustainable transformation." As stated by the United Nations General Assembly, the three pillars of sustainable development are economic development, social development, and environmental protection, and it has been verified that the Inditex group is undertaking all three.

Of the aforementioned challenges that companies will have to face, Inditex is confronting all of them, one of which is related to technology. This involves focusing on the creation of garments that are more eco-efficient by using more environmentally-friendly raw materials, thereby reducing water consumption. Another aspect that the company is making a strong effort to avoid is the offshoring of production.

Furthermore, in line with what sustainability is intended to involve, the aim of Inditex is for everything related to sustainability to extend throughout the entire value chain, from the factories to the shops.

The staggering success of this group in terms of its management approach has also proven to be a sustainable model, as "Inditex has created an integrated chain that starts from the purchase of fabrics, and continues through the manufacturing process, logistics and operations in the shops. At all of these stages, the agents involved are given a great deal of flexibility to increase or decrease production according to consumer preferences" (ABC, 2019).

The second objective was to determine the level of consistency between what was communicated and what was actually carried out. It is important to remember that "the backbone of sustainable fashion, and the main factor that makes consumers choose this model, is the consistent and transversal nature with which they develop their activity" (Fernández, 2019, p. 2).

To this end, a wide range of initiatives are being undertaken, several of which have been mentioned in the previous section. The most noteworthy of these are the following: years ago, the group launched the fashion line known as "Join Life: working towards sustainability," which represents their entire concept of sustainability; plastic bags have already been eliminated from shops and, in some countries, they now charge for paper bags; the money raised from the sale of these bags is allocated to environmental projects; and since 2022, the aim has been for 100% of its shops to be powered by renewable energy.

Regarding other initiatives, along with the training available to employees, as well as specific technical education, Inditex has focused on the promotion of learning in two very important areas of the company: sustainability; and diversity and inclusion. As an example, in collaboration with the University of Leeds, which is an international benchmark in the textile sector, they have developed "The sustainable fashion school," aimed primarily at training teams who work in the areas of purchase and design in the latest innovations in sustainability. By 2022, approximately 1,000 people were participating in the programme (*El Economista*, 2022).

Zara also has a second-hand clothes donation programme at the following website (https://www.zara.com/es/es/help-center/ClothesCollectionProgram). In this way, Inditex is promoting the circular economy, due to the fact that reusing and recycling are two key starting points in helping reduce the consumption of resources. "Each person in Spain generates an average of ten kilos of textile waste per year" (*Asitex* report 2019, in Riezu, 2021, pg. 85).

Another way the group is introducing its products into the circular economy is by extending the lifespan of its garments. To do so, in 2022 they launched a platform that offers repair services, sales among individuals, and donations, which is known as "Zara Pre-Owned." This type of programme has already been in operation for some time in the UK. Moreover, it arrived in France last September, and in Germany shortly afterward (Diaz, 2023).

Conclusion

The focus on sustainability is undoubtedly one of the most important trends in recent years. In first world countries, a change has been observed in the textile industry involving the redefinition of its business model toward the production of clothing that takes into account the environment and respect for human rights, resulting in more durable and higher quality products.

This change is being driven by several factors, yet the most important is increased awareness among the population regarding the environmental, along with the social risks posed by the "fast fashion" business model, especially among young people who are more aware of such issues. Therefore, the growing concern among consumers in relation to sustainability and the circular economy is being reflected in the strategies and business models of fashion companies. In fact, for these firms to win over and retain the new generations, they must evolve toward models based on ethics, sustainability, and the circular economy.

The transition toward sustainability must encompass the entire value chain -from top management and economic rationale to consumer relationships and product lifecycle management. Sustainability must become a tool for innovation. If sustainability were truly implemented, less would have to be produced, the cost per garment would have to be increased, and consumers would have to be made aware of the need to buy fewer garments.

In the competitive environment in which textile brands operate, Zara has found it necessary to adapt to this new scenario. One of the reasons, among others, is that in recent years the dangers of climate change have become increasingly evident, and the environment has become a determining factor when it comes to influencing consumer purchase decisions.

The authors have observed that the adoption of sustainable practices is one of the main objectives of the Inditex group. However, this is not something that the company has been doing since it was founded. Although it could be argued that sustainability is not part of the DNA of its brand, the company became aware of this need early on and have tried to turn it into a competitive advantage. Sustainability is part of the group's overall strategy, ranging from product design to shop management, both in the short and long term. As such, there is an obvious concern for future generations. This is evidenced by the fact that their environmental objectives, which started as early as 2001 when they signed the UN Global Compact, will extend until 2050.

At first glance, fast fashion and sustainability may seem incompatible. However, this chapter demonstrates Inditex´s commitment to sustainability through innovative solutions. They have proven their intentions by taking action in a variety of ways. One example is the group's aid programme for community projects in which it collaborates with more than 400 non-profit organisations, and from which 8.7 million people have benefitted directly.

The group's business model represents the "flexible fashion" approach based on the ability to respond quickly and anticipate customer desires. This model also makes the company more sustainable because it produces according to what they know they are going to sell, thereby avoiding surpluses and reducing their carbon footprint.

Other issues that should be addressed include offering greater transparency to consumers by clearly stating the sustainable materials they use in producing their garments. Going even further, as Zara is aware of its strong influence as a prescriber, the company could act as a means of dissemination in an attempt to educate others regarding sustainability issues. More could be done, and more should be done, but any kind of initiative, however small and individual, will open the path toward sustainability in the fashion sector.

We must not forget that our obligation as consumers is to be aware and consequent in our role, because "rethinking the textile industry model we have means rethinking the societal model we want" (Riezu, 2021, p. 64).

References

Alianza de las Naciones Unidas para una moda sostenible (2019). ONU, programa para el medio ambiente. Kenia, Nairobi. Marzo, 2019. Disponible en: https://www.unep.org/es/noticias-y-reportajes/comunicado-de-prensa/la-alianza-de-la-onu-para-la-moda-sostenible-abordara-el.

Alonso Álvarez, L. (2000). Vistiendo a 3 continentes: la ventaja competitiva del grupo Inditex. 1963-1999. *Revista de Historia Industrial*, nº 18, pp. 157-182

Asamblea General de las Naciones Unidas (s.f.). Disponible en https://www.un.org/es/ga/president/65/issues/sustdev.shtml.

Carrera-Gallissà, E. (2017). Los retos sostenibilistas del sector textil. "Revista de Química e Industria Textil," 1 marzo, núm. 220, p. 20-32.

Cristófol Rodríguez, C., Mcquillan, K., y Segarra-Saavedra, J. (2021). La comunicación de la sostenibilidad como herramienta de ventas y de cambio social: fast fashion vs. slow fashion. *Revista de Comunicación de la SEECI,* 54, 17-37. doi: https://doi.org/10.15198/seeci.2021.54.e667.

Díaz, M. P. (2023). Así es la plataforma "Zara Pre-Owned" con ropa de segunda mano que Inditex traerá en esta fecha a España." 4.10.2023. El Confidencial. Disponible en https://www.elconfidencial.com/empresas/2023-10-04/fecha-zara-pre-owned-ropa-segunda-mano-2023_3747784/.

Fernández Sánchez, D. (2019). La moda sostenible un nicho emergente dentro del sector textil (trabajo de fin de grado). Grado en Pub. Y RRPP. Segovia: Universidad de Valladolid. https://uvadoc.uva.es/bitstream/handle/10324/37310/TFG-N.%201195.pdf?sequence=1&isAllowed=y.

El Economista (2022). Inditex potencia el desarrollo profesional de sus empleados. Ecobrands, unidad branded content de El Economista. 12.05.2022. Disponible en: https://www.eleconomista.es/branded-content/noticias/11734901/04/22/Inditex-potencia-el-desarrollo-profesional-de-sus-empleados.html.

Ellison, J. (2023). The Zara woman: an exclusive interview with Marta Ortega Pérez. Financial Times. 29-March-2023. Disponible en: https://www.ft.com/content/f5e10605-3c9d-4517-86f5-2e7570bf16f0.

Gazzola, P., Pavione, E., Pezzeti, R. & Grechi, D. (2020). Trends in the Fashion Industry. The Perception of Sustainability and Circular Economy: A Gender/Generation Quantitative Approach. MDPI. *Sustainability Journal* 12 (7). doi: 10.3390/su12072809.

Grupo Inditex (s.f.). Inditex, Web corporativa. Disponible en https://www.inditex.com/itxcomweb/es/home.

Hinojosa, M. y Vizcarra, A. (2019). ¿Cómo afecta el concepto de desarrollo sostenible a las empresas Fast Fashion?. Facultad de Ciencias Empresariales y Económicas. Repositorio Institucional, Universidad de Lima, Perú. Disponible en: https://hdl.handle.net/20.500.12724/10869.

Inditex (2021). Resumen del año. Disponible en: https://static.inditex.com/annual_report_2021/es/resumen-del-ano.html.

Lipsky-Karasz, E. (2021). Why Marta Ortega Pérez is the secret to Zara´s success. *Wall Street Journal Magazine.* Aug. 31, 2021. Recuperado en: https://www.wsj.com/articles/why-marta-ortega-perez-is-the-secret-to-zaras-success-11630413099.

Martín López, R. (2019). Comunicación de la sostenibilidad de las principales marcas de fast fashion españolas e italianas: Zara, Mango, Calcedonia y OVS. Diferencias entre el punto de venta online y el punto de venta físico. *Repositori Universitat Jaume* I, pp. 123-151. http://dx.doi.org/10.6035/2174-0992.2019.18.8.

Martínez, J. (2020). Zara renueva su colección "Join Life." En Fashion united. 26-Feb-2020. Disponible en: https://fashionunited.es/noticias/moda/zara-renueva-su-coleccion-sostenible-join-life/2020022632235.

Museo del Traje. Centro de Investigación del Patrimonio Etnológico (2023). Asociación para la gestión colectiva del residuo textil en España. 12.01.2023. Disponible en: https://www.culturaydeporte.gob.es/mtraje/en/museo/prensa/notas-de-prensa/np-historico/2023/asociacion.html.

Naciones Unidas. World Commission on Environment (1987). El desarrollo sostenible, una guía sobre nuestro futuro común: El informe de la Comisión Mundial sobre el Medio Ambiente y el Desarrollo. Oxford: University Press (pp. 1- 416). Disponible en: https://www.ecominga.uqam.ca/PDF/BIBLIOGRAPHIE/GUIDE_LECTURE_1/CMMAD-Informe-Comision-Brundtland-sobre-Medio-Ambiente-Desarrollo.pdf.

Ramírez Barredo, B., Guerrero González-Valerio, B., & Martín Critikián, D. (2023). Zara Joins the Trends: Analysis of Its Content Creation Within the Framework of Its Business Strategy. In R. Pettinger, B. Gupta, A. Roja, & D. Cozmiuc (Eds.), *Handbook of Research on Digitalization Solutions for Social and Economic Needs* (pp. 274-289). IGI Global. https://doi.org/10.4018/978-1-6684-4102-2.ch01.

Riezu, M. (2021). *La moda justa.* Una invitación a vestir con ética. Barcelona: editorial Anagrama.

Sánchez Vicente, T. (2019). Zara cambia el concepto de "moda rápida" por el de "flexible". En ABC economy. Disponible en: https://www.abc.es/economia/abci-zara-cambia-concepto-moda-rapida-flexible-201901110217_noticia.html.

Sitaro, T. D. (2020). Fast fashion and Sustainability. The case of Inditex-Zara. Forham University. Senior Theses, 46. https://research.library.fordham.edu/international_senior/46.

Thomas, D. (2020). Fashionopolis. El precio de la moda rápida y el futuro de la ropa. Barcelona: editorial Superflua.

United Nations. Sustainable development goals. Disponible en: https://www.un.org/sustainabledevelopment/

Zambrana, M. (2018). De la moda rápida a la moda sostenible. La transformación del consumidor. (trabajo fin de máster). Madrid: Universidad Pontificia de Comillas. Disponible en: https://repositorio.comillas.edu /rest/bitstreams/215010/retrieve.

Chapter 16

Ultraviolet Light: Non-Visual Effects of Light and Catalysis to Enhance Physical and Psychological Well-Being

Daniel Arranz-Paraíso[1]
Miguel Ángel de Miguel Paraíso[2],*
and Sandra Arranz Paraíso[3]
[1]R&D Development Manager at Pinisan SL. C/Gran Canaria, Madrid, Spain
[2]Rey Juan Carlos University, Madrid, Spain
[3]Universidad Autónoma de Madrid, Departamento de Psicología Básica, Madrid, Spain

Abstract

Living organisms consist of all substances they acquire from their surrounding environment, whether organic (carbohydrates, lipids, proteins, nucleic acids, simple organic compounds) or inorganic (mineral salts and metals). This chapter will focus on the presence of pollutants transported through the air and the possibility of their elimination to prevent the potential induction of physical or psychological illness in human beings. These pollutants can have diverse natures, both organic and inorganic, and may include microorganisms such as viruses, bacteria, and fungi. Inhalation of these components can induce pathologies (infections, mutagenesis, mental alterations) depending on individuals' idiosyncrasies. The epigenetic, metabolomic, and anatomical conditions of individuals determine their sensitivity to potentially toxic or infectious compounds. The organism is a combination of physical and mental aspects, and stability between the two is necessary for proper functioning. Therefore, the relationship between environmental pollution and psychological problems resulting from interaction with potentially toxic components has been the subject of study.

Keywords: pollutant, VOCs, microorganism, HEPA, PM2.5, Ultraviolet light, TiO_2, toxic compounds

---

* Corresponding Author's Email: miguelangel.demiguel@urjc.es

In: Psycho-Environmental Variables That Ensure People's Well-Being and Health …
Editors: Roberto Alonso González Lezcano and Guadalupe Cantarero García
ISBN: 979-8-89530-831-8
© 2025 Nova Science Publishers, Inc.

Introduction

In the air, there are suspensions of particles that differ according to their ability to penetrate the deeper regions of the pulmonary epithelium. Microorganisms, particularly viruses, can penetrate deeper into the lungs due to their small size. The deeper these particles penetrate, the greater their potential for vascular permeation into the blood increasing the risk of developing pathologies. However, it is not always necessary for particles to reach the lower respiratory system to cause adverse effects. For instance, pollen, dust mite antigens, and animal hair can trigger allergies upon contact with the upper respiratory tract (nostrils, pharynx, and larynx). Similarly, some microorganisms, depending on their biological cycle and growth niche, can cause diseases in the upper respiratory tract, such as rhinoviruses.

The first consideration is which components of the air can induce alterations: organic and inorganic compounds, and microorganisms. Organic compounds can be of both natural origin (such as methane generated from ruminants' digestion or essential oils releasing terpenes) and human or artificial origin (such as industrial emissions, dry cleaning, tobacco smoke, and evaporation of organic solvents) [1–9]. Volatile Organic Compounds (VOCs) are a complex group of chemical substances that can pose direct health risks, as they are generally carcinogenic and may lead to respiratory and neurological issues [10, 11]. An association has been established between these pollutants and cancer, considering them as biomarkers for cancer diagnosis [12] due to the high risk associated with exposure [13]. Some VOCs, such as benzene and its derivatives, have been identified as carcinogens with mechanisms including endocrine disruption and direct action [14]. Controlling the concentrations of volatile organic compounds is important because they are significant precursors in the formation of ground-level ozone, a major atmospheric pollutant [15].

VOCs are particularly relevant in sensitive environments such as hospitals and facilities responsible for cleaning and disinfecting clothing [16–19]. The hospital population is vulnerable and more susceptible to the pathological effects of pollutants due to their existing conditions and the confined environment where they receive treatment. The most sensitive individuals include those with respiratory diseases, especially in special units such as Intermediate Respiratory Care Units (IRCU) or Intensive Care Units (ICU). Increased pollutants in their environment can trigger complications. Other sensitive populations include neonates, particularly premature infants, patients undergoing major surgeries, and those with diseases or treatments that induce immunosuppression, such as transplants or HIV/AIDS. These groups are more susceptible to nosocomial infections and require the use of aggressive cleaning products [20–22].

Pharmaceutical and biotechnological research and development (R&D) departments or laboratory quality assurance departments also have high ambient VOC concentrations due to organic solvents. Analytical methods like high-performance liquid chromatography (HPLC) and ultra-high-performance liquid chromatography (UHPLC) are essential for analyzing VOCs. VOCs play a significant role in the pharmaceutical industry, particularly in the synthesis of organic compounds and the development of analytical methods [23–36]. These compounds are crucial for extracting and analyzing various substances, including polyphenols, volatile oils, and other bioactive compounds [37, 38].

The pharmaceutical industry's dependence on solvents and their emissions raises concerns about environmental impact and carbon footprint [39, 40]. Consequently, there is growing emphasis on developing eco-friendly and solvent-free reactions to minimize environmental impacts [32, 41]. Continuous solvent recovery systems and solvent-efficient processes, such as vapor-assisted tumbling (VAT), are being explored to address sustainability concerns [42]. In analytical methods, HPLC and UHPLC are fundamental for studying the quality of food, pharmaceuticals, and nutraceuticals to determine active ingredients, detect product adulteration, and control narcotic trafficking [26, 27, 36]. HPLC methods have also been developed to detect pesticide residues in soil and crops, demonstrating their importance in ensuring product safety and quality [43].

The use of air-purifying plants, such as Sansevieria Laurentii, has gained attention for their potential in eliminating VOCs, particularly formaldehyde, from indoor air [44, 45]. These plants have been found to be more effective than air purifiers in reducing VOCs, especially formaldehyde [44]. Sansevieria trifasciata, or the snake plant, also has reported anti-diabetic activity, indicating potential bioactive properties [46]. To achieve healthier urban and industrial environments, the potential of plants in phytoremediation has been explored, showing their ability to purify contaminants in soil, water, and air [47]. Extracts from these plants have been effective in reducing bacteria and fungi levels in indoor environments [48].

The effectiveness of air purification systems, both electrical and biological, has been extensively studied to verify their efficacy in reducing indoor air pollutants [49,50]. Natural air-purifying plants like Sansevieria spp. offer a sustainable and environmentally friendly alternative for managing indoor air quality, aligning with the 2030 Agenda's goals to improve air quality and reduce resource use without relying on electrical energy [47].

Inorganic compounds are another significant group of pollutants that can impact human health in various ways [51]. Air pollution is a complex mixture of gases and particulate matter that can lead to neurotoxicity, among other pathologies. The air contains various inorganic elements such as iron oxides, calcium, silicon, carbon oxides, sulfur, and nitrogen [52]. Sources of these inorganic components include coal combustion, biomass burning, vehicle emissions, and industrial processes. Governments are implementing improvement processes to ensure a better environment for future generations [52–54].

Inorganic elements in the air can take forms such as suspended solids, PM10 particles, PM2.5 particles, and water-soluble inorganic ions [55–57]. Exposure to these components is linked to numerous diseases and adverse health effects, including neurodevelopmental disorders, neurodegenerative diseases, respiratory conditions like asthma, and lung cancer such as asbestosis [58]. Cardiovascular diseases, low birth weight, child development issues, diabetes, and dementia have also been associated with inorganic air pollutants [51, 59–62].

Inhaled particulate matter, including both inorganic and organic fractions, is associated with oxidative stress and inflammation. Both the organic fraction (polycyclic aromatic hydrocarbons, PAHs) and the inorganic fraction (metals) generate reactive oxygen species and cause oxidative stress, linked to the activation of the Nrf2 transcription factor driven by redox imbalance [63].

The pollution resulting from the natural breakdown of synthetic structures needs to be studied to produce relevant environmental impact reports. For example, perovskite solar cells are highly unstable when exposed to moisture and temperature, which they constantly face in solar energy applications [64]. This instability must be considered, as increased pollution from organic or inorganic microparticles is not acceptable in the pursuit of green energy [65].

Initiatives to reduce the negative effects of inorganic elements and improve air quality are underway. Current efforts involve revolutionizing sectors like individual mobility, industry, freight transport, and indoor thermal conditioning of buildings. Plans include refurbishing old buildings to improve insulation levels in walls and windows [66–68]. The reduction of anthropogenic emissions during the COVID-19 lockdown positively impacted air quality worldwide, with significant decreases in PM2.5 concentrations and secondary inorganic aerosols [69–72].

Industrial and adjacent residential areas face higher risks of environmental pollution from VOCs and heavy metals. Heavy metals, particularly concerning near iron and steel factories and car manufacturing plants, pose risks due to their release into the atmosphere. The accumulation of heavy metals in the air is a risk factor for adverse health effects for workers and nearby residents [73, 74]. Sources of heavy metal pollution include industrial emissions and high concentrations of industrial vehicles [75–78]. Mining activities and mineral processing also contribute to heavy metal pollution [79].

Heavy metal pollution extends beyond the atmosphere, affecting soil near industrial sites [80]. Soil contamination from industrial activities, such as tannery operations, is a global crisis, particularly in developing countries [81]. Soil pollution with heavy metals poses ecological risks and can have far-reaching environmental consequences. Historically, industries like hat-making and gold extraction have been dangerous due to mercury use [82–86].

Historical building materials have included highly polluting substances such as asbestos, a mineral fiber used for its heat resistance and durability. However, the disintegration of asbestos-containing materials releases silica-based fibers into the air, posing significant health risks [87]. Asbestos in buildings has been linked to severe occupational diseases and deaths [88]. Asbestos-related diseases have long latent periods, complicating early diagnosis [89]. The association between mesothelioma histological subtypes and asbestos exposure is well established, with crocidolite asbestos fibers found in most mesothelioma cases [90].

Other materials used in modern construction are also not entirely risk-free. Rock or glass fiber insulation materials can pose health risks, as mineral wool contains carcinogenic fibers similar to asbestos [91]. The production of mineral wool has been associated with occupational health risks, including skin diseases due to allergies [92]. Disintegration of these materials during installation can release hazardous fibers, causing respiratory diseases and other health problems [93].

The third major group of air and surface pollutants is microorganisms. Nosocomial contamination in hospitals and care centers is a critical issue that challenges healthcare systems worldwide. Nosocomial infections, or healthcare-associated infections (HAIs), are acquired during a patient's stay in a healthcare facility and can be caused by bacteria, viruses, or fungi. These infections can lead to prolonged hospital stays, increased healthcare costs, and mortality [94]. The risk increases with the artificial selection of specimens resistant to clinical treatments. Transmission routes include contaminated surfaces, air, medical equipment, and healthcare workers' hands [95]. Effective infection control measures are crucial to protect patients and healthcare workers and reduce the spread of infections [96, 97].

Microorganisms can spread through the air, contributing to infections in various settings. Different types of microorganisms have been linked to nosocomial infections. For example, Pseudomonas aeruginosa is associated with hospital-acquired infections and can survive in various environments, including soil and water [98]. Acinetobacter baumannii is another pathogen linked to healthcare-associated infections and is known for its resistance to multiple antibiotics [99]. Effective air filtration systems and regular cleaning protocols are essential in controlling these infections and maintaining a safe environment in healthcare settings [100, 101].

In addition to surface contamination, the role of hospital wastewater in the dissemination of pathogens has also been recognized as a concern. Hospital effluents containing microbiological and chemical contaminants can contribute to environmental pollution and the spread of antibiotic resistance [102, 103]. Therefore, the characterization and treatment of hospital wastewater is essential for controlling the impact of hospital contaminants on the environment [102]. The impact of nosocomial contamination extends beyond patient health, affecting healthcare systems, healthcare workers, and the broader community. Contaminated blood cultures, for example, can lead to prolonged hospital stays, unnecessary antibiotic therapy, and increased healthcare costs [104–106]. Furthermore, the risk of occupational transmission of infections among healthcare workers underscores the need for comprehensive infection control measures to protect the healthcare workforce [107].

To alleviate the above, several systems have been developed that can remove pollutants of all kinds. Among the best known are the air purification systems that became widespread in domestic use during the Covid pandemic. High Efficiency Particulate Air (HEPA) filters are ideal for their effectiveness in capturing small particles such as PM2.5 and some airborne viruses [108]. These filtration systems have been proven to outperform electrostatic air purifiers, which rely on ionic processes for filtration [109]. Additionally, the use of air purifiers equipped with HEPA filters has been shown to help control allergic diseases by reducing pollen and contaminant particles [110–112].

Some HEPA air purifiers are equipped with ultraviolet (UV) light for additional air purification. For example, a study demonstrated that a TiO2/zeolite filter with UV illumination exhibited high photo-regeneration efficiency, indicating the potential of UV light in air purification [112]. Moreover, some air purifiers incorporate activated carbon filters, known for absorbing volatile organic compounds (VOCs) [113]. The combination of HEPA filters and activated carbon filters in air purifiers provides a comprehensive solution for capturing suspended particles and VOCs, thereby improving indoor air quality. All of this is based on the use of HEPA filters, which have been widely used in critical medical settings, such as surgical operating rooms, to prevent the spread of airborne bacterial and viral organisms, emphasizing their importance in healthcare environments and in laminar flow hoods where cells are cultured [114].

There are other advancements, such as a melamine sponge with a copper-organic framework as a multifunctional filter for air purifiers, indicating the potential of innovative materials in air filtration systems [115]. Additionally, the development of washable ceramic catalytic filters with a long lifespan for air purification presents a promising solution for the removal of PM2.5 and other pollutants [116].

The challenge with these filters is that due to their narrow pores, they require high energy to force air through them. This often makes their use impractical due to noise, vibrations, and energy consumption. This has led to the development of other technologies that focus on combining filters with coarser pores along with UV and metallic alloys. To effectively eliminate VOCs and microorganisms, avoiding the above problems, the use of ultraviolet (UV) irradiation in combination with titanium alloys, silver, and other minerals has been extensively studied. A series of metallic cycles combining oxidizing systems and catalysts is generated through irradiation. UV rays alone induce the generation of hydroxyl radicals, which are effective in degrading VOCs [117]. Based on this, it has been demonstrated that the use of semiconductor materials such as TiO_2, along with UV sources, efficiently decomposes VOCs through oxidation reactions, resulting in the production of harmless byproducts [118]. Photocatalytic research on materials with the combined use of metals under deep UV irradiation has sparked interest in indoor VOCs removal [119]. The photocatalytic properties of TiO2 have been widely recognized for their ability to initiate the oxidation of VOCs, leading to their degradation [120]. Another aspect explored is the application of doped TiO2 for the photocatalytic oxidation of formaldehyde, indicating the widespread use of titanium dioxide for treating VOCs [121].

Additionally, the activation of persulfate by TiO2-Fe3O4 nanocomposites under UV-LED irradiation has been demonstrated for the removal of reactive red 198, emphasizing the potential of advanced materials in combination with UV light for pollutant degradation [122]. It is very important to know new methods of elimination of red 198 because it is a dye very used in textile industry with a high solubility in water, being a pollutant of difficult elimination due to its capacity to be distributed in great volumes of water. Lastly, it has been shown that the use of UV-C irradiation can regenerate VOCs filters through the photocatalytic activity of TiO2, highlighting the potential of UV-based technologies in air purification systems [112]. This regeneration extends the lifespan of these filtering systems, improving their effectiveness.

In recent years, excellent antibacterial activity and biological effects have been observed in copper-bearing titanium alloys, making them advantageous for tissue engineering applications [123]. This can be leveraged in modern architectural systems, creating systems that can continuously purify water or air without the need for heat sources or toxic products such as sodium hypochlorite for its ability to eliminate bacterial biofilms [124–126]. The eco-friendly and economical photocatalytic water purification process, employing semiconductors under UV rays, is considered highly suitable for degrading and eliminating organic contaminants in water [127]. Ozone micro/nanobubbles with catalytic processes have also been widely utilized in the treatment of refractory organic wastewater, showcasing the diverse applications of UV-based processes for environmental pollution control [128].

Objectives

The aim of this chapter is to focus on the primary air pollutants, their sources, and their effects on the health of living beings. Based on this, various existing solutions and future developments to improve or mitigate these environmental pollutants have been explored. All of these solutions can be implemented in architectural systems. Specifically, the objectives of this chapter are:

a. Air components that cause health problems.
b. Health risks of VOCs:
c. Vulnerability to VOCs in hospitals and pharmaceutical facilities:
d. Sustainable practices in the pharmaceutical industry: reduce VOC emissions, develop eco-friendly solvents, implement solvent-free reactions, continuously recover solvents, use solvent-efficient processes.
e. Air-purifying plants.
f. Effectiveness of air purification systems:

g. Health problems caused by inorganic pollutants: Alzheimer's, Parkinson's, Asthma, COPD, lung cancer, cardiovascular diseases.
h. Initiatives to reduce inorganic pollution.
i. Impact of nosocomial contamination.

Material and Methods

1. *Initial Search:*
   - A comprehensive literature search was performed in the PubMed, Web of Science, and Scopus databases.
2. *The following keywords were used:*
   - "Hospital VOCs"
   - "Ultraviolet light"
   - "HEPA filters and metal actives filters"
   - "Pollution, microparticles, origin, restriction laws"
   - "Inhalation of microparticles, VOCs, diseases and possible pathologies"

   Keywords were combined using Boolean operators "AND" and "OR."
   A total of 547 articles were retrieved.
3. *Duplicate Removal:*
   - Duplicates were removed from the different databases.
   - The removal of duplicates was manually verified to ensure accuracy.
   - A reduction to 214 unique articles was achieved.
4. *Filtering Date:*
   - Only articles published between January 1, 2019 and December 31, 2023 were selected.
   - The publication date of each article was verified.
   - A final collection of 151 articles was obtained.
5. *Abstract Assessment:*
   - A critical reading of the abstracts of the 151 selected articles was performed.
   - The thematic relevance of each abstract was assessed with respect to the systematic review.
   - 132 articles that met the pre-established relevance criteria were selected.
6. *Methodological Quality Assessment:*
   - A specific methodology was applied to evaluate the methodological quality of the 132 articles.
   - Aspects such as study design, sample size, analysis methodology, and presentation of results were evaluated.
   - 128 articles that met the methodological quality criteria were selected.
7. *Analysis and Synthesis of Information:*
   - The information collected in the 128 selected articles will be analyzed.
   - The research findings will be synthesized to answer the questions of the systematic review.

Discussion

Air pollution is one of the most pressing global issues, and it is expected to worsen over the coming years. This pollution not only affects humans but also animals, plants, and the ecosystem as a whole. Both human and animal activities contribute to this pollution, releasing various types of particles into the environment. For these reasons, it is crucial to develop and implement new systems capable of reducing pollution and preventing illnesses that arise from continuous exposure to these harmful environmental agents.

The main source of pollution continues to be the combustion of fossil fuels for transportation, heating, and other applications. Additionally, breaking and transmission systems still rely on friction, contributing to pollution. While electrification offers some solutions, it is not a complete fix, as much of our electricity is generated by burning fuels, and solar panel degradation also leads to pollution. Evaluating the trade-offs of battery-powered electricity is crucial, considering the environmental impact of mineral extraction and material usage. In planning new urban environments, these factors must be addressed realistically, as the disposal of inorganic compounds from degraded solar panels also poses health risks.

The near future will focus on developing new materials that can insulate buildings from the elements without producing potentially carcinogenic inorganic pollutants. When comparing the health risks of asbestos to the diseases caused by the breakdown of rock or fiberglass insulation, it becomes clear that both pose significant health hazards. Asbestos exposure is well-documented and linked to severe health conditions, while the disintegration of rock or fiberglass insulation materials also presents occupational health risks. It is, therefore, critical to assess and manage the use of these materials in construction and insulation to minimize potential health threats.

Another key issue to consider in creating low-pollution environments is the serious risk of deflagration in batteries used to store energy in vehicles and homes equipped with solar panels or renewable energy systems. Even a slight amount of moisture can trigger explosions and deflagrations, endangering people nearby and polluting the environment with heavy metals released into the air, soil, and water.

To progress toward a healthier future, it is essential to develop systems that can eliminate, for example, the contamination generated in research and development laboratories working with pathogenic viruses. The need for such systems became particularly apparent during the COVID-19 pandemic. Existing systems must be strengthened to prevent the release of these harmful agents into the environment. This requires exploring new filtration systems, catalysis methods, and technologies that can virtually eliminate emissions. Many emissions results from reagents that release volatile organic compounds (VOCs) into the air. Special attention should be given to air regeneration, filtering, and catalytic systems designed to create safe environments in hospitals and healthcare centers. Already, there are systems on the market that combine ultraviolet radiation with metal alloys and PM2.5 filters, which not only remove physical pollutants but also catalytically eliminate both organic and inorganic pollutants larger than PM 2.5, as well as neutralize VOCs from natural or human sources.

Air, like water, must be kept as pure as possible. In the future, we may see the development of air purification plants, rooms, or integrated air purification systems to ensure clean air in homes, hospitals, and workplaces. The rising prevalence of cancer and allergies underscores the need for significant interventions to ensure high life expectancy and public health.

Integrated systems with filters, UV light, and metallic catalytic mechanisms may well become the defining technological revolution of the second third of the 21st century. These systems will be essential in eliminating pollutants from all sources, thanks to the integration of advanced technologies.

Conclusion

- Growing concern about air pollution: Air pollution is a major and growing problem, affecting not only humans, but also animals, plants and the ecosystem. The main source of pollutants is the burning of fossil fuels used for transport and heating, as well as the use of certain technologies.
- Challenges of electrification: Although electrification is raised, the real situation is that it may not be a complete solution, as electricity generation still involves the burning of fuels and poses environmental challenges, such as pollution from the degradation of solar panels. The need to balance the costs and benefits of using electricity from batteries is emphasized. Especially for the architecture of new cities, planning should be done in order to easily and economically replace obsolete technologies in both energy generation and storage. An example would be to make it possible to replace solar panels installed on pavements without having to destroy their perimeter area.
- Health risks in building materials: The text stresses the importance of carefully considering the development of new materials for building insulation. It compares the health risks associated with traditional materials such as asbestos with those of rock or fiberglass used in insulation, highlighting the need to manage the use of these materials to minimize potential health risks.
- The use of the non-visual effects of UV radiation should be studied and developed to make the best use of its harmful effects against prokaryotic cells, VOCs and other particulate matter that cause or may cause harm to humans and animals. Ultraviolet light, particularly from LED sources, offers an economical solution with minimal electrical consumption and reduced penetration into the living tissues of higher organisms. It is a well-developed technology that can prevent toxic discharges into water and air. And it can even improve the quality of life by increasing the shelf life or spoilage time of food by sterilizing it.
- The importance of pollution control in healthcare facilities: the development and implementation of advanced systems, such as filtration, catalysis and air regeneration technologies, to remove pollutants generated in medical and research environments remain a key area for further development. The focus should also be on ensuring safe environments in hospitals and health care centers, with a revolution in existing technologies combining ultraviolet radiation and metal alloys for the effective removal of pollutants.

References

[1] Lee-Rangel, H. A., Roque-Jiménez, J. A., Cifuentes-López, R. O., Álvarez-Fuentes, G., Cruz-Gómez, A. D. la, Martínez-García, J. A., Arévalo-Villalobos, J. I., & Chay-Canul, A. J. (2022). *Evaluation of Three Marine Algae on Degradability, In Vitro Gas Production, and CH_4 and CO_2 Emissions by Ruminants. Fermentation,* 8(10), 511. https://doi.org/10.3390/fermentation8100511.

[2] Sadgrove, N. J., Padilla-González, G. F., & Phumthum, M. (2022). *Fundamental Chemistry of Essential Oils and Volatile Organic Compounds, Methods of Analysis and Authentication. Plants*, 11(6), 789. https://doi.org/10.3390/plants11060789.

[3] Tangpao, T., Charoimek, N., Teerakitchotikan, P., Leksawasdi, N., Jantanasakulwong, K., Rachtanapun, P., Seesuriyachan, P., Phimolsiripol, Y., Chaiyaso, T., Ruksiriwanich, W., Jantrawut, P., Van Doan, H., Cheewangkoon, R., & Sommano, S. R. (2022). *Volatile Organic Compounds from Basil Essential Oils: Plant Taxonomy, Biological Activities, and Their Applications in Tropical Fruit Productions. Horticulturae*, 8(2), 144. https://doi.org/10.3390/horticulturae8020144.

[4] Eun, D. M., Han, Y. S., Park, S. H., Yoo, H. S., Le, Y. T. H., Jeong, S., Jeon, K. J., & Youn, J. S. (2022). *Analysis of VOCs Emitted from Small Laundry Facilities: Contributions to Ozone and Secondary Aerosol Formation and Human Risk Assessment. International Journal of Environmental Research and Public Health,* 19(22), 15130. https://doi.org/10.3390/ijerph192215130.

[5] Xue, Y., Wang, L., Liu, S., Huang, Y., Chen, L., Cui, L., Cheng, Y., & Cao, J. (2022). *High impact of vehicle and solvent emission on the ambient volatile organic compounds in a major city of northwest China. Chinese Chemical Letters*, 33(5), 2753–2756. https://doi.org/10.1016/j.cclet.2021.11.013.

[6] Ghouas, H., Haddou, B., Canselier, J. P., & Gourdon, C. (2022). *Wastewater Pollution Prevention for volatile organic compounds (Benzene, Toluene, Ethylbenzene, and Xylene) using cloud point extraction and regeneration of surfactant by evaporation. Euro-Mediterranean Journal for Environmental Integration*, 7(1), 1–12. https://doi.org/10.1007/s41207-022-00292-9.

[7] Xu, Z., Zou, Q., Jin, L., Shen, Y., Shen, J., Xu, B., Qu, F., Zhang, F., Xu, J., Pei, X., Xie, G., Kuang, B., Huang, X., Tian, X., & Wang, Z. (2023). *Characteristics and sources of ambient Volatile Organic Compounds (VOCs) at a regional background site, YRD region, China: Significant influence of solvent evaporation during hot months. Science of The Total Environment*, 857, 159674. https://doi.org/10.1016/j.scitotenv.2022.159674.

[8] Etemadi, A., Abnet, C. C., Dawsey, S. M., & Freedman, N. D. (2023). *Biomarkers of Tobacco Carcinogenesis in Diverse Populations: Challenges and Opportunities. Cancer Epidemiology, Biomarkers & Prevention*, 32(3), 289–291. https://doi.org/10.1158/1055-9965.EPI-22-1289.

[9] Sambiagio, N., Berthet, A., Wild, P., Sauvain, J. J., Auer, R., Schoeni, A., Rodondi, N., Feller, M., Humair, J. P., Berlin, I., Breider, F., Grandjean, D., & Hopf, N. B. (2022). *Associations between urinary biomarkers of oxidative stress and biomarkers of tobacco smoke exposure in smokers. Science of The Total Environment,* 852, 158361. https://doi.org/10.1016/j.scitotenv.2022. 158361.

[10] Huang, Y., Lin, W., Huang, T., Li, Z., Zhang, Z., Xiao, R., Yang, X., Lian, S., Pan, J., Ma, J., Wang, W., Sun, L., Li, J., & Guan, B. (2022). *Ultrafast Response Optical Microfiber Interferometric VOC Sensor Based on Evanescent Field Interaction with ZIF-8/Graphene Oxide Nanocoating. Advanced Optical Materials,* 10(3). https://doi.org/10.1002/adom.202101561.

[11] Sakunkoo, P., Phonphinyo, S., Maneenin, N., Jirapornkul, C., Limmongkon, Y., Rayubkul, J., Thongtip, S., & Sangkham, S. (2021). *Comparison of Volatile Organic Compound Concentrations in Ambient Air among Different Source Areas around Khon Kaen, Thailand. Atmosphere*, 12(12), 1694. https://doi.org/10.3390/atmos12121694.

[12] Shaffie, A., Soliman, A., Eledkawy, A., Fu, X.-A., Nantz, M. H., Giridharan, G., van Berkel, V., & El-Baz, A. (2022). *Lung Cancer Diagnosis System Based on Volatile Organic Compounds (VOCs) Profile Measured in Exhaled Breath. Applied Sciences*, 12(14), 7165. https://doi.org/10.3390/ app12147165.

[13] Khajeh Hoseini, L., Jalilzadeh Yengejeh, R., Mohammadi Rouzbehani, M., & Sabzalipour, S. (2022). *Health risk assessment of volatile organic compounds (VOCs) in a refinery in the southwest of Iran using SQRA method. Frontiers in Public Health*, 10. https://doi.org/10.3389/fpubh.2022.978354.

[14] Goldberg, M. S., Zapata-Marin, S., Labrèche, F., Ho, V., Lavigne, E., Valois, M. F., & Parent, M. E. (2022). *Ambient exposures to selected volatile organic compounds and the risk of prostate cancer in Montreal. Environmental Epidemiology*, 6(6), e231. https://doi.org/10.1097/EE9.000 0000000000231.

[15] Guan, Y., Zhang, Y., Zhang, Y., Wang, X., Han, J., Song, W., Hou, L., & Duan, E. (2020). *Pollution Characteristics and Key Reactive Species of Volatile Organic Compounds in Beijing-Tianjin-Hebei Area, China. Aerosol and Air Quality Research*, 20(9), 1886–1897. https://doi.org/10.4209/aaqr.2019.11.0595.

[16] Riveron, T. P., Wilde, M. J., Ibrahim, W., Carr, L., Monks, P. S., Greening, N. J., Gaillard, E. A., Brightling, C. E., Siddiqui, S., Hansell, A. L., & Cordell, R. L. (2023). *Characterisation of volatile organic compounds in hospital indoor air and exposure health risk determination. Building and Environment*, 242, 110513. https://doi.org/10.1016/j.buildenv.2023.110513.

[17] Parveen, N., Chowdhury, S., & Goel, S. (2022). *Environmental impacts of the widespread use of chlorine-based disinfectants during the COVID-19 pandemic. Environmental Science and Pollution Research*, 29(57), 85742–85760. https://doi.org/10.1007/s11356-021-18316-2.

[18] Kumar Nirala, N., Chopra, L., & Manikanika. (2023). *Review of Indoor Air Pollution Cause and Remedy. IOP Conference Series: Earth and Environmental Science,* 1110(1), 012056. https://doi.org/10.1088/1755-1315/1110/1/012056.

[19] Virji, M. A., Bowers, L. N., & LeBouf, R. F. (2022). *Inhalation and Skin Exposure to Chemicals in Hospital Settings.* In *Handbook of Indoor Air Quality (pp. 1–36). Springer Singapore.* https://doi.org/10.1007/978-981-10-5155-5_60-1.

[20] Epelle, E. I., Macfarlane, A., Cusack, M., Burns, A., Okolie, J. A., Vichare, P., Rolland, L., & Yaseen, M. (2023). *Ozone Decontamination of Medical and Nonmedical Devices: An Assessment of Design and Implementation Considerations. Industrial & Engineering Chemistry Research*, 62(10), 4191–4209. https://doi.org/10.1021/acs.iecr.2c03754.

[21] Ibrahim, F., Samsudin, E. Z., Ishak, A. R., & Sathasivam, J. (2022). *Hospital indoor air quality and its relationships with building design, building operation, and occupant-related factors: A mini-review. Frontiers in Public Health*, 10. https://doi.org/10.3389/fpubh.2022.1067764.

[22] Gaynor, J. W., Graham, E. M., Bhandari, D., Fenchel, M., Bradman, A., Klepczynski, B., Collier, H., Ittenbach, R. F., Reese, Christopher. M., & Blount, B. C. (2023). P*erioperative exposure to volatile organic compounds in neonates undergoing cardiac surgery. The Journal of Thoracic and Cardiovascular Surgery*. https://doi.org/10.1016/j.jtcvs.2023.07.049.

[23] Kianinia, M., & Abdoli, S. M. (2021). *The Design and Optimization of Extractive Distillation for Separating the Acetone/ n -Heptane Binary Azeotrope Mixture. ACS Omega*, 6(34), 22447–22453. https://doi.org/10.1021/acsomega.1c03513.

[24] Mizzi, L., Chatzitzika, C., Gatt, R., & Valdramidis, V. (2020). *HPLC Analysis of Phenolic Compounds and Flavonoids with Overlapping Peaks. Food Technology and Biotechnology,* 58(1), 1–12. https://doi.org/10.17113/ftb.58.01.20.6395.

[25] George, J., Nguyen, T., Williams, D., Hardner, C., Sanewski, G., & Smyth, H. E. (2023). *Review of the Aroma Chemistry of Pineapple (Ananas comosus). Journal of Agricultural and Food Chemistry*, 71(9), 4069–4082. https://doi.org/10.1021/acs.jafc.2c08546.

[26] Zhu, Y., Yin, Q., & Yang, Y. (2021). *A comparative study of HPLC-DAD and UPLC-UV methods for simultaneous determination of 11 polyphenols in Moringa oleifera leaves. Tropical Journal of Pharmaceutical Research,* 20(11), 2371–2379. https://doi.org/10.4314/tjpr.v20i11.20.

[27] Calle, A., Curi-Borda, C. K., Gutiérrez, C., Salcedo, L., Flores, Y., & Almanza, G. R. (2023). *Quantification and in vitro photo-protective studies of phenolic compounds from Baccharis papillosa Rusby. Journal of Pharmacy & Pharmacognosy Research*, 11(1), 33–46. https://doi.org/10.56499/jppres22. 1477_11.1.33.

[28] Fetisov, V., Pshenin, V., Nagornov, D., Lykov, Y., & Mohammadi, A. H. (2020). *Evaluation of Pollutant Emissions into the Atmosphere during the Loading of Hydrocarbons in Marine Oil Tankers in the Arctic Region. Journal of Marine Science and Engineering*, 8(11), 917. https://doi.org/10.3390/jmse8110917.

[29] Swain, S. P., Prasad, N., Reddy, L., Subrahmanyam, G., & Mohanty, S. (2021). *Solvent-Free Single-Pot Mannich Reaction and Detoxification of Industrial Hazardous Waste Methyl Mercaptan Gas. Chemistry Select,* 6(5), 1088–1092. https://doi.org/10.1002/slct.202004447.

[30] Lu, Y., Wang, J., Shen, G., Liu, J., Zhu, H., Zhao, J., & He, S. (2021). *Rapid Determination and Quality Control of Pharmacological Volatiles of Turmeric (Curcuma longa L.) by Fast Gas Chromatography–Surface Acoustic Wave Sensor. Molecules*, 26(19), 5797. https://doi.org/10.3390/molecules 26195797.

[31] Ueta, I., Takenaka, R., Fujimura, K., Yoshimura, T., Narukami, S., Mochizuki, S., & Maeda, T. (2020). *Simultaneous Extraction and Determination of Volatile Organic Compounds and Semi-volatile Organic Compounds in Indoor Air Using Multi-bed Solid Phase Extraction Device. Analytical Sciences,* 36(9), 1071–1074. https://doi.org/10.2116/analsci.20P022.

[32] Shores, B. T., Sieg, P. E., Nicosia, A. T., Hu, C., Born, S. C., Shvedova, K., Sayin, R., Testa, C. J., Wu, W., Takizawa, B., Ramanujam, S., & Mascia, S. (2020). *Design of a Continuous Solvent Recovery System for End-to-End Integrated Continuous Manufacturing of Pharmaceuticals. Organic Process Research & Development,* 24(10), 1996–2003. https://doi.org/10.1021/acs. oprd.0c00092.

[33] Mitran, E. C., Sandulache, I. M., Lite, C. M., & Radu, L. G. (2021). *Textile Museum Collections. SIM Method Validation for the Assessment of Pesticides. Materiale Plastice*, 58(3), 1–10. https://doi.org/10.37358/MP.21.3.5498.

[34] Chhanikar, P. T., Gupta, K. R., & Umekar, M. J. (2021). *Derivatizing Reagents for Detection of Organic Compounds By HPLC. Asian Journal of Applied Chemistry Research,* 1–13. https://doi.org/10.9734/ajacr/2021/v9i230207.

[35] Hodges, M. D., & Fitzgerald, N. (2020). *Investigating the Potential of an In-Situ Method for Monitoring the Malting of Barley Using Solid Phase Microextraction with a Portable Gas Chromatography Mass Spectrometry Instrument. Beverages*, 6(4), 72. https://doi.org/10.3390/beverages6040072.

[36] Rosbottom, I., Cheng, T. N. H., & Heng, J. Y. Y. (2020). *Computational Analysis of the Solid-State and Solvation Properties of Carbamazepine in Relation to its Polymorphism. Chemical Engineering & Technology*, 43(6), 1152–1159. https://doi.org/10.1002/ceat.202000056.

[37] García-Seval, V., Martínez-Alfaro, C., Saurina, J., Núñez, O., & Sentellas, S. (2022). *Characterization, Classification and Authentication of Spanish Blossom and Honeydew Honeys by Non-Targeted HPLC-UV and Off-Line SPE HPLC-UV Polyphenolic Fingerprinting Strategies. Foods*, 11(15), 2345. https://doi.org/10.3390/foods11152345.

[38] Ribeiro, V. P., Arruda, C., Mejía, J. A. A., Candido, A. C. B. B., dos Santos, R. A., Magalhães, L. G., & Bastos, J. K. (2021). *Brazilian southeast brown propolis: gas chromatography method development for its volatile oil analysis, its antimicrobial and leishmanicidal activities evaluation. Phytochemical Analysis,* 32(3), 404–411. https://doi.org/10.1002/pca.2988.

[39] Booth, A., Jager, A., Faulkner, S. D., Winchester, C. C., & Shaw, S. E. (2023). *Pharmaceutical Company Targets and Strategies to Address Climate Change: Content Analysis of Public Reports from 20 Pharmaceutical Companies. International Journal of Environmental Research and Public Health*, 20(4), 3206. https://doi.org/10.3390/ijerph20043206.

[40] Ray, A., Sharma, S., & Sadasivam, B. (2021). *Carbovigilance: curtailing the global pharmaceutical carbon footprint. Future Healthcare Journal,* 8(3), e683–e685. https://doi.org/10.7861/fhj.2021-0071.

[41] Youssef, S. H., Abdella, S., & Garg, S. (2022). *Development and Validation of a Novel Tool for Assessing the Environmental Impact of 3D Printing Technologies: A Pharmaceutical Perspective. Pharmaceutics*, 14(5), 933. https://doi.org/10.3390/pharmaceutics14050933.

[42] Stirk, A. J., Souza, F. E. S., Gerster, J., Mir, F. M., Karadeolian, A., & Rey, A. W. (2022). *Formation of pharmaceutical salts and cocrystals via vapour-assisted tumbling (VAT) – a solvent efficient process. Green Chemistry*, 24(4), 1505–1514. https://doi.org/10.1039/D1GC03683A.

[43] Stefanut, M. N., Dobrescu, M., Cata, A., Fitigau, F. I., Osser, G., Lile, I. E., Bondar, L. I., & Ienascu, I. M. del C. (2021). *HPLC-DAD method for detection of some pesticide residues in soil and crops cultivated in Banat county. Journal of Science and Arts*, 21(1), 307–314. https://doi.org/10.46939/J.Sci.Arts-21.1-b07.

[44] Sokhal, A., & Narayan, U. (2020). *Plants are More Effective in Absorbing Volatile Organic Compounds from the Atmosphere than Air Purifiers. Journal of Student Research,* 9(2). https://doi.org/10.47611/jsrhs.v9i2.1047.

[45] Bandehali, S., Miri, T., Onyeaka, H., & Kumar, P. (2021). *Current State of Indoor Air Phytoremediation Using Potted Plants and Green Walls. Atmosphere,* 12(4), 473. https://doi.org/10.3390/atmos12040473.

[46] Oomariyah, N., & Dijk, G. van. (2022). *The Bioavailability Prediction and Screening Phytochemicals of Sansevieria Trifasciata Leaves Extract. MATEC Web of Conferences,* 372, 02003. https://doi.org/10.1051/matecconf/ 202237202003.

[47] Ratnawati, R., & Faizah, F. (2020). *Phytoremediation of Mercury Contaminated Soil with the Addition of Compost. Journal of Engineering and Technological Sciences,* 52(1), 66–80. https://doi.org/ 10.5614/j.eng.technol.sci.2020.52.1.5.

[48] Rachmaniyah, R., Rusmiati, R., & Khambali, K. (2022). *The use of Sansevieria sp. and Cymbopogon nardus extracts on humidifier modification to reduce airborne germs. International Journal of Public Health Science*, 11(4), 1407. https://doi.org/10.11591/ijphs.v11i4.21381.

[49] Lee, J. J., Hwang, H., Hong, S. C., & Lee, J. Y. (2021). *Effect of Air Purification Systems on Particulate Matter and Airborne Bacteria in Public Buses. Atmosphere,* 13(1), 55. https://doi.org/ 10.3390/atmos13010055.

[50] Basińska, M., Michałkiewicz, M., & Ratajczak, K. (2021). *Effect of Air Purifier Use in the Classrooms on Indoor Air Quality—Case Study. Atmosphere,* 12(12), 1606. https://doi.org/10.3390/ atmos12121606.

[51] Cory-Slechta, D. A., Merrill, A., & Sobolewski, M. (2023). *Air Pollution–Related Neurotoxicity Across the Life Span. Annual Review of Pharmacology and Toxicology,* 63(1), 143–163. https://doi.org/10.1146/annurev-pharmtox-051921-020812.

[52] Zagorodnov, S. Y. (2020). *Component composition of atmospheric dusts as a characteristic of environmental pollution. IOP Conference Series: Earth and Environmental Science*, 548(7), 072069. https://doi.org/10.1088/1755-1315/548/7/072069.

[53] Liang, J., Zhang, Q., Chen, Z., Zheng, Z., Yang, C., & Ma, Q. (2021). *The combustion and emission characteristics of diesel-ethanol blends with THF as cosolvents in a diesel engine operating with EGR. Fuel*, 298, 120843. https://doi.org/10.1016/j.fuel.2021.120843.

[54] Jbaily, A., Zhou, X., Liu, J., Lee, T.-H., Kamareddine, L., Verguet, S., & Dominici, F. (2022). *Air pollution exposure disparities across US population and income groups. Nature*, 601(7892), 228–233. https://doi.org/10.1038/s41586-021-04190-y.

[55] Madhav, S., Ahamad, A., Singh, A. K., Kushawaha, J., Chauhan, J. S., Sharma, S., & Singh, P. (2020). *Water Pollutants: Sources and Impact on the Environment and Human Health. Sensors in Water Pollutants Monitoring: Role of Material* (pp. 43–62). https://doi.org/10.1007/978-981-15-0671-0_4.

[56] Qiao, B., Chen, Y., Tian, M., Wang, H., Yang, F., Shi, G., Zhang, L., Peng, C., Luo, Q., & Ding, S. (2019). *Characterization of water soluble inorganic ions and their evolution processes during PM2.5 pollution episodes in a small city in southwest China. Science of The Total Environment*, 650, 2605–2613. https://doi.org/10.1016/j.scitotenv.2018.09.376.

[57] Villanueva, F., Ródenas, M., Ruus, A., Saffell, J., & Gabriel, M. F. (2022). *Sampling and analysis techniques for inorganic air pollutants in indoor air. Applied Spectroscopy Reviews*, 57(7), 531–579. https://doi.org/10.1080/05704928.2021.2020807.

[58] Veit, D. (2022). *Asbestos. In Fibers* (pp. 381–401). *Springer International Publishing*. https://doi.org/ 10.1007/978-3-031-15309-9_12.

[59] Eckard, M. L., Marvin, E., Conrad, K., Oberdörster, G., Sobolewski, M., & Cory-Slechta, D. A. (2023). *Neonatal exposure to ultrafine iron but not combined iron and sulfur aerosols recapitulates air pollution-induced impulsivity in mice. NeuroToxicology*, 94, 191–205. https://doi.org/ 10.1016/j.neuro.2022.12.004.

[60] Flood-Garibay, J. A., Angulo-Molina, A., & Méndez-Rojas, M. Á. (2023). *Particulate matter and ultrafine particles in urban air pollution and their effect on the nervous system. Environmental Science: Processes & Impacts,* 25(4), 704–726. https://doi.org/10.1039/D2EM00276K.

[61] Thiankhaw, K., Chattipakorn, N., & Chattipakorn, S. C. (2022). *PM2.5 exposure in association with AD-related neuropathology and cognitive outcomes. Environmental Pollution,* 292, 118320. https://doi.org/10.1016/j.envpol.2021.118320.

[62] Mata, T. M., Felgueiras, F., Martins, A. A., Monteiro, H., Ferraz, M. P., Oliveira, G. M., Gabriel, M. F., & Silva, G. V. (2022). *Indoor Air Quality in Elderly Centers: Pollutants Emission and Health Effects. Environments*, 9(7), 86. https://doi.org/10.3390/environments9070086.

[63] Pardo, M., Qiu, X., Zimmermann, R., & Rudich, Y. (2020). *Particulate Matter Toxicity Is Nrf2 and Mitochondria Dependent: The Roles of Metals and Polycyclic Aromatic Hydrocarbons. Chemical Research in Toxicology*, 33(5), 1110–1120. https://doi.org/10.1021/acs.chemrestox.0c00007.

[64] Liang, J., & Qi, Y. B. (2021). *Recent progress on all-inorganic metal halide perovskite solar cells. Materials Today Nano,* 16, 100143. https://doi.org/10.1016/j.mtnano.2021.100143.

[65] Mazumdar, S., Zhao, Y., & Zhang, X. (2021). *Stability of Perovskite Solar Cells: Degradation Mechanisms and Remedies. Frontiers in Electronics*, 2. https://doi.org/10.3389/felec.2021.712785.

[66] Šekularac, N., Ivanović-Šekularac, J., Petrovski, A., Macut, N., & Radojević, M. (2020). *Restoration of a Historic Building in Order to Improve Energy Efficiency and Energy Saving—Case Study—The Dining Room within the Žiča Monastery Property. Sustainability*, 12(15), 6271. https://doi.org/10.3390/su12156271.

[67] Karim, A. N., Johansson, P., & Kalagasidis, A. S. (2020). *Super insulation plasters in renovation of buildings in Sweden: energy efficiency and possibilities with new building materials. IOP Conference Series: Earth and Environmental Science,* 588(4), 042050. https://doi.org/10.1088/1755-1315/588/4/042050.

[68] Del Curto, D., & Cinieri, V. (2020). *Aerogel-Based Plasters and Energy Efficiency of Historic Buildings. Literature Review and Guidelines for Manufacturing Specimens Destined for Thermal Tests. Sustainability*, 12(22), 9457. https://doi.org/10.3390/su12229457.

[69] Ravindra, K., Singh, T., Vardhan, S., Shrivastava, A., Singh, S., Kumar, P., & Mor, S. (2022). *COVID-19 pandemic: What can we learn for better air quality and human health? Journal of Infection and Public Health*, 15(2), 187–198. https://doi.org/10.1016/j.jiph.2021.12.001.

[70] Bluhm, R., Polonik, P., Hemes, K. S., Sanford, L. C., Benz, S. A., Levy, M. C., Ricke, K. L., & Burney, J. A. (2022). *Disparate air pollution reductions during California's COVID-19 economic shutdown. Nature Sustainability,* 5(6), 509–517. https://doi.org/10.1038/s41893-022-00856-1.

[71] Bakola, M., Hernandez Carballo, I., Jelastopulu, E., & Stuckler, D. (2022). *The impact of COVID-19 lockdown on air pollution in Europe and North America: a systematic review. European Journal of Public Health,* 32(6), 962–968. https://doi.org/10.1093/eurpub/ckac118.

[72] Mehmood, K., Mushtaq, S., Bao, Y., Saifullah, Bibi, S., Yaseen, M., Khan, M. A., Abrar, M. M., Ulhassan, Z., Fahad, S., & Petropoulos, G. P. (2022). *The impact of COVID-19 pandemic on air pollution: a global research framework, challenges, and future perspectives. Environmental Science and Pollution Research,* 29(35), 52618–52634. https://doi.org/10.1007/s11356-022-19484-5.

[73] Salih, Z., & Aziz, F. (2020). *Heavy Metal Accumulation in Dust and Workers' Scalp Hair as a Bioindicator for Air Pollution from a Steel Factory. Polish Journal of Environmental Studies,* 29(2), 1805–1813. https://doi.org/10.15244/pjoes/109724.

[74] KOÇ, İ. (2021). *Using Cedrus atlantica's annual rings as a biomonitor in observing the changes of Ni and Co concentrations in the atmosphere. Environmental Science and Pollution Research*, 28(27), 35880–35886. https://doi.org/10.1007/s11356-021-13272-3.

[75] Li, Z., Lu, W., & Huang, J. (2020). *Monitoring, Diffusion and Source Speculation Model of Urban Soil Pollution. Processes*, 8(11), 1339. https://doi.org/10.3390/pr8111339.

[76] Yoo, J. S., & Lee, Y. Z. (2022). *A Study on the Skin Adhesion Test of Fine Particles by Brake Pad Friction. Lubricants*, 10(12), 338. https://doi.org/10.3390/lubricants10120338.

[77] Kravchenko, O., Barta, D., Gerlici, J., Kravchenko, K., Rybicka, I., & Zigo, A. (2023). *Environmental Problems Associated with Vehicle Braking and Their Solutions. In TRANSBALTICA XIII: Transportation Science and Technology* (pp. 258–267). *Springer International Publishing.* https://doi.org/10.1007/978-3-031-25863-3_24.

[78] Saha, D., Sharma, D., & Satapathy, B. K. (2023). *Challenges pertaining to particulate matter emission of toxic formulations and prospects on using green ingredients for sustainable eco-friendly automotive*

brake composites. Sustainable Materials and Technologies, 37, e00680. https://doi.org/10.1016/j.susmat.2023.e00680.

[79] Benibo, A. G., Sha'Ato, R., Wuana, R. A., & Itodo, A. U. (2020). *Assessment of Ambient Air Quality around Ihetutu Minefield, Ishiagu, Nigeria. Journal of Chemical Society of Nigeria,* 45(6). https://doi.org/10.46602/jcsn. v45i6.554.

[80] Korzeniowska, J., & Krąż, P. (2020). *Heavy Metals Content in the Soils of the Tatra National Park Near Lake Morskie Oko and Kasprowy Wierch—A Case Study (Tatra Mts, Central Europe). Minerals,* 10(12), 1120. https://doi.org/10.3390/min10121120.

[81] Tisha, S. M., Chowdhury, T. R., & Hossain, M. D. (2021). *Heavy Metal Contamination and Ecological Risk Assessment in the Soil of Tannery Industry at Savar. Chemical Engineering Research Bulletin,* 106–113. https://doi.org/10.3329/cerb.v22i1.54308.

[82] Bâlon, P., Boissard, G., Cailleau, C., Belbeze, S., Hubé, D., Vincq, C., Brunet, J.-F., Lion, F., Zornig, C., Coftier, A., & Ollivier, P. (2022). *Relating mercury occurrence in soil gases at establishments hosting children to historical mercury-using activities in Paris, France. Science of The Total Environment,* 814, 152388. https://doi.org/10.1016/j.scitotenv.2021.152388.

[83] Zhao, M., Li, Y., & Wang, Z. (2022). *Mercury and Mercury-Containing Preparations: History of Use, Clinical Applications, Pharmacology, Toxicology, and Pharmacokinetics in Traditional Chinese Medicine. Frontiers in Pharmacology,* 13. https://doi.org/10.3389/fphar.2022. 807807.

[84] Malone, A., Figueroa, L., Wang, W., Smith, N. M., Ranville, J. F., Vuono, D. C., Alejo Zapata, F. D., Morales Paredes, L., Sharp, J. O., & Bellona, C. (2023). *Transitional dynamics from mercury to cyanide-based processing in artisanal and small-scale gold mining: Social, economic, geochemical, and environmental considerations. Science of The Total Environment,* 898, 165492. https://doi.org/10.1016/j.scitotenv.2023.165492.

[85] Cheng, Y., Watari, T., Seccatore, J., Nakajima, K., Nansai, K., & Takaoka, M. (2023). *A review of gold production, mercury consumption, and emission in artisanal and small-scale gold mining (ASGM). Resources Policy,* 81, 103370. https://doi.org/10.1016/j.resourpol.2023.103370.

[86] Soe, P. S., Kyaw, W. T., Arizono, K., Ishibashi, Y., & Agusa, T. (2022). *Mercury Pollution from Artisanal and Small-Scale Gold Mining in Myanmar and Other Southeast Asian Countries. International Journal of Environmental Research and Public Health,* 19(10), 6290. https://doi.org/10.3390/ijerph19106290.

[87] Berry, T.-A., Belluso, E., Vigliaturo, R., Gieré, R., Emmett, E. A., Testa, J. R., Steinhorn, G., & Wallis, S. L. (2022). *Asbestos and Other Hazardous Fibrous Minerals: Potential Exposure Pathways and Associated Health Risks. International Journal of Environmental Research and Public Health,* 19(7), 4031. https://doi.org/10.3390/ijerph19074031.

[88] Rodriguez Elizalde, R. (2022). *Asbestos Presence in 20th Century Buildings. Journal of Engineering and Applied Sciences Technology,* 1–14. https://doi.org/10.47363/JEAST/2022(4)152.

[89] Abbasi, M., Mostafa, S., Vieira, A. S., Patorniti, N., & Stewart, R. A. (2022). *Mapping Roofing with Asbestos-Containing Material by Using Remote Sensing Imagery and Machine Learning-Based Image Classification: A State-of-the-Art Review. Sustainability,* 14(13), 8068. https://doi.org/10.3390/su14138068.

[90] Vorster, T., Mthombeni, J., teWaterNaude, J., & Phillips, J. I. (2022). *The Association between the Histological Subtypes of Mesothelioma and Asbestos Exposure Characteristics. International Journal of Environmental Research and Public Health,* 19(21), 14520. https://doi.org/10.3390/ijerph192114520.

[91] Sattler, T., Pomberger, R., Schimek, J., & Vollprecht, D. (2020). *Mineral wool waste in Austria, associated health aspects and recycling options. Detritus,* 9, 174–180. https://doi.org/10.31025/2611-4135/2020.13904.

[92] Kupczewska-Dobecka, M., Konieczko, K., & Czerczak, S. (2020). *Occupational risk resulting from exposure to mineral wool when installing insulation in buildings. International Journal of Occupational Medicine and Environmental Health,* 33(6), 757–769. https://doi.org/10.13075/ijomeh.1896.01637.

[93] Moitra, S., Farshchi Tabrizi, A., Idrissi Machichi, K., Kamravaei, S., Miandashti, N., Henderson, L., Mukherjee, M., Khadour, F., Naseem, M. T., Lacy, P., & Melenka, L. (2020). *Non-Malignant*

Respiratory Illnesses in Association with Occupational Exposure to Asbestos and Other Insulating Materials: Findings from the Alberta Insulator Cohort. International Journal of Environmental Research and Public Health, 17(19), 7085. https://doi.org/10.3390/ijerph17197085.

[94] Kazemifar, A. M., Yahyaee, A., Seddighi, M., & Soleimannejad, M. (2020). *The Prevalence and Risk Factors of Nosocomial Infections in the Intensive Care Unit of a Hospital in Iran. The Journal of Qazvin University of Medical Sciences,* 24(4), 356–365. https://doi.org/10.32598/JQUMS.24.4.5.

[95] Chen, L., Zhao, J., Peng, J., Li, X., Deng, X., Geng, Z., Shen, Z., Guo, F., Zhang, Q., Jin, Y., Wang, L., & Wang, S. (2020). *Detection of SARS-CoV-2 in saliva and characterization of oral symptoms in COVID-19 patients. Cell Proliferation,* 53(12). https://doi.org/10.1111/cpr.12923.

[96] Wang, Y., Wang, Y., Chen, Y., & Qin, Q. (2020). *Unique epidemiological and clinical features of the emerging 2019 novel coronavirus pneumonia (COVID-19) implicate special control measures. Journal of Medical Virology,* 92(6), 568–576. https://doi.org/10.1002/jmv.25748.

[97] Pan, S.-J., Hou, Y., Yang, Y.-P., Wang, G.-G., Chen, X.-Y., Qian, W.-Y., Tung, T.-H., & Hu, X.-M. (2022). *Relationship between nosocomial infections and coronavirus disease 2019 in the neurosurgery unit: clinical characteristics and outcomes from a Chinese Tertiary-Care Hospital. BMC Infectious Diseases*, 22(1), 836. https://doi.org/10.1186/s12879-022-07845-x.

[98] Chen, J.-C., Munir, M. T., Aviat, F., Lepelletier, D., Le Pape, P., Dubreil, L., Irle, M., Federighi, M., Belloncle, C., Eveillard, M., & Pailhoriès, H. (2020). *Survival of Bacterial Strains on Wood (Quercus petraea) Compared to Polycarbonate, Aluminum and Stainless Steel. Antibiotics*, 9(11), 804. https://doi.org/10.3390/antibiotics9110804.

[99] Bowler, P., Murphy, C., & Wolcott, R. (2020). *Biofilm exacerbates antibiotic resistance: Is this a current oversight in antimicrobial stewardship? Antimicrobial Resistance & Infection Control*, 9(1), 162. https://doi.org/ 10.1186/s13756-020-00830-6.

[100] Čović, I., Vasilj, I., Hrkać, A., & Perković, R. (2021). *Knowledge and attitude on prevention of nosocomial infections of students of university of mostar faculty of health studies. Zdravstveni Glasnik,* 14, 73–82. https://doi.org/10.47960/2303-8616.2021.14.73.

[101] Lyu, X., Hu, J., Xu, X., Xianyu, Y., & Dong, W. (2021). *Factors influencing risk perception and nosocomial infection prevention practices of frontline nurses during the COVID-19 pandemic. BMC Nursing,* 20(1), 78. https://doi.org/10.1186/s12912-021-00591-6.

[102] Fatimazahra, S., Latifa, M., Laila, S., & Monsif, K. (2023). *Review of hospital effluents: special emphasis on characterization, impact, and treatment of pollutants and antibiotic resistance. Environmental Monitoring and Assessment*, 195(3), 393. https://doi.org/10.1007/s10661-023-11002-5.

[103] Achak, M., Alaoui Bakri, S., Chhiti, Y., M'hamdi Alaoui, F. E., Barka, N., & Boumya, W. (2021). *SARS-CoV-2 in hospital wastewater during outbreak of COVID-19: A review on detection, survival and disinfection technologies. Science of The Total Environment,* 761, 143192. https://doi.org/10.1016/j.scitotenv.2020.143192.

[104] Liaquat, S., Baccaglini, L., Haynatzki, G., Medcalf, S. J., & Rupp, M. E. (2021). *Clinical consequences of contaminated blood cultures in adult hospitalized patients at an institution utilizing a rapid blood-culture identification system. Infection Control & Hospital Epidemiology*, 42(8), 978–984. https://doi.org/10.1017/ice.2020.1337.

[105] Klucher, J. M., Davis, K., Lakkad, M., Painter, J. T., & Dare, R. K. (2022). *Risk factors and clinical outcomes associated with blood culture contamination. Infection Control & Hospital Epidemiology,* 43(3), 291–297. https://doi.org/10.1017/ice.2021.111.

[106] Farrell, M., Bram, S., Gu, H., Mathew, S., Messer, E., Hayes, E., & Srinivasan, M. (2020). *Impact of Contaminated Blood Cultures on Children, Families, and the Health Care System. Hospital Pediatrics,* 10(10), 836–843. https://doi.org/10.1542/hpeds.2020-0146.

[107] Chisompola, N. K., Kamanga, K. M., & Matafwali, P. V. (2020). Risk *Factors for Occupational Transmission of Tuberculosis among Healthcare Workers in Zambia. International Journal of tropical disease & Health*, 59–65. https://doi.org/10.9734/ijtdh/2020/v41i1130335.

[108] Ueki, H., Ujie, M., Komori, Y., Kato, T., Imai, M., & Kawaoka, Y. (2022). *Effectiveness of HEPA Filters at Removing Infectious SARS-CoV-2 from the Air. MSphere,* 7(4). https://doi.org/ 10.1128/msphere.00086-22.

[109] Hassan Al-abdalall, A., Abdullah Al-dakheel, S., & Abdulhadi Al-Abkari, H. (2020). *Impact of Air-Conditioning Filters on Microbial Growth and Indoor Air Pollution. In Low-temperature Technologies. IntechOpen*. https://doi.org/10.5772/intechopen.88548.

[110] Park, K. H., Sim, D. W., Lee, S. C., Moon, S., Choe, E., Shin, H., Kim, S. R., Lee, J.-H., Park, H. H., Huh, D., & Park, J.-W. (2020). *Effects of Air Purifiers on Patients with Allergic Rhinitis: a Multicenter, Randomized, Double-Blind, and Placebo-Controlled Study. Yonsei Medical Journal*, 61(8), 689. https://doi.org/10.3349/ymj.2020.61.8.689.

[111] Deshpande, A. A., & Rehman, M. A. A. (2022). *Design and Fabrication of Economical Industrial Air Filter. SAMRIDDHI : A Journal of Physical Sciences, Engineering and Technology,* 14(01 SPL), 138–144. https://doi.org/10.18090/samriddhi.v14spli01.25.

[112] Kim, S., Kim, S., & Lee, S. (2022). *Renewable Activated Carbon Filters Bearing Photocatalytic Particles for Volatile Organic Compound Removal. ChemPlusChem,* 87(1). https://doi.org/10.1002/cplu.202100486.

[113] Sokhal, A., & Narayan, U. (2020). *Plants are More Effective in Absorbing Volatile Organic Compounds from the Atmosphere than Air Purifiers. Journal of Student Research,* 9(2). https://doi.org/10.47611/jsrhs.v9i2.1047.

[114] Mohammed, A. M., A Saleh, I., H Ibrahim, Y., & RG Mohamed, N. (2022). *Theory and technology of air filtration: review. Material Science & Engineering International Journal,* 6(1), 6–12. https://doi.org/10.15406/ mseij.2022.06.00173.

[115] Le, V. C. T., Thanh, T. N., Kang, E., Yoon, S., Mai, H. D., Sheraz, M., Han, T. U., An, J., & Kim, S. (2022). *Melamine sponge-based copper-organic framework (Cu-CPP) as a multi-functional filter for air purifiers. Korean Journal of Chemical Engineering,* 39(4), 954–962. https://doi.org/10.1007/s11814-021-1000-4.

[116] Kwon, H. J., Yang, D. S., Koo, M. S., Ji, S. M., Jeong, J., Oh, S., Kuk, S. K., Heo, H., Ham, D. J., Kim, M., Choi, H., Lee, J.-M., Shur, J.-W., Lee, W.-J., Bin, C.-O., Timofeev, N., Wu, H., Wang, L., Lee, T., Lee, H. C. (2023). *Long-lifetime water-washable ceramic catalyst filter for air purification. Nature Communications,* 14(1), 520. https://doi.org/10.1038/s41467-023-36050-w.

[117] Syafrudin, M., Kristanti, R. A., Yuniarto, A., Hadibarata, T., Rhee, J., Al-onazi, W. A., Algarni, T. S., Almarri, A. H., & Al-Mohaimeed, A. M. (2021). *Pesticides in Drinking Water—A Review. International Journal of Environmental Research and Public Health,* 18(2), 468. https://doi.org/10.3390/ijerph18020468.

[118] Serhane, Y., Bouzaza, A., Wolbert, D., & Assadi, A. A. (2023). *New UV-LED frontal flow photocatalytic reactor for VOCs treatment: Compactness, intensification and optimization studies. Chemical Engineering Journal,* 451, 138784. https://doi.org/10.1016/j.cej.2022.138784.

[119] Lee, J.-H., Doan, T. A., Park, Y. J., Hoa, H. T. M., Phuong, P. H., Le, D. T., Hung, N. H., Tran, Q. T., Lee, H.-S., Ryu, J. H., Yoo, J.-Y., & Cuong, T. V. (2020). *Synthesis and Photocatalytic Activity of β-Ga2O3 Nanostructures for Decomposition of Formaldehyde under Deep Ultraviolet Irradiation. Catalysts*, 10(10), 1105. https://doi.org/10.3390/catal10101105.

[120] Bakbolat, B., Daulbayev, C., Sultanov, F., Beissenov, R., Umirzakov, A., Mereke, A., Bekbaev, A., & Chuprakov, I. (2020). *Recent Developments of TiO2-Based Photocatalysis in the Hydrogen Evolution and Photodegradation: A Review. Nanomaterials,* 10(9), 1790. https://doi.org/10.3390/nano10091790.

[121] Sun, Y., Feng, B., Li, Q., Tian, C., Ma, L., & Li, Z. (2022). *The Application of Bi-Doped TiO 2 for the Photocatalytic Oxidation of Formaldehyde. Crystal Research and Technology*, 57(6). https://doi.org/10.1002/crat.202100231.

[122] Rahimi, S., Mohammadi, F., Ghodsi, S., Mohammadi, M., & Karimi, H. (2023). *Activation of persulfate by TiO 2 -Fe 3 O 4 nanocomposite for reactive red 198 degradation along with modeling and optimization approach. Environmental Health Engineering and Management*, 10(2), 165–177. https://doi.org/10.34172/EHEM.2023.19.

[123] Yan, J., Huang, W., Kuang, H., Wang, Q., & Li, B. (2022). *The effect of etched 3D printed Cu-bearing titanium alloy on the polarization of macrophage. Frontiers in Materials,* 9. https://doi.org/10.3389/fmats.2022.941311.

[124] Baig, U., Ansari, M. A., Gondal, M. A., Akhtar, S., Khan, F. A., & Falath, W. S. (2020). *Single step production of high-purity copper oxide-titanium dioxide nanocomposites and their effective*

antibacterial and anti-biofilm activity against drug-resistant bacteria. Materials Science and Engineering: C, 113, 110992. https://doi.org/10.1016/j.msec.2020.110992.

[125] Bisht, N., Dwivedi, N., Kumar, P., Venkatesh, M., Yadav, A. K., Mishra, D., Solanki, P., Verma, N. K., Lakshminarayanan, R., Ramakrishna, S., Mondal, D. P., Srivastava, A. K., & Dhand, C. (2022). *Recent advances in copper and copper-derived materials for antimicrobial resistance and infection control. Current Opinion in Biomedical Engineering,* 24, 100408. https://doi.org/10.1016/j.cobme.2022.100408.

[126] Astasov-Frauenhoffer, M., Koegel, S., Waltimo, T., Zimmermann, A., Walker, C., Hauser-Gerspach, I., & Jung, C. (2019). *Antimicrobial efficacy of copper-doped titanium surfaces for dental implants. Journal of Materials Science: Materials in Medicine,* 30(7), 84. https://doi.org/10.1007/s10856-019-6286-y.

[127] Yousef, A., Zouli, N. I., Maafa, I. M., Hadidi, H. M., Sallam, S., Moosa, M., & El-Halwany, M. M. (2022). *Fabrication of heterojunction MnTiO 3 –TiO 2 -decorated carbon nanofibers via electrospinning as an effective multifunctional photocatalyst. Materials Science-Poland*, 40(2), 289–305. https://doi.org/10.2478/msp-2022-0028.

[128] Xiao, W., Zhang, H., Wang, X., Wang, B., Long, T., Deng, S., & Yang, W. (2022). *Interaction Mechanisms and Application of Ozone Micro/Nanobubbles and Nanoparticles: A Review and Perspective. Nanomaterials,* 12(12), 1958. https://doi.org/10.3390/nano12121958.

Index

L

M

N

O

P

R

S

T

U

V

W